Minimally Invasive Image-Guided Spine Interventions

Editor

MAJID KHAN

NEUROIMAGING CLINICS OF NORTH AMERICA

www.neuroimaging.theclinics.com

Consulting Editor
SURESH K. MUKHERJI

November 2019 • Volume 29 • Number 4

ELSEVIER

1600 John F. Kennedy Boulevard • Suite 1800 • Philadelphia, Pennsylvania, 19103-2899

http://www.neuroimaging.theclinics.com

NEUROIMAGING CLINICS OF NORTH AMERICA Volume 29, Number 4
November 2019 ISSN 1052-5149, ISBN 13: 978-0-323-70884-5

Editor: John Vassallo (j.vassallo@elsevier.com)
Developmental Editor: Casey Potter

Neuroimaging Clinics of North America (ISSN 1052-5149) is published quarterly by Elsevier Inc., 360 Park Avenue South, New York, NY 10010-1710. Months of issue are February, May, August, and November. Business and editorial offices: 1600 John F. Kennedy Blvd., Suite 1800, Philadelphia, PA 19103-2899. Business and editorial offices: 6277 Sea Harbor Drive, Orlando, FL 32887-4800. Periodicals postage paid at New York, NY, and additional mailing offices. Subscription prices are USD 397 per year for US individuals, USD 653 per year for US institutions, USD 100 per year for US students and residents, USD 451 per year for Canadian individuals, USD 832 per year for Canadian institutions, USD 525 per year for international individuals, USD 832 per year for international institutions and USD 260 per year for Canadian and foreign students and residents. To receive student/resident rate, orders must be accompanied by name of affiliated institution, date of term, and the *signature* of program/residency coordinator on institution letterhead. Orders will be billed at individual rate until proof of status is received. Foreign air speed delivery is included in all *Clinics* subscription prices. All prices are subject to change without notice. POSTMASTER: Send address changes to *Neuroimaging Clinics of North America*, Elsevier Health Sciences Division, Subscription **Customer Service, 3251 Riverport Lane, Maryland Heights, MO 63043. Telephone: 1-800-654-2452 (U.S. and Canada); 314-447-8871 (outside U.S. and Canada). Fax: 314-447-8029. E-mail: journalscustomer service-usa@elsevier.com (for print support); journalsonlinesupport-usa@elsevier.com (for online support)**.

Reprints. For copies of 100 or more of articles in this publication, please contact the Commercial Reprints Department, Elsevier Inc., 360 Park Avenue South, New York, NY 10010-1710. Tel.: 212-633-3874; Fax: 212-633-3820; E-mail: reprints@elsevier.com.

Neuroimaging Clinics of North America is covered by *Excerpta Medical/EMBASE,* the RSNA Index of Imaging Literature, *MEDLINE/PubMed (Index Medicus),* MEDLINE/MEDLARS, SciSearch, Research Alert, and Neuroscience Citation Index.

Printed in the United States of America.

PROGRAM OBJECTIVE

The goal of *Neuroimaging Clinics of North America* is to keep practicing radiologists and radiology residents up to date with current clinical practice in radiology by providing timely articles reviewing the state of the art in patient care.

TARGET AUDIENCE

Practicing radiologists, radiology residents, and other healthcare professionals who utilize neuroimaging findings to provide patient care.

LEARNING OBJECTIVES

Upon completion of this activity, participants will be able to:
1. Review commonly used spinal MR imaging protocols and associated common artifacts.
2. Discuss image guided approaches for the treatment of common spine pain generators.
3. Recognize recent advances in minimally invasive, percutaneous image-guided thermal ablation for management of spinal metastases.

ACCREDITATION

The Elsevier Office of Continuing Medical Education (EOCME) is accredited by the Accreditation Council for Continuing Medical Education (ACCME) to provide continuing medical education for physicians.

The EOCME designates this journal-based CME activity for a maximum of 12 *AMA PRA Category 1 Credit*(s)™. Physicians should claim only the credit commensurate with the extent of their participation in the activity.

All other healthcare professionals requesting continuing education credit for this enduring material will be issued a certificate of participation.

DISCLOSURE OF CONFLICTS OF INTEREST

The EOCME assesses conflict of interest with its instructors, faculty, planners, and other individuals who are in a position to control the content of CME activities. All relevant conflicts of interest that are identified are thoroughly vetted by EOCME for fair balance, scientific objectivity, and patient care recommendations. EOCME is committed to providing its learners with CME activities that promote improvements or quality in healthcare and not a specific proprietary business or a commercial interest.

The planning committee, staff, authors and editors listed below have identified no financial relationships or relationships to products or devices they or their spouse/life partner have with commercial interest related to the content of this CME activity:

Israh Akhtar, MD; Timothy J. Amrhein, MD; John A. Arrington, MD; Matteo Bellini, MD; Yian Chen, MD; Michael Anthony Erdek, MD, MA; Wende Nocton Gibbs, MD, MA; Linda Gray, MD; Troy A. Hutchins, MD; Gaurav Jindal, MD; Alison Kemp; Matthew Kiczek, DO; Peter G. Kranz, MD; Sergiy V. Kushchayev, MD; Pradeep Kuttysankaran; Michael D. Malinzak, MD, PhD; Varsha Manucha, MD; Miriam E. Peckham, MD; Mark C. Preul, MD; Lubdha M. Shah, MD; Amirali Modir Shanechi, MD; Teresa Tang, MD; Oleg M. Teytelboym, MD; Anderanik Tomasian, MD; John Vassallo; Philip C. Wiener, DO; Chiara Zini, MD, PhD.

The planning committee, staff, authors and editors listed below have identified financial relationships or relationships to products or devices they or their spouse/life partner have with commercial interest related to the content of this CME activity:

Amish Doshi, MD: participates in speakers bureau for Merit Medical Systems.

Philippe Gailloud, MD: is a consultant/advisor for Cerenovus and receives research support from Siemens Medical Solutions USA, Inc.

Jack W. Jennings, MD, PhD: is a consultant/advisor for Medtronic and Galil Medical, Inc.

Majid Khan, MBBS, MD: is a consultant/advisor for Stryker and MedWaves, Inc.

Stefano Marcia, MD: is a consultant/advisor for Techlamed.

Suresh K. Mukherji, MD, MBA, FACR: is a consultant/advisor for iSchemaView, Inc.

UNAPPROVED/OFF-LABEL USE DISCLOSURE

The EOCME requires CME faculty to disclose to the participants:
1. When products or procedures being discussed are off-label, unlabelled, experimental, and/or investigational (not US Food and Drug Administration [FDA] approved); and
2. Any limitations on the information presented, such as data that are preliminary or that represent ongoing research, interim analyses, and/or unsupported opinions. Faculty may discuss information about pharmaceutical agents that is outside of FDA-approved labelling. This information is intended solely for CME and is not intended to promote off-label use of these medications. If you have any questions, contact the medical affairs department of the manufacturer for the most recent prescribing information.

TO ENROLL

To enroll in the *Neuroimaging Clinics of North America* Continuing Medical Education program, call customer service at 1-800-654-2452 or sign up online at http://www.theclinics.com/home/cme. The CME program is available to subscribers for an additional annual fee of USD 244.40.

METHOD OF PARTICIPATION

In order to claim credit, participants must complete the following:

1. Complete enrolment as indicated above.
2. Read the activity.
3. Complete the CME Test and Evaluation. Participants must achieve a score of 70% on the test. All CME Tests and Evaluations must be completed online.

CME INQUIRIES/SPECIAL NEEDS

For all CME inquiries or special needs, please contact elsevierCME@elsevier.com.

NEUROIMAGING CLINICS OF NORTH AMERICA

SERIES OF RELATED INTEREST

MRI Clinics of North America
www.Mri.theclinics.com
PET Clinics
www.pet.theclinics.com
Radiologic Clinics of North America
www.Radiologic.theclinics.com

THE CLINICS ARE AVAILABLE ONLINE!
Access your subscription at:
www.theclinics.com

Contributors

CONSULTING EDITOR

SURESH K. MUKHERJI, MD, MBA, FACR
Clinical Professor, Marian University, Director
of Head & Neck Radiology, ProScan Imaging,
Regional Medical Director, Envision Physician
Services, Indianapolis, Indiana, USA

EDITOR

MAJID KHAN, MBBS, MD
Associate Professor, Russell H. Morgan
Department of Radiology, Division of
Neuroradiology/Neuro-Intervention Radiology,
The Johns Hopkins Hospital, Director of Non-
Vascular Spine Interventions, Department of
Neuro-Intervention Radiology, Baltimore,
Maryland, USA

AUTHORS

ISRAH AKHTAR, MD
Director of Cytology, Cytopathology
Fellowship Program Director, Professor,
Department of Pathology, University of
Mississippi Medical Center, Jackson,
Mississippi, USA

TIMOTHY J. AMRHEIN, MD
Associate Professor, Department of
Radiology, Director of Spine Intervention,
Division of Neuroradiology, Duke University
Medical Center, Durham, North Carolina,
USA

JOHN A. ARRINGTON, MD
Department of Radiology, Moffitt Cancer
Center, Tampa, Florida, USA

MATTEO BELLINI, MD
Unit of Neuroimaging and Neurointervention,
Ahead of Minimal Invasive Spinal Treatments,
Department of Neurological and Motory
Sciences, Hospital "Santa Maria alle Scotte,"

Azienda Ospedaliera Universitaria Senese,
Siena, Italy

YIAN CHEN, MD
Assistant Professor, Department of
Anesthesiology and Critical Care Medicine,
Johns Hopkins School of Medicine, Baltimore,
Maryland, USA

AMISH DOSHI, MD
Associate Professor of Radiology, Icahn
School of Medicine at Mount Sinai, New York,
New York, USA

MICHAEL ANTHONY ERDEK, MD, MA
Associate Professor, Department of
Anesthesiology and Critical Care Medicine,
Johns Hopkins School of Medicine, Berman
Institute of Bioethics, Baltimore, Maryland,
USA

PHILIPPE GAILLOUD, MD
Division of Interventional Neuroradiology, The
Johns Hopkins Hospital, Baltimore, Maryland,
USA

WENDE NOCTON GIBBS, MD, MA
Neuroradiology Section, Assistant Professor, Department of Radiology, Mayo Clinic Arizona, Phoenix, Arizona, USA

LINDA GRAY, MD
Associate Professor, Department of Radiology, Division of Neuroradiology, Duke University Medical Center, Durham, North Carolina, USA

TROY A. HUTCHINS, MD
Associate Professor, Department of Radiology, University of Utah, Salt Lake City, Utah, USA

JACK W. JENNINGS, MD, PhD
Mallinckrodt Institute of Radiology, St Louis, Missouri, USA

GAURAV JINDAL, MD
Associate Professor, Division of Interventional Neuroradiology, Department of Radiology, University of Maryland Medical Center, Baltimore, Maryland, USA

MAJID KHAN, MBBS, MD
Associate Professor, Russell H. Morgan Department of Radiology, Division of Neuroradiology/Neuro-Intervention Radiology, The Johns Hopkins Hospital, Director of Non-Vascular Spine Interventions, Department of Neuro-Intervention Radiology, Baltimore, Maryland, USA

MATTHEW KICZEK, DO
Instructor, Russell H. Morgan Department of Radiology and Radiological Science, Johns Hopkins School of Medicine, Baltimore, Maryland, USA

PETER G. KRANZ, MD
Associate Professor, Department of Radiology, Chief, Division of Neuroradiology, Duke University Medical Center, Durham, North Carolina, USA

SERGIY V. KUSHCHAYEV, MD
Assistant Professor, Department of Radiology, Moffitt Cancer Center, Tampa, Florida, USA; Department of Radiology, Johns Hopkins Hospital, Baltimore, Maryland, USA

MICHAEL D. MALINZAK, MD, PhD
Assistant Professor, Department of Radiology, Division of Neuroradiology, Duke University

Medical Center, Durham, North Carolina, USA

VARSHA MANUCHA, MD
Associate Professor, Director of Surgical Pathology, Department of Pathology, University of Mississippi Medical Center, Jackson, Mississippi, USA

STEFANO MARCIA, MD
Ahead Diagnostic and Interventional Radiology Unit, Hospital "Santissima Trinità," ATS Sardegna ASSL, Cagliari, Italy

MIRIAM E. PECKHAM, MD
Assistant Professor, Department of Radiology, University of Utah, Salt Lake City, Utah, USA

MARK C. PREUL, MD
Department of Neurosurgery, Barrow Neurological Institute, St. Joseph's Hospital and Medical Center, Phoenix, Arizona, USA

LUBDHA M. SHAH, MD
Professor, Department of Radiology, University of Utah, Salt Lake City, Utah, USA

AMIRALI MODIR SHANECHI, MD
Instructor, Russell H. Morgan Department of Radiology and Radiological Science, Johns Hopkins School of Medicine, Baltimore, Maryland, USA

TERESA TANG, MD
Fellow, Department of Anesthesiology and Critical Care Medicine, Johns Hopkins School of Medicine, Baltimore, Maryland, USA

OLEG M. TEYTELBOYM, MD
Department of Radiology, Mercy Catholic Medical Center, Darby, Pennsylvania, USA

ANDERANIK TOMASIAN, MD
Department of Radiology, University of Southern California, Los Angeles, California, USA

PHILIP C. WIENER, DO
Einstein Healthcare Network, Philadelphia, Pennsylvania, USA

CHIARA ZINI, MD, PhD
Unit of Radiology, Hospital "Santa Maria Annunziata," Azienda USL Toscana Centro, Florence, Italy

Contents

> Sacral fractures result from high-impact trauma or in the form of insufficiency or pathologic fractures, resulting from osteoporosis, radiation therapy, or malignancy. In the emergency setting, the escalating use of computed tomography has substantially increased diagnosis of sacral fractures, which are frequently occult on radiographs. Radiologists should be familiar with and create reports using the most current fracture classification systems, because this improves communication with the treatment team and optimizes patient care. Sacroplasty is a safe, minimally invasive treatment option for many types of sacral fractures. It provides rapid and durable pain relief, with a low incidence of complications.

> The vertebral column is the most common site of osseous metastasis, and percutaneous minimally invasive thermal ablation is becoming an important contributor to multidisciplinary treatment algorithms. Continuously evolving minimally invasive image-guided percutaneous spine thermal ablation procedures have proven safe and effective in management of selected patients with spinal metastases to achieve pain palliation and/or local tumor control. This article details the armamentarium available and the most recent advances in minimally invasive, percutaneous image-guided thermal ablation for management of spinal metastases.

> This article reviews image-guided approaches for the treatment of common spine pain generators. The following treatment targets are discussed: epidural space (interlaminar and transforaminal approaches), facet joint, sacroiliac joint, and synovial cysts.

> In addition to basic image-guided injections, there are many advanced procedures to address the challenges of spine pain. Patients with debilitating symptoms are offered relief, a shorter recovery period, and fewer potential complications. Pain arises from numerous sites along the spine, presenting as spine pain or radiculopathy. This article is an overview of advanced techniques in this rapidly progressing field, including neuromodulation, radiofrequency thermocoagulation, discography, intradiscal thermocoagulation, and percutaneous image-guided lumbar decompression; and it highlights etiologic factors and their relationship to therapeutic technique and clinical evidence.

> Low back pain, radicular leg pain, and lumbar spinal stenosis are the most common of all chronic pain disorders. Discogenic pain is related to distress of annular fibers and tears, whereas spinal stenosis is related to reduction of the spinal canal

dimensions and compression of the neural elements; radicular pain is mainly related to disc herniation and is initially managed conservatively. The percutaneous minimally invasive approach in discogenic and radicular pain is designed to reduce the volume of the nucleus pulposus in patients with failure of medical and physical treatment prolonged for at least 6 weeks.

Foreword
Spine Intervention

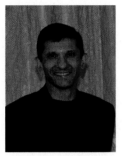

Suresh K. Mukherji, MD, MBA, FACR
Consulting Editor

Spine intervention has been a fascinating field for me as I have seen the procedures evolve from simple lumbar punctures to complex ablative therapies in a relatively short period of time. It has been very challenging to keep up with the technological advances and accepted clinical applications, which is why we decided to devote a specific issue of *Neuroimaging Clinics* to this specific topic.

I was delighted when Dr Majid Khan from Johns Hopkins University accepted our invitation to guest edit this very important issue. This issue provides a wonderful combination of anatomy, pathology, and minimally invasive treatment options for a variety of spine disorders. There are specific articles devoted to bony and vascular anatomy of the spine, spine-augmentation techniques, tumor ablation, vascular interventional techniques, neuromodulation, epidural steroid injections, sacroiliac and facet joint injections, selective nerve root blocks, implanted drug-delivery systems, and epidural blood and fibrin patches for cerebrospinal fluid leaks.

I want to personally thank Dr Khan and the article contributors. All of the authors are recognized experts in the area of spinal imaging, and their magnificent contributions are reflective of their vast expertise and stellar international reputations.

There are numerous physicians who are involved with managing patients with various types of back pain, including anesthesiologists, neurosurgeons, orthopedic surgeons, neuroradiologists, body radiologists, and musculoskeletal-interventional radiologists. I am confident that all of these providers will benefit from this issue, whether they are are in private practice or in an academic setting. Thank you again to Dr Khan and all of the article authors for your outstanding contributions.

Suresh K. Mukherji, MD, MBA, FACR
Clinical Professor, Marian University
Director of Head & Neck Radiology
ProScan Imaging, Regional Medical Director,
Envision Physician Services
Indianapolis, Indiana, USA

E-mail address:
sureshmukherji@hotmail.com

Neuroimag Clin N Am 29 (2019) xiii
https://doi.org/10.1016/j.nic.2019.07.013
1052-5149/19/© 2019 Published by Elsevier Inc.

Preface
Spine Intervention

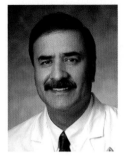

Majid Khan, MBBS, MD
Editor

Minimally invasive, image-guided, spine-interventional radiology has evolved over time from being simply a diagnostic modality primarily used for biopsies to one that is currently being considered in the treatment paradigm for complex spine pathologic conditions.

We must constantly progress our methods and push our research and clinical teams to discover and execute newer and more efficient ways of minimally invasive techniques; we are under tremendous pressure from allied specialties, such as neurosurgery and orthopedic surgeries, which are devising more minimally invasive surgical options.

Moreover, osteoporosis and obesity are on the rise, thus significantly increasing the number of vertebral compression fractures and prompting the early onset of back pain and early development of spine degenerative changes. Although the advent of improved cancer chemotherapy and targeted radiation has resulted in greater patient longevity, we are simultaneously seeing the greater incidence of both spinal and extraspinal metastases, which require a multidisciplinary treatment approach in which interventional radiology forms an integral part.

In the 1990s to 2000s, we witnessed the introduction of spine tumor ablation techniques with substantial improvements in vertebral cement augmentation devices, which has enabled these modalities to be recognized as part of the treatment paradigm for osseous spine metastases. Now, spine neuromodulation and insertion of pain pumps for pain palliation are done routinely for patients with chronic pain, and such advances have led to a decrease in oral narcotic usage and have somewhat allayed rampant narcotic abuse at a time when narcotic abuse has become a national crisis.

This issue is meant to familiarize the readers with the extensive and ever-expanding list of image-guided, spine-intervention procedures that are now available, used mostly as an adjunct and sometimes as an alternate treatment method to conventional treatment modalities in the spine. It explains in detail anatomic and vascular spine anatomy through clinical evaluation, pharmacologic requirements, and indications and contraindications of specific procedures. In addition, it covers a broad range of spine procedures discussed by experts in each field, including spine-augmentation techniques, tumor ablation, vascular interventional techniques, neuromodulation, epidural steroid injections, sacroiliac and facet joint injections, selective nerve root blocks, implanted drug-delivery systems, and epidural blood and fibrin patches for spontaneous cerebrospinal fluid leaks. Some of the described procedures, such as percutaneous treatment of lumbar stenosis and treatment of disc degeneration, are not being presently performed in the United States, but, expected to develop further in the next few years, they will gain attention in the United States.

This issue is useful to all physicians who treat back pain, including pain anesthesiologists, neurosurgeons, and orthopedic surgeons and neuroradiologists, body radiologists, and musculoskeletal-interventional radiologists. Also, several of these procedures will prove very useful for general radiologists, particularly in private-practice settings.

I have established advanced spine intervention programs at 2 large academic university hospitals

Neuroimag Clin N Am 29 (2019) xv–xvi
https://doi.org/10.1016/j.nic.2019.07.012
1052-5149/19/© 2019 Published by Elsevier Inc.

and have observed firsthand the fast-paced growth in this field with ever-increasing patient referrals, and, for instance, Fellows are being hired every year to specifically start spine intervention programs in both academic and private practice settings.

This issue is the latest opportunity for the image-guided interventional community to implement these procedures and work closely with other clinical services to improve the quality of life of our deserving patients. I sincerely hope this work will be useful in helping others establish and grow a minimally invasive, spine-interventional practice. It has been a tremendously rewarding field for me and allows me to connect the diagnostic and interventional services to help our patients from both perspectives.

Majid Khan, MBBS, MD
Russell H. Morgan Department of Radiology
Division of Neuroradiology/Neuro-Intervention
Radiology
Johns Hopkins University Hospital
7220 Bloomberg Building
1800 Orleans Street
Baltimore, MD 21287, USA

E-mail address:
mkhan9@jhmi.edu

Spine Anatomy Imaging
An Update

Amirali Modir Shanechi, MD[a],*, Matthew Kiczek, DO[a], Majid Khan, MBBS, MD[a],
Gaurav Jindal, MD[b]

KEYWORDS

• Normal spinal anatomy • Spinal anatomy • Spinal MR imaging • Spinal CT • CT myelography

KEY POINTS

• MR imaging provides excellent detail of spinal anatomy including the intraspinal contents, neural foramina, joints, ligaments, intervertebral discs and bone marrow.
• CT better demonstrates the fine osseous detail of the spine and has an important role in the assessment of trauma as well as preoperative planning.
• CT myelography remains an alternative to MR imaging in those with contraindications or in the assessment of spinal CSF leak.
• This article illustrates normal spinal anatomy as defined by MR imaging and includes correlative CT and CT myelography images.

INTRODUCTION

Over the past few decades, spinal MR imaging has largely replaced computed tomography (CT) and CT myelography in the assessment of intraspinal pathologic conditions at institutions where MR imaging is available. Given its high-contrast resolution, MR imaging allows the differentiation of the several adjacent structures comprising the spine. Conventional CT remains a complementary imaging modality to MR imaging because of its high-resolution depiction of osseous anatomy and has a central role in operative planning or the evaluation of traumatic injury. CT myelography remains an alternative to MR imaging in those with contraindications to MR imaging or in the assessment of leak of cerebrospinal fluid (CSF) from the spine. This article illustrates normal spinal anatomy as defined by MR imaging, describes commonly used spinal MR imaging protocols (**Tables 1–3**), and discusses associated common artifacts.

Correlative CT and CT myelography images are also included.

SPINAL MR IMAGING TECHNIQUES

Sagittal and axial MR images should be acquired through the cervical, thoracic, and lumbar segments of the spine, as they are generally considered complementary, and imaging the spine in only 1 plane may result in misinterpretation. The addition of coronal images may also be useful, especially in patients with scoliosis. Stacked axial images and/or angled images through the discs can be obtained, and are often useful when the indication for imaging is pain, degenerative change, and/or radiculopathy.[1] Although imaging in the axial plane is a matter of personal preference, using only angled axial images through the discs may be inadequate, because portions of the spinal canal will not be imaged axially. Slice thickness from 3 to 4 mm is generally optimal for

Disclosure: A.M. Shanechi and M. Kiczek have nothing to disclose. M. Khan is a consultant for Stryker Medical Corporation and Avecure Medwaves Corporation. G. Jindal: Grant funding from Stryker and Medtronic unrelated to this publication.
[a] Russell H. Morgan Department of Radiology and Radiological Science, Johns Hopkins University School of Medicine, 600 North Wolfe Street, Phipps B100, Baltimore, MD 21287, USA; [b] Division of Interventional Neuroradiology, Department of Radiology, University of Maryland Medical Center, 22 South Greene Street, Baltimore, MD 21201, USA
* Corresponding author.
E-mail address: amodirs1@jhmi.edu

Neuroimag Clin N Am 29 (2019) 461–480
https://doi.org/10.1016/j.nic.2019.08.001
1052-5149/19/© 2019 Elsevier Inc. All rights reserved.

Table 1
Cervical spine MR imaging protocols

Sequence	Localizer	FLAIR	T2	T2	GRE	T1	T1	STIR	Enhanced T1	Enhanced T1
Plane	3 plane	Sagittal	Sagittal	Axial	Axial	Sagittal	Axial	Sagittal	Sagittal	Axial
Coil type	Neck	Neck	Neck	Neck	Neck	Neck	Neck	Neck	Neck	Neck
Thickness, mm	10	3	3	3	3	3	3	3	3	3
TR, ms	24	1700	3530	4210	32	653	649	4400	653	649
TE, ms	6	12	106	111	14	10	11	74	10	11
Flip angle	30	150	180	150	5	170	150	150	170	150
NEX	1	1	2	2	1	2	2	1	2	2
Matrix	128 × 256	250 × 384	269 × 384	240 × 320	216 × 320	269 × 384	205 × 256	192 × 256	269 × 384	205 × 256
FOV read, mm	300	260	240	200	200	240	240	240	240	240
FOV phase, mm	100	100	100	75	75	200	100	100	100	100
Comments								Trauma, Mets	If indicated	If indicated

Abbreviations: FLAIR, fluid-attenuated inversion-recovery imaging; FOV, field of view; GRE, gradient-recalled echo; Mets, metastases; NEX, number of excitations; STIR, short tau inversion recovery; TE, echo time; TR, repetition time.

Table 2
Thoracic spine MR imaging protocols

Sequence	Localizer	T1	T2	T2	STIR	Enhanced T1	Enhanced T1
Plane	3 plane	Sagittal	Sagittal	Axial	Sagittal	Sagittal	Axial
Coil type	Spine	Spine	Spine	Spine	Spine	Spine	Spine
Thickness, mm	10	4	4	4	4	4	4
TR, ms	20	641	3000	7360	3220	670	579
TE, ms	6	17	100	106	74	14	13
Flip angle	30	180	150	150	180	150	130
NEX	1	1	2	1	2	2	2
Matrix	128 × 256	256 × 256	307 × 384	192 × 256	256 × 256	269 × 384	230 × 256
FOV read, mm	380	300	320	200	320	320	200
FOV phase, mm	100	100	100	100	100	100	100
Comments					Trauma, Mets	If indicated	If indicated

Abbreviations: FOV, field of view; Mets, metastases; STIR, short tau inversion recovery; TE, echo time; TR, repetition time.

imaging of the spine. Axial gradient-echo images through the cervical spine are typically 2 mm thick.[2]

To depict the fine anatomic detail in the spine, high spatial resolution is a priority because of the small size of the cervical spine relative to the human body and because of the relatively superficial position of the spine within the human body. The use of surface coils, typically phased array receiver coils, helps to maximize signal-to-noise ratio and spatial resolution. Increasing phase-encoding steps results in a larger matrix and higher spatial resolution as a result, but also leads to increased imaging acquisition time, which increases the possibility of motion-related image degradation. Among the other factors affecting spinal imaging are matrix size, field of view, gradient moment nulling motion compensation, pulse triggering and gating, bandwidth, and phase-encoding axis.[3]

The pulse sequences used are determined by the clinical indications for the examination based

Table 3
Lumbar spine MR imaging protocols

Sequence	Localizer	T1 FLAIR	T2	T2	T1	STIR	Enhanced T1	Enhanced T1
Plane	3 plane	Sagittal	Sagittal	Axial	Axial	Sagittal	Sagittal	Axial
Coil type	Spine	Spine	Spine	Spine	Spine	Spine	Spine	Spine
Thickness, mm	10	4	4	4	4	4	4	4
TR, ms	3.27	1600	3150	4250	500	4560	657	539
TE, ms	1.64	12	95	106	14	79	12	14
Flip angle	55	150	180	150	90	180	90	90
NEX	2	1	2	1	1	2	2	1
Matrix	115 × 256	256 × 256	256 × 256	218 × 256	205 × 256	192 × 256	192 × 256	192 × 256
FOV read, mm	450	280	280	200	200	280	280	200
FOV phase, mm	100	100	100	100	100	100	75	100
Comments						Trauma, Mets	If indicated	If indicated

Abbreviations: FLAIR, fluid-attenuated inversion-recovery imaging; FOV, field of view; Mets, metastases; STIR, short tau inversion recovery; TE, echo time; TR, repetition time.

on the following major categories: degenerative disease including radicular symptomatology, trauma, cord compression/bony metastases, and infection.[4] Spin-echo and fast spin-echo sequences are the most common sequences used in spinal MR imaging. Short tau inversion recovery (STIR) imaging is useful to assess the bone marrow[5] and also in cases of infectious,[6] inflammatory,[7] and neoplastic[8] lesions. STIR imaging is also useful in the workup of trauma, to assess for ligamentous injury[9] and changes because of hemorrhage and/or edema. Contrast-enhanced imaging should be used, unless contraindicated, for indications including evaluation of the postoperative spine, suspected infection, or intradural or nontraumatic cord lesions.[10] Abnormalities within the epidural space identified during unenhanced evaluation for metastases and/or cord compression can be better delineated using contrast-enhanced images.[10]

Gradient-recalled echo (GRE), or gradient-echo, sequences allow for delineation of bone and disc margins, provide excellent contrast between the spinal cord and surrounding subarachnoid space, and allow clear visualization of the neural foramina and exiting nerve roots. Gradient-echo axial images are used in the cervical and thoracic spine to detect spinal canal and foraminal stenoses,[11] and serve as an important complement to long repetition time spin-echo imaging, given the faster acquisition time of GRE. As a result, GRE images are less susceptible to patient motion artifact. Although signal-to-noise ratio is increased with GRE, fat is of low signal intensity on GRE sequences compared with T1-weighted spin-echo imaging; as a result, morphologic detail defined by fat is not as well demonstrated on GRE images as on spin-echo images.[12]

Proton density images can be obtained simultaneously (repetition time [TR] 2000–3000 ms or greater, echo time [TE] 20–90 ms) when obtaining T1-weighted images and can also be derived from an earlier (first) echo while generating T2-weighted images. Proton density images of the spine are not routinely obtained but can provide valuable information concerning normal and pathologic spinal morphology.[5]

NORMAL SPINAL ANATOMY BASICS

The cervical spine comprises the first 7 superior vertebrae of the spinal column. The first and second segments of the cervical spine are unique. The other cervical vertebrae are similar in size and configuration. The first segment, C1, also known as the atlas, is ring shaped and consists of anterior and posterior arches and lateral articular masses. It lacks a central vertebral body. The second segment, C2, also known as the axis, is also ring shaped and has a superiorly oriented odontoid process, also known as the dens, which lies posterior to the anterior arch of C1. The normal distance between the dens and anterior arch of C1 is approximately 3 mm in adults and 4 mm in children.[13] There are prominent tubercles along the medial aspects of the lateral masses of C1 from which extend the transverse portion of the cruciate/cruciform ligament, that is, the transverse ligament, which confines the odontoid process of C2 posteriorly and delineates the anterior and posterior compartments. This relationship allows free rotation of C1 on C2 and provides for stability during upper cervical spinal flexion, extension, and lateral bending. The transverse ligament is covered posteriorly by the tectorial membrane. The alar ligaments are paired wing-like structures connecting the lateral aspects of the odontoid process with the occipital condyles. The thin apical ligament of the odontoid process directly anchors the tip of the odontoid process to the clivus in the anterior aspect of the foramen magnum. The tip of the odontoid process is anterior to the lower medulla. A line of low T1-weighted signal intensity seen through the base of the dens, with a correlative area of sclerosis on CT, represents the subdental synchondrosis, present in many healthy individuals; it may be distinguished from a fracture because the synchondrosis does not extend to the adjacent cortical bone (**Figs. 1** and **2**).

Unique to the cervical spine, the bilateral uncovertebral joints, also referred to as Luschka joints, are formed by articulation of the uncinate process of the inferior vertebral body with the uncus of the superior vertebral body (see **Fig. 2**; **Figs. 3** and **4**). The uncus is a cup-shaped groove on the posterior/inferior aspect of each cervical vertebral body (except C1), whereas the uncinate processes are located bilaterally on the posterosuperior aspects of the cervical vertebral bodies (except for C1 and C2). The cervical vertebrae also form transverse foramina bilaterally through which the vertebral arteries pass. Although the C7 vertebral body forms transverse foramina, the vertebral arteries usually enter the foramina at C6. The vertebral arteries are circular low signal structures owing to the flow-void phenomenon (see **Fig. 3C**). The spinous processes of the cervical spine are short and have bifid tips. Compared with the lumbar discs, the discs of the cervical and thoracic spine are much thinner and the outermost portion of the anulus is not as thick. The

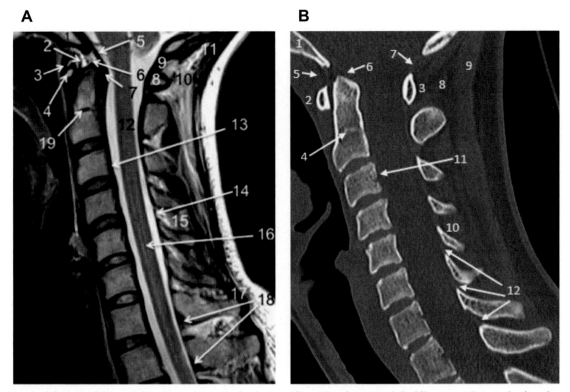

Fig. 1. (*A*) Sagittal T2-weighted image, cervical spine. 1, Clivus; 2, atlanto-occipital ligament; 3, anterior longitudinal ligament; 4, anterior arch C1; 5, superior fascicle of cruciform ligament/tectorial membrane; 6, apical ligament; 7, transverse ligament (of cruciform ligament); 8, posterior arch C1; 9, posterior occipital-atlantal membrane; 10, nuchal ligament; 11, semispinalis capitis muscle; 12, cervical spinal cord; 13, posterior longitudinal ligament/anterior thecal sac dura; 14, posterior dural sac; 15, interspinous ligament; 16, gray matter along central canal; 17, supraspinous ligament; 18, ligamentum flavum; 19, dental synchondrosis (disc anlage). (*B*) Sagittal CT image, cervical spine. 1, Clivus; 2, anterior arch C1; 3, posterior arch C1; 4, dental synchondrosis (disc anlage); 5, anterior longitudinal ligament; 6, tectorial membrane; 7, posterior occipital-atlantal membrane; 8, nuchal ligament; 9, semispinalis capitis muscle; 10, interspinous ligament; 11, posterior longitudinal ligament; 12, ligamentum flavum.

cervical spine is depicted in images in **Figs. 1–4**, **Figs. 5** and **6**.

Given the anterolateral-directed obliquity of the cervical neural foramina, oblique sagittal views are required to view cross-sectional sagittal anatomy of the neural foramina of the cervical spine.[14,15] In MR imaging, these images are obtained by using an axial image to first assess optimal angulation of the oblique sagittal plane through the foramina. Similar reconstructions can be performed with CT at the scanner based on the raw data. Alternatively, given the relatively routine availability of thin-section reconstructions, reformations in any plane, including the oblique sagittal plane through the foramina, can now be performed at the reading station on the picture archiving and communication system.

Throughout the spine, the intervertebral canals, or neural foramina, contain the nerve root and its sleeve, the dorsal root ganglion, fat, and blood vessels. The neural foramina are bounded anteriorly by the vertebral bodies and disc, superiorly and inferiorly by the pedicles, and posteriorly by the facet joints, which are covered by the ligamentum flavum (see **Fig. 3**).[16] The segmental osseous structures of the spine include the vertebral bodies and their appendages, including the pedicles, the articular pillars, laminae, and transverse and spinous processes. The major ligaments of the spine are the anterior longitudinal ligament, posterior longitudinal ligament, and ligamentum flavum (**Fig. 7**).[16] The spinal canal contains the thecal sac enclosed by the dura mater and surrounded by the epidural space, which contains epidural fat and a large venous plexus. Within the thecal sac are the spinal cord, conus medullaris, and cauda equina, surrounded by freely flowing CSF within the subarachnoid space. The conus medullaris normally terminates near the L1 vertebral level.[16] In the

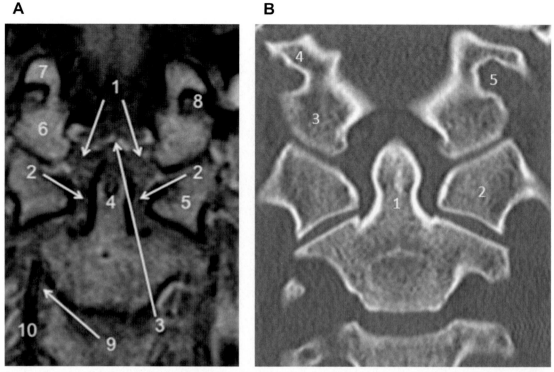

Fig. 2. (*A*) Coronal T1-weighted image, craniocervical junction. 1, Alar ligament; 2, transverse ligament (of cruciform ligament); 3, apical ligament; 4, dens; 5, lateral mass C1; 6, occipital condyle; 7, jugular tubercle of occipital bone; 8, hypoglossal canal; 9, uncinate process C3; 10, vertebral artery. (*B*) Coronal CT image, craniocervical junction. 1, Dens; 2, lateral mass C1; 3, occipital condyle; 4, jugular tubercle of occipital bone; 5, hypoglossal canal.

supine position, the nerve roots of the cauda equina in the lumbar spine are clustered in the dependent/posterior aspect of the spinal canal (**Figs. 8** and **9**).

The posterior border of nearly all of the vertebral bodies is flat or slightly concave when viewed in axial section, and the discs do not normally extend beyond the margins of the adjacent

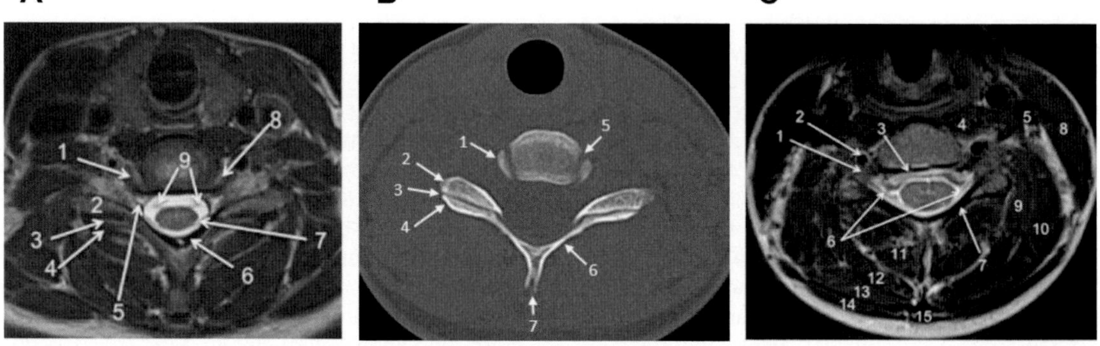

Fig. 3. (*A*) Axial T2-weighted image, lower cervical spine. 1, Uncinate process C7; 2, superior articular process C7; 3, apophyseal (facet) joint; 4, inferior articular process C6; 5, foraminal vein; 6, ligamentum flavum/cortex of lamina; 7, dorsal rootlet C7; 8, uncovertebral joint; 9, ventral rootlets C7. (*B*) Axial CT image, lower cervical spine. 1, Uncinate process C7; 2, superior articular process C7; 3, apophyseal (facet) joint; 4, inferior articular process C6; 5, uncovertebral joint; 6, lamina C6; 7, spinous process C6. (*C*) Axial T2-weighted image, mid-cervical spine. 1, Dorsal root ganglion; 2, vertebral artery; 3, posterior longitudinal ligament/anterior thecal sac dura; 4, longus colli muscle; 5, internal jugular vein; 6, dorsal rootlets; 7, lamina; 8, sternocleidomastoid muscle; 9, longissimus capitis muscle; 10, levator scapulae muscle; 11, semispinalis colli muscle; 12, semispinalis capitis muscle; 13, splenius capitis muscle; 14, trapezius muscle; 15, nuchal ligament.

A   **B**

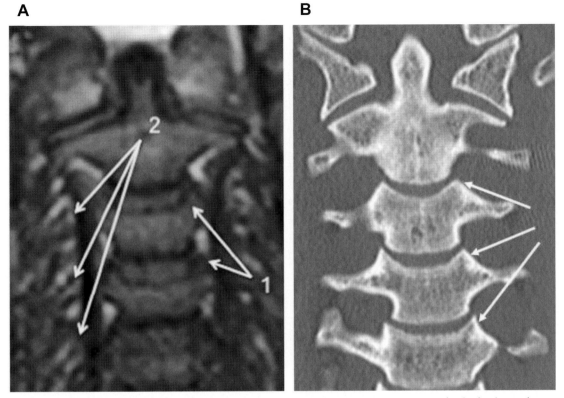

Fig. 4. (*A*) Coronal T1-weighted image, cervical spine. 1, Uncinate processes; 2, segmental spinal veins and nerve roots. (*B*) Coronal CT image, cervical spine. Arrows point to uncinate processes.

vertebral bodies.[16] However, with exaggerated extension, 1- to 2-mm budging may occur in some histologically normal discs.[17–19] The posterior margins of the discs tend to be slightly concave in the upper lumbar spine, straight at the L4/5 level, and slightly convex at the lumbosacral spinal junction. This appearance should not be confused with pathologic bulging. The axial appearance of the L5 vertebral body is biconcave, and iliolumbar ligaments emanate laterally from L5, characteristics that allow distinction of this vertebral segment from others when viewed in the axial plane (see **Fig. 9**). The spinal canal is round in the upper lumbar region and transitions to a triangular configuration in the lower lumbar region. Posterior epidural fat is consistently present in the posterior part of the spinal canal, whereas the anterior epidural fat is most prominent in the L5-S1 region (see **Fig. 8**).[16]

The bony canals of the neural foramina are normally well seen en face in the lumbar region using standard sagittal images (**Fig. 10**), because the orientation of the neural foramina in the lumbar spine is nearly directly lateral as opposed to

the anterolateral angle of the neural foramina of the cervical spine. This is distinct from the anterior obliquity required to optimally visualize the neural foramina of the cervical spine in the sagittal plane.

NORMAL SPINAL ANATOMY, T1-WEIGHTED MR IMAGING

T1-weighted images (TR 300–500 ms, TE 20–30 ms) in the sagittal plane are obtained as the preliminary survey pulse sequence for analyzing the cervical, thoracic, and lumbar spine. Sagittal and axial T1-weighed sequences provide the anatomic detail with which to begin a survey of the spine.

On T1-weighted images, high signal intensity is demonstrated in mature bone marrow and the epidural fat. The normal bone marrow signal is usually homogeneous, but may be heterogeneous and normally changes with aging.[20] The basivertebral venous channel is seen on the midline sagittal images as a high signal within the posterior aspect of the vertebral body owing to fat surrounding the vein with correlative area of

A

B

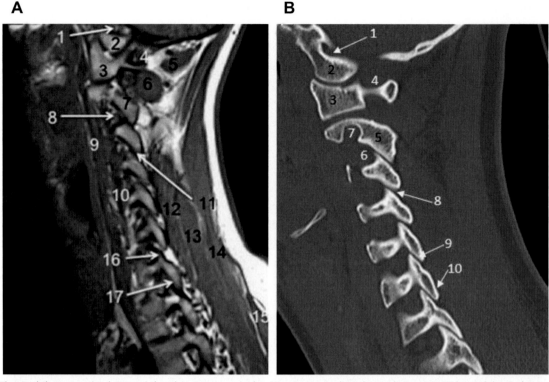

Fig. 5. (*A*) Parasagittal T1-weighted image, cervical spine. 1, Hypoglossal canal; 2, occipital condyle; 3, lateral mass C1; 4, vertebral artery; 5, rectus capitis posterior major muscle; 6, obliquus capitis inferior muscle; 7, articular pillar C2; 8, C3 dorsal root ganglion; 9, longus coli (cervicis) muscle; 10, vertebral artery; 11, apophyseal (facet) joint C3-4; 12, multifidis muscle; 13, semispinalis cervicis muscle; 14, splenius capitis muscle; 15, trapezius muscle; 16, superior articular process; 17, inferior articular process. (*B*) Parasagittal CT image, cervical spine. 1, Hypoglossal canal; 2, occipital condyle; 3, lateral mass C1; 4, groove for vertebral artery C1; 5, articular pillar C2; 6, C3 dorsal root ganglion location; 7, foramen transversarium C2 (contains vertebral artery); 8, apophyseal (facet) joint C3-C4; 9, superior articular process; 10, inferior articular process.

radiolucency on CT (see **Fig. 8**).[10] Peripherally, bone marrow is surrounded by low signal, proton-poor cortical bone, making it indistinguishable from the adjacent low T1-weighted signal intensity of the annulus fibrosus, spinal ligaments, and dura (see **Fig. 6**).[21] The relatively poor distinction between these structures on spin-echo imaging of the cervical and thoracic spine is attributable to little anterior epidural fat compared with that in the lumbar spine (see **Figs. 6** and **8**). Spin-echo imaging often also poorly differentiates cortical osteophytes from disc material. The anterior and posterior longitudinal ligaments adhere to the fibers of the annulus and appear on midsagittal images as an uninterrupted band of very low signal intensity on all pulse sequences (see **Figs. 8** and **10**).[21]

The intervertebral discs demonstrate slightly less signal than the adjacent vertebral bodies and differentiation of the centrally located nucleus pulposis and peripheral annulus fibrosis of the discs cannot be made precisely on T1-weighted images (see **Figs. 8** and **10**).

CSF demonstrates low signal on T1-weighted images and provides contrast with the adjacent, relatively higher signal intensity spinal cord and nerve roots within the spinal canal. The periphery of the spinal canal is lined by high signal-intensity epidural fat (see **Fig. 9**). The nerve roots and dorsal ganglia occupy the upper portion of the neural foramina, also referred to as the subpedicular notch (see **Fig. 10**), and appear as rounded low signal structures surrounded by high signal fat in the neural foramina. The nerve roots can be followed through the neural foramina on sagittal images. Epidural veins appear as signal voids anterosuperior to the nerves. It is important to distinguish the ventral internal longitudinal vein from the adjacent nerve and ganglion (see **Figs. 6**, **9**, and **10**). Each intervertebral canal can be divided arbitrarily into superior and inferior portions. The superior portion of the canal contains

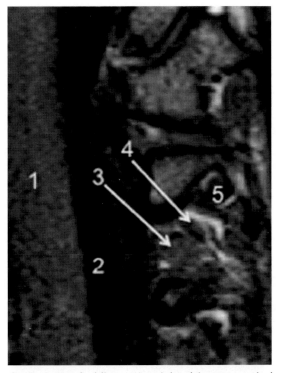

Fig. 6. Coronal oblique T1-weighted image, cervical spine. 1, Cervical spinal cord; 2, subarachnoid space; 3, dorsal root ganglion; 4, superior foraminal vein; 5, vertebral artery.

the dorsal root ganglion, veins, and epidural fat. The inferior portion contains the nerves, which lie below the disc level close to the superior articular process of the facet joint.[2]

The facet joints appear as linear structures with intermediate signal owing to the presence of intra-articular hyaline cartilage and synovial fluid (see **Fig. 9**).[22] The facet joint is formed by the concave surface of the superior articular process and the convex surface of the inferior articular process (see **Fig. 10**). The superior facet is located antero-laterally and faces posteromedially. The inferior facet is located posteromedially and faces antero-laterally. This differs in the cervical spine, where the superior and inferior articular processes are fused on either or both sides to form articular pillars, columns of bone that project laterally from the junction of the pedicle and lamina. The bony processes of the spine are better delineated on CT as compared with MR imaging. The ligamentum flava, which bilaterally cover the inner surface of the lamina and the anterior aspects of the facet joints, are intermediate in signal intensity and are distinguishable from the adjacent high signal central epidural fat and adjacent peripheral low signal lamina (see **Fig. 9**; **Fig. 11**).

NORMAL SPINAL ANATOMY, T2-WEIGHTED MR IMAGING

The parameters of T2-weighted imaging include a TR of 2000 to 3000 ms and a TE of 60 to 120 ms; the acquisition time is 2 to 3 times longer than that of T1-weighted imaging, rendering T2-weighted imaging more susceptible to motion artifact and greater noise.

In general, T2-weighted images reveal greater contrast differentiation among structures in

A   **B**

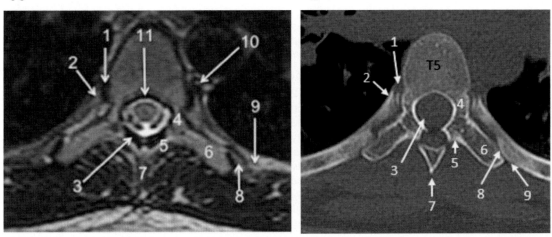

Fig. 7. (*A*) Axial T2-weighted image, thoracic spine. 1, Costovertebral joint; 2, head of rib; 3, ligamentum flavum; 4, pedicle; 5, lamina; 6, transverse process; 7, spinous process; 8, costotransverse joint; 9, tubercle of rib; 10, hemi-azygous vein; 11, posterior longitudinal ligament. (*B*) Axial CT image, thoracic spine. 1, Costovertebral joint; 2, head of rib; 3, ligamentum flavum; 4, pedicle T5; 5, lamina T5; 6, transverse process T5; 7, spinous process T4; 8, costotransverse joint; 9, tubercle of rib.

A   **B**

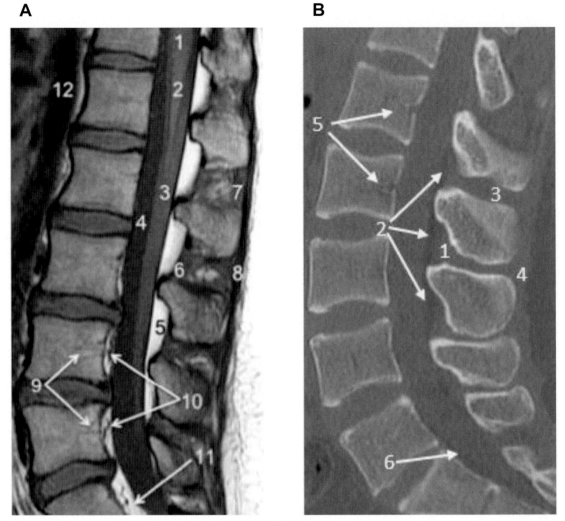

Fig. 8. (A) Sagittal T1-weighted image, lumbar spine. 1, Spinal cord; 2, conus medullaris; 3, cauda equina; 4, subarachnoid space; 5, posterior epidural fat; 6, ligamentum flavum; 7, interspinous ligament; 8, supraspinous ligament; 9, basivertebral venous plexus; 10, epidural venous plexus; 11, anterior epidural fat; 12, aorta. (B) Sagittal CT image, lumbar spine. 1, Ligamentum flavum; 2, posterior epidural fat; 3, interspinous ligament; 4, supraspinous ligament; 5, basivertebral venous plexus; 6, anterior epidural fat.

comparison with T1-weighted images. With T2 weighting, the proton-poor cortical bone demonstrates low signal intensity and the bone marrow remains fairly high in signal intensity because of its fat content. The basivertebral veins may be of even higher signal intensity because of flow phenomena and should not be mistaken for a fracture (**Fig. 12**). The channel of the basivertebral vein is usually of intermediate signal on the T2-weighted image. The normally hydrated nucleus pulposus composed of water and proteoglycans shows high T2-weighted signal centrally, with lower signal from the less-hydrated annulus fibrosis (see **Fig. 12**). The annulus fibrosis is composed

of fibrocartilage centrally, whereas the outer fibers are made up of concentrically oriented collagen fibers. The annulus is anchored to the adjacent vertebral bodies by Sharpey fibers, which are normally not visible by MR imaging.

CSF demonstrates high signal intensity because of its long T2-weighted relaxation time, which allows sensitive identification of surrounding intraspinal structures such as the spinal cord and nerve roots that are intermediate in signal intensity (see **Fig. 12**; **Figs. 13–15**). When the patient is supine, as in most cases of spinal imaging, the mid-thoracic spinal cord is positioned within the central/anterior aspect of the

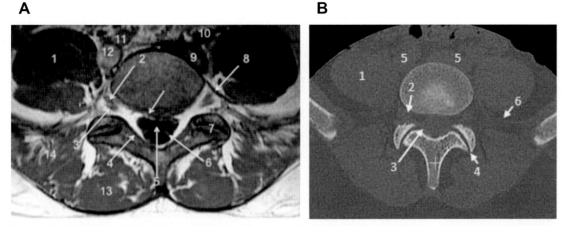

Fig. 9. (*A*) Axial T1-weighted image, lumbar spine at L5-S1. 1, Psoas muscle; 2, L5 nerve root, ventral ramus; 3, L5 nerve root, dorsal ramus; 4, ligamentum flavum; 5, subarachnoid space; 6, nerve roots of cauda equina; 7, facet joint; 8, iliolumbar ligament (signifies L5 vertebral level); 9, left external iliac vein; 10, left external iliac artery; 11, right external iliac artery; 12, right external iliac vein; 13, transversospinalis (multifidis) muscle; 14, erector spinae muscle group. (*B*) Axial CT image, lumbar spine at L5-S1. 1, Psoas muscle; 2, L5 nerve root; 3, ligamentum flavum; 4, facet joint; 5, iliac vasculature; 6, iliolumbar ligament.

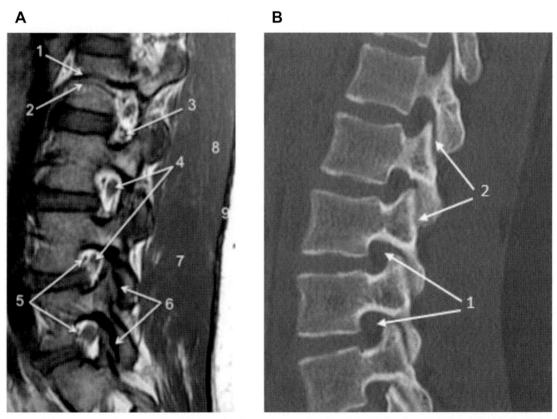

Fig. 10. (*A*) Parasagittal T1-weighted image, lumbar spine. 1, Lumbar vein; 2, lumbar artery; 3, inferior foraminal veins; 4, dorsal root ganglia; 5, superior foraminal veins; 6, facet joints; 7, transversospinalis (multifidis) muscle; 8, erector spinae muscle group; 9, thoracolumbar fascia, posterior layer. (*B*) Parasagittal CT image, lumbar spine. 1, Dorsal root ganglia/lumbar nerve roots; 2, facet joints.

A   **B**

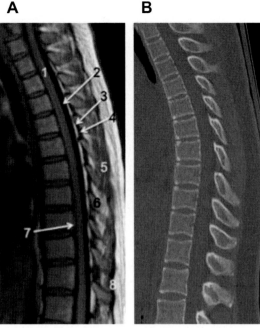

Fig. 11. (A) Sagittal T1-weighted image, thoracic spine. 1, Thoracic spinal cord; 2, subarachnoid space; 3, posterior epidural fat; 4, ligamentum flavum; 5, transversospinalis (multifidus) muscle; 6, spinous process; 7, epidural vein; 8, supraspinous ligament. (B) Correlative Sagittal CT image, thoracic spine. The posterior epidural fat and the ligamentum flavi can be seen.

spinal canal owing to the normally mild thoracic kyphosis (see **Fig. 12**). CSF often has patchy areas of low signal because of turbulence of flow and/or other flow artifacts related to pulsation effects; these can be particularly troublesome in images with longer echo delays and in those acquired using high magnetic field strength systems (see **Fig. 14**).

T2* images intensify structures with long T2 relaxation times, such as CSF, the nucleus pulposis, and facet joint cartilage. On T2* images, the high signal intensity of the venous plexus posterior to the vertebral body separates the posterior longitudinal ligament and cortical bone of the vertebral body. T2* imaging also allows differentiation of the gray and white matter of the spinal cord. Gray matter appears as a butterfly-shaped region of high signal intensity centrally within the spinal cord when using this technique.[23]

NORMAL SPINAL BONE MARROW MR IMAGING

The axial skeleton contains red marrow, a major site of hematopoiesis throughout life. There is normally a gradual conversion of red marrow to fatty marrow in the appendicular skeleton, which

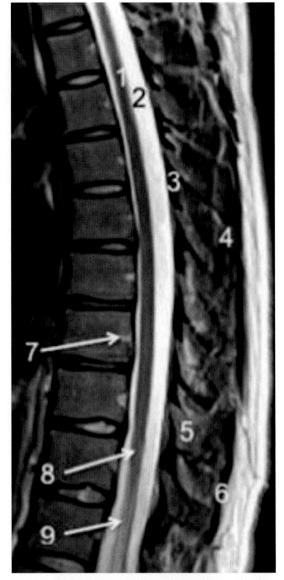

Fig. 12. Sagittal T2-weighted image, thoracic spine. 1, Thoracic spinal cord; 2, subarachnoid space; 3, ligamentum flavum; 4, transversospinalis (multifidus) muscle; 5, spinous process; 6, supraspinous ligament; 7, basivertebral vein; 8, conus medullaris; 9, cauda equina.

is completed by approximately 25 years of life. The red marrow in the vertebrae also normally undergoes conversion of fatty marrow, although more subtly than in the appendicular skeleton. The fat content of the vertebral body varies with age, degeneration of adjacent discs, therapy, such as radiation, and increased hematopoiesis in processes such as sickle cell disease or other diseases affecting the bone marrow.[20] In younger patients, high signal fatty marrow can be seen as linear areas adjacent to the

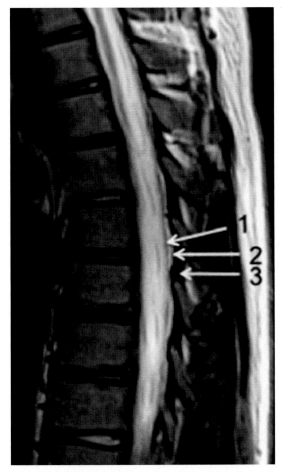

Fig. 13. Parasagittal T2-weighted image, thoracic spine. 1, Posterior thecal sac dura; 2, posterior epidural fat; 3, ligamentum flavum.

basivertebral vein. With advancing age, fatty marrow may appear band-like, triangular, or multifocal, and may take up relatively large areas of the vertebral body in patients older than 40 years.[20] There is significant variability in the marrow pattern among adults and even within an individual.[20,24]

Ricci and colleagues[25] identified several patterns of marrow distribution in the spine. In pattern 1, the vertebral body demonstrates uniformly low signal on T1-weighted images except for linear areas of high, fatty signal surrounding the basivertebral vein. In pattern 2, band-like and triangular areas of high signal are found near the end plates and corners of the vertebral body, possibly related to mechanical stress near the end plates. In pattern 3, there are diffusely distributed areas of high signal from fat measuring a few millimeters (pattern 3a) or relatively well-marginated areas on the range of 1 cm (pattern 3b).

In the cervical spine, pattern 1 is found predominantly in patients younger than 40 with patterns 2 and 3 in those who are older than 40 years. Patterns 2 and 3 generally develop earliest in the lumbar spine, followed by the thoracic spine, and lastly in the cervical spine.[25] Overall, there is continued gradual replacement of hematopoietic marrow with fatty marrow that continues until death. Healthy elderly individuals have marked high signal throughout the vertebral body, reflecting the predominance of fatty marrow. Large variations exist, however, secondary to differences among individuals and responses to mechanical stress.[25]

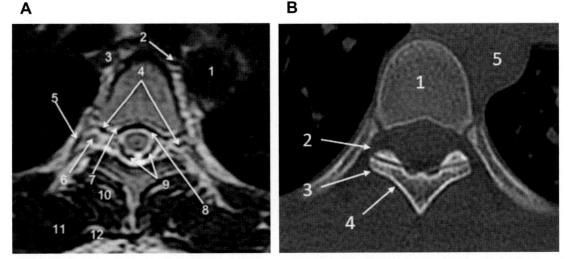

Fig. 14. (A) Axial T2-weighted image, thoracic spine. 1, Aorta; 2, hemiazygous vein; 3, azygous vein; 4, foraminal veins; 5, thoracic intercostal vein; 6, dorsal root ganglion; 7, basivertebral veins, slow flow; 8, posterior longitudinal ligament; 9, CSF flow artifacts; 10, transversospinalis (multifidis) muscle; 11, longissimus dorsi muscle; 12, trapezius muscle. (B) Axial CT image, thoracic spine. 1, T8 vertebral body; 2, T9 superior articular process; 3, T8 inferior articular process; 4, T8 right lamina; 5, aorta.

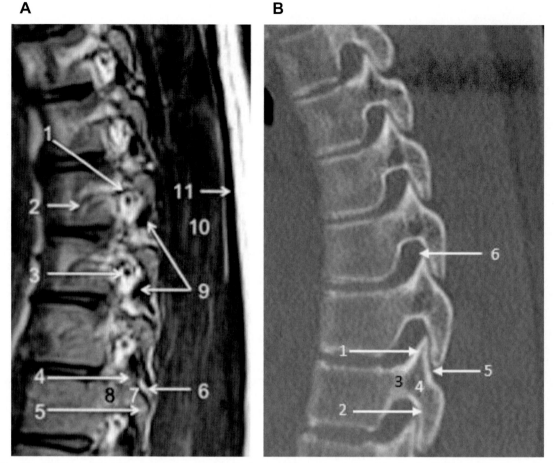

Fig. 15. (*A*) Parasagittal T2 weighted image, thoracic neural foramen. 1, Foraminal vein; 2, Thoracic paravertebral intercostal vein and artery; 3, Foraminal nerve root; 4, Superior articular process; 5, Inferior articular process; 6, Facet joint; 7, Pars interarticularis; 8, Pedicle; 9, Ligamentum flavum; 10, Erector spinae muscle group; 11, Trapezius muscle. (*B*) Parasagittal CT image, thoracic neural foramen. 1, Superior articular process; 2, Inferior articular process; 3, Pedicle; 4, Pars interarticularis; 5, Facet joint; 6, Neuroforamen with foraminal nerve root.

Chemical shift artifact, used extensively in imaging of the adrenal glands and the liver, can be used to assess the bone marrow of the spine in certain instances. In-phase/opposed-phase imaging assesses for the presence of fat and water in a voxel of tissue. The technique takes advantage of the fact that water and fat protons precess at different frequencies and without a refocusing pulse; when there are both fat and water protons in a given voxel, there will be some signal intensity loss on images that are obtained when the protons are in their opposed phase. The utility of chemical shift imaging lies in that cases of spinal neoplastic disease, normal fat-containing marrow is replaced with tumor, which can result in lack of signal suppression on the opposed-phase images. There have been a few reports that have described in-phase/opposed-phase imaging of the spinal bone marrow.[26–28]

MYELOGRAPHY

Myelography is a minimally invasive technique that allows better visualization of the intrathecal contents by administering a positive contrast agent. A lumbar puncture is performed and contrast is delivered percutaneously into the intrathecal space typically through a 22-gauge spinal needle. This technique allows evaluation of the spine in individuals who would otherwise benefit from an MR imaging but are unable to receive one because of some contraindication or the presence of hardware which would otherwise produce artifact and subsequently degrade the examination.

Before the current use of water-soluble nonionic contrast agents, agents such as air and lipiodol were used in conjunction with radiography to help image spinal tumors as early as the 1920s.[29] Lipiodol came with multiple complications including chronic adhesive arachnoiditis.[30] In the 1940s, pantoopaque was used, which still gave rise to cases of arachnoiditis and other complications.[29] Use of plain radiographs for imaging was used until the 1970s when CT began to increase in usage.[29]

Common indications for the utilization of this technique would be in postsurgical patients, those with spinal stenosis and contraindication to MR imaging, radiation therapy treatment planning, and spinal CSF leak evaluation. The bony anatomy on imaging is the same as exemplified on normal CT. On fluoroscopy, after injection of subarachnoid contrast material, the contrast should spread out in the thecal space in a rostral-caudal manner, with positive outlining of the cauda equina nerve roots. On fluoroscopy, the bony anatomic landmarks and the positive contrast in the spine should appear as in **Fig. 16**. With subsequent performance of a CT myelogram, the intrathecal contents including the spinal cord and nerve roots can be well visualized (**Fig. 17**).

An advanced imaging technique used with myelography is dual energy CT with isolation of the CSF

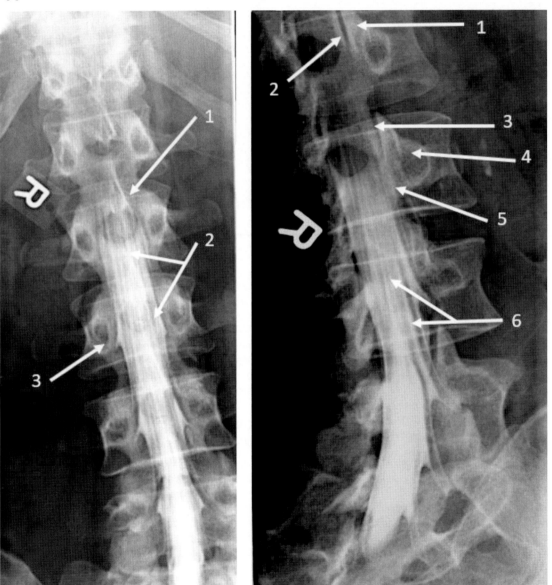

A **B**

Fig. 16. (*A*) AP spot fluoroscopic image. 1, Spinous process; 2, cauda equina nerve roots outlined by contrast; 3, pedicle. (*B*) Oblique spot fluoroscopic image. 1, Inferior articular process; 2, superior articular process; 3, facet joint; 4, pedicle; 5, pars interarticularis; 6, contrast outlining cauda equina nerve roots.

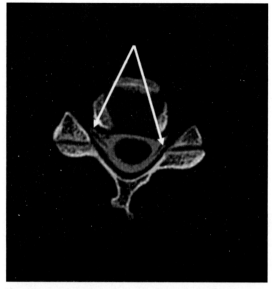

Fig. 17. Axial postcontrast cervical CT myelogram. Arrows point to the nerve roots outlined by intrathecal contrast.

column or using a bone subtracting algorithm to help better visualize the intrathecal space. These methods can be particularly useful in cases of subtle CSF leak or identifying focal areas of CSF diverticula. As is shown in **Fig. 18**, the intrathecal contrast column can be subtracted from the surrounding tissues. In **Fig. 19**, utilizing a CT algorithm to extract the bone is shown to be useful in focusing on the thecal sac and evaluating for areas of leak.

MR IMAGING FINDINGS OF VERTEBRAL HEMANGIOMAS

Hemangiomas, composed of angiomatoid fibroadipose tissue interspersed among tortuous thin-walled sinuses, are the most common benign tumors of the spine, seen in 10% or more of healthy adults.[31] They are most common in the thoracic spine followed by the lumbar spine, and are relatively rare in the cervical spine.[31] They tend to be well-circumscribed tumors within the vertebral bodies, demonstrating high signal intensity on both T1-weighted and T2-weighted images. T1 shortening is produced by the fatty component, whereas T2 prolongation is produced by the angiomatous component. The very low signal of the bony trabeculae, which can classically be seen on CT and result in the classic "polka dot" or "corduroy" appearance, is overshadowed on MR imaging by the signals from the internal elements described previously. Focal fatty infiltration, a common marrow variant, may be confused with hemangiomas on T1-weighted images;

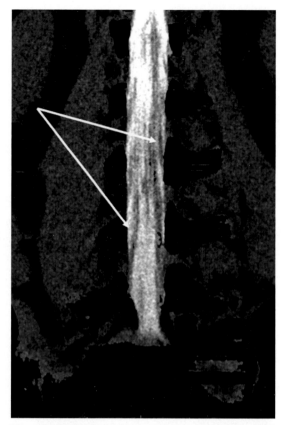

Fig. 18. Coronal dual energy CT myelogram with bone subtraction algorithm. Arrows point to the clearly outlined nerve roots of the cauda equina.

however, the expected corresponding decrease in signal intensity on T2-weighted images serves to distinguish focal fat from the normally high T2-weighted signal of hemangiomas.[32] Hemangiomas may sometimes have a paucity of fatty elements, which may render these lesions isointense or hypointense on T1-weighted images.[32]

NORMAL MR IMAGING OF INTERVERTEBRAL DISCS

In the neonate, the nucleus pulposis is a highly gelatinous, translucent, relatively large, ovoid structure. The anulus fibrosus consists of dense fibers organized as concentric lamellae similar to tree rings. In the second decade of life, the outer portion of the disc is replaced by solid tissue and the anulus becomes more dense. In adults, the nucleus pulposis consists of amorphous fibrocartilage and the anulus becomes even more dense. The demarcation between the nucleus and anulus becomes less distinct with age. In adults, a transversely oriented band of low signal intensity in the

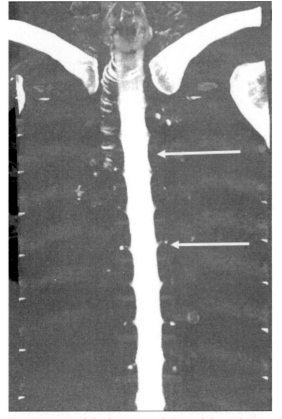

Fig. 19. Coronal dual energy subtracted thoracic myelogram. Arrow points to the intrathecal contrast column. Arrowhead highlights small outpouchings at the nerve roots.

midportion of the disc represents a fibrous plate visible on MR imaging. Concentric tears of the annulus are seen in normal discs, and transverse tears, although a manifestation of degenerative disease, are not infrequently seen in asymptomatic adults.[17,19]

Intervertebral herniation of disc material may remodel the vertebral end plate or may extend into the vertebral body. Such herniations are typically referred to as Schmorl nodes.[31] This type of herniation is presumed to have little clinical significance, and it has been observed as early as the second decade of life.

There are abnormalities and normal variants that may mimic the appearance of an extruded or sequestered disc on MR imaging. These include synovial cysts, dilated nerve root sleeves (arachnoid diverticulae), perineural cysts, conjoined nerve roots, nerve sheath tumors, and foreign material such as bullet fragments, metallic hardware, and cement from vertebroplasties. Dilated nerve root sleeves demonstrate signal characteristics identical to CSF, which should allow for differentiation of these from disc material.[4]

COMMON NORMAL SPINAL MR IMAGING ARTIFACTS

The most common source of artifact in MR imaging occurs secondary to patient motion. Whereas random movement leads to blurring, periodic motion, such as with CSF pulsation, cardiac motion, and respiratory motion, leads to ghosting artifacts in the form of image harmonics along the phase-encoding direction because phase information is acquired over an entire scan (minutes), whereas frequency information is acquired over a single frequency readout (milliseconds).[21]

CSF flow-related phenomena can be divided into time-of-flight (TOF) effects and turbulent flow, which produces dark signal. TOF effects are divided into TOF signal loss resulting in dark CSF signal and flow-related enhancement producing bright CSF signal. TOF loss typically occurs in spin-echo or fast spin-echo imaging when protons do not experience both the initial radiofrequency pulse and the subsequent radiofrequency refocusing pulse. TOF loss effects are more pronounced (darker signal) with faster proton velocity, thinner slices, longer TE, and an imaging plane perpendicular to flow. GRE techniques are less susceptible to TOF loss because of the short TE.

Typical locations for TOF losses include the lateral ventricles just superior to the foramen of Monro, the third ventricle, the fourth ventricle, and within the cervical and thoracic spinal canal. Given the positive relationship between CSF velocity and TOF losses, this effect is magnified in individuals with an underlying abnormally hyperdynamic state, such as hydrocephalus. In addition, laminar flow results in peripherally located protons moving at a slower velocity and leads to a reduction in TOF losses. Turbulent flow results in a broader spectrum of proton velocities and a wide range of flow directions that are not seen in typical laminar flow. This results in more rapid dephasing and signal loss termed "intravoxel dephasing." A commonly encountered CSF flow artifact is the signal void in the dorsal subarachnoid space on sagittal T2-weighted images of the thoracic spine owing to a combination of the respiratory-related and cardiac-related pulsatile CSF flow superimposed on cranially directed bulk CSF flow and turbulent flow from CSF moving from the ventral subarachnoid space to the dorsal subarachnoid space (see **Fig. 14; Fig. 20**).

Another common artifact that occurs normally on MR imaging relates to chemical shift and occurs because water and fat protons resonate at slightly different frequencies because of the

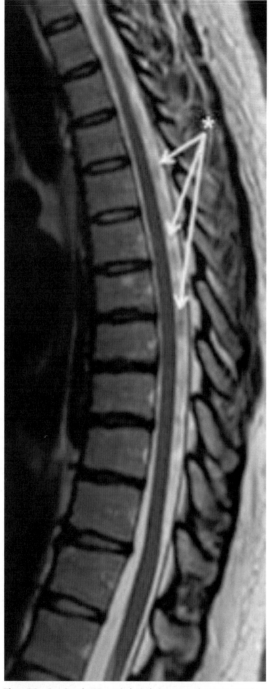

Fig. 20. Sagittal T2-weighted image demonstrating CSF pulsation artifact within the posterior aspect of the thecal sac (*asterisk*).

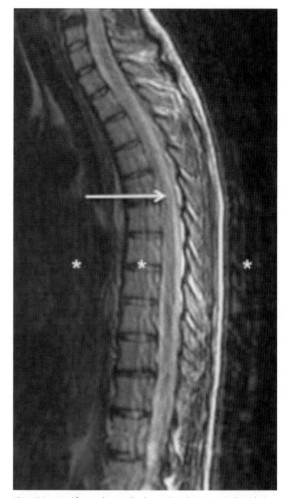

Fig. 21. Artifact degraded sagittal T2-weighted image, thoracic spine. Truncation artifacts (*asterisk*). Truncation artifact simulating spinal cord syrinx (*solid white arrow*).

effects of their local magnetic environment. The most common type of chemical shift artifact occurs along the frequency-encoding axis and results in a spatial misregistration.[33] In the spine, this artifact is manifested as artifactual black lines along the frequency-encoding axis and are most evident in the sagittal T1-weighted images where they produce asymmetric thicknesses of the vertebral end plates. The hyaline cartilage end plate is usually difficult to visualize on MR imaging owing to overlap from chemical shift artifact.[34] Phase-encoding and frequency-encoding gradients may be reversed for imaging the spine in the sagittal plane to avoid chemical shift artifacts in the end plates and discs from the discovertebral interfaces.[34] Chemical shift is proportional to the magnetic field strength.

Truncation artifact, known as Gibb phenomenon, is seen as bands parallel to the spinal cord. This occurs at the interface of CSF and spinal cord because of high-contrast boundaries and is related to acquisition parameters, such as field of view and voxel size (**Fig. 21**).[35,36]

SUMMARY

Spinal MR imaging is an excellent tool for identifying details of spinal anatomy, including the intraspinal contents, neural foramina, joints, ligaments, intervertebral discs, and bone marrow. The cortical bony structures of the spine, as elsewhere in the body, are generally better imaged using CT. Conventional and CT myelography is an alternative to MR imaging in those with contraindications to MR imaging or in the evaluation of spinal CSF leaks. Motion-related and flow-related artifacts may occur during spinal MR imaging and should not be mistaken for a pathologic condition. As advancements continue to be made in both MR imaging hardware and software, spinal MR imaging can continue to expand its role in the delineation of normal and abnormal spinal anatomy.

REFERENCES

1. Brown BM, Schwartz HR, Frank E, et al. Preoperative evaluation of cervical radiculopathy and myelopathy by surface-coil MR imaging. AJNR Am J Neuroradiol 1988;9:859–66.
2. Norman D, Mills CM, Grant-Zawadzki M, et al. Magnetic resonance imaging of the spinal cord and canal: potentials and limitations. AJR Am J Roentgenol 1983;141:1147–52.
3. Chan WP, Lang P, Genant HK, et al. MRI of the musculoskeletal system. Philadelphia: W.B. Saunders Company; 1994.
4. Kaplan PA, Helms CA, Dussault R, et al. Musculoskeletal MRI. Philadelphia: W.B. Saunders Company; 2001.
5. Demaerel P, Sunaert S, Wilms G. Sequences and techniques in spinal MR imaging. JBR-BTR 2003; 86:221–2.
6. Dagirmanjian A, Schils J, McHenry MC. MR imaging of spinal infections. Magn Reson Imaging Clin N Am 1999;7:525–38.
7. Maksymowych WP, Crowther SM, Dhillon SS, et al. Systematic assessment of inflammation by magnetic resonance imaging in the posterio elements of the spine in ankylosing spondylitis. Arthritis Care Res 2010;62:4–10.
8. Myslivecek M, Nekula J, Bacovsky J, et al. Multiple myeloma: predictive value of tc-99m mibi scintigraphy and MRI in its diagnosis and therapy. Nucl Med Rev Cent East Eur 2008;11:12–6.
9. Williams RL, Hardman JA, Lyons K. MR imaging of suspected acute spinal instability. Injury 1998;29: 109–13.
10. Breger RK, Williams AL, Daniels DL, et al. Contrast enhancement in spinal MR imaging. AJNR Am J Neuroradiol 1989;10:633–7.
11. Hedberg MC, Drayer BP, Flom RA, et al. Gradient echo (GRASS) MR imaging in cervical radiculopathy. AJNR Am J Neuroradiol 1988;9:145–51.
12. Wang M, Dai Y, Han Y, et al. Susceptibility weighted imaging in detecting hemorrhage in acute cervical spinal cord injury. Magn Reson Imaging 2011;29: 365–73.
13. Parke WW, Sherk HH. Normal adult anatomy. In: Sherk HH, editor. The cervical spine. Philadelphia: JB Lippincott; 1989. p. 11.
14. Yenerich DO, Haughton VM. Oblique plane MR imaging of the cervical spine. J Comput Assist Tomogr 1986;10:823.
15. Modic MT, Masaryk TJ, Ross JS, et al. Cervical radiculopathy: value of oblique MR imaging. Radiology 1987;163:227.
16. Drake RL, Vogl AW, Mitchell AW, et al. Gray's atlas of anatomy. Philadelphia: Churchill Livingstone; 2007.
17. Boden S, Davis D, Dina T, et al. Abnormal magnetic resonance scans of the lumbar spine in asymptomatic subjects: a prospective investigation. J Bone Joint Surg Am 1990;72:403–8.
18. Yu S, Haughton V, Sether LA. Anulus fibrosus in bulging intervertebral disks. Radiology 1988;169: 761–3.
19. Jensen M, Brant-Zawadski M, Obuchowski N, et al. Magnetic resonance imaging of the lumbar spine in people without back pain. N Engl J Med 1995;331: 69–73.
20. Dooms GC, Fisher MR, Hricack H, et al. Bone marrow imaging: magnetic resonance studies related to age and sex. Radiology 1985;155:429–32.
21. Reicher MA, Gold RH, Halbach VV, et al. MR imaging of the lumbar spine: anatomic correlations and the effects of technical variations. Am J Roentgenol 1986;147:891–8.
22. Czervionke LF, Daniels DL, Ho PSP, et al. Cervical neural foramina: correlative anatomic and MR imaging study. Radiology 1988;169:753.
23. Czervionke LF, Daniels DL, Ho PSP, et al. The MR appearance of gray and white matter in the cervical spinal cord. AJNR Am J Neuroradiol 1988;9:557–62.
24. Loevner L, Tobey JD, Yousem DM. MR imaging characteristics of cranial bone marrow in adult patients with underlying systemic disorders compared with healthy control subjects. AJNR Am J Neuroradiol 2002;23(2):248–54.
25. Ricci C, Cova M, Kang YS, et al. Normal age-related patterns of cellular and fatty bone marrow distribution in the axial skeleton: MR imaging study. Radiology 1990;177:83–8.
26. Eito K, Waka S, Naoko N, et al. Vertebral neoplastic compression fractures: assessment by dual-phase chemical shift imaging. J Magn Reson Imaging 2004;20:1020–4.
27. Baker LL, Goodman SB, Perkash I, et al. Benign versus pathologic compression fractures of vertebral

bodies: assessment with conventional spin-echo, chemical-shift, and STIR MR imaging. Radiology 1990;174:495–502.

28. Erly WK, Oh ES, Outwater EK. The utility of in-phase/opposed-phase imaging in differentiating malignancy from acute benign compression fractures of the spine. AJNR Am J Neuroradiol 2006; 27:1183–8.

29. Pomerantz SI. Myelography: modern techniques and indications. In: Masdeu JC, Gilberto González R, editors. Handbook of clinical neurology. Amsterdam: Elsevier; 2016. p. 193–208.

30. Hoeffner EG, Mukherji SK, Srinivasan A, et al. Neuroradiology back to the future: head and neck imaging. AJNR Am J Neuroradiol 2012; 33(11):2026–32.

31. Schmorl G, Junghanns H. The human spine in health and disease. NewYork: Grune and Stratton; 1959. p. 12.

32. Laredo JD, Reizine D, Bard M, et al. Vertebral hemangiomas: radiologic evaluation. Radiology 1986; 161:183.

33. Bronskill MJ, McVeigh ER, Kucharazyk W, et al. Syrinx-like artifacts on MR images of the spinal cord. Radiology 1988;166:485–8.

34. Bellon EM, Haacke EM, Coleman PE, et al. MR artifacts: a review. Am J Roentgenol 1986;147:1271–81.

35. Pusey E, Lufkin R, Brown R, et al. Magnetic resonance imaging artifacts: mechanisms and clinical significance. Radiographics 1986;6:891–911.

36. Czervionke LF, Czervionke JM, Daniels DL, et al. Characteristic features of MR truncation artifacts. AJNR Am J Neuroradiol 1988;9:815–24.

Percutaneous Vertebroplasty
A History of Procedure, Technology, Culture, Specialty, and Economics

Sergiy V. Kushchayev, MD[a,b,]*, Philip C. Wiener, DO[c],
Oleg M. Teytelboym, MD[d], John A. Arrington, MD[a], Majid Khan, MBBS, MD[a],
Mark C. Preul, MD[e]

KEYWORDS

- Percutaneous vertebroplasty • Polymethyl methacrylate (PMMA) • Vertebral biomechanics
- Kyphoplasty

KEY POINTS

- Percutaneous vertebroplasty (VP) became one of the fastest emerging techniques in spine surgery.
- VP was the synthesis of information gained from spinal biopsy developments, the inception of bio-materials used in surgery, and unique health care climate within France and the United States.
- Designed as a revolutionary technique, VP was determined to safely and effectively treat vertebral body fractures with minimal side effects experienced by the patient and was rapidly adopted and marketed in the United States.
- Development of VP stood at the vanguard of percutaneous spinal surgery procedures.

INTRODUCTION

Progression of surgical technology is the result of many factors, and a "better procedure" adoption is often not the result of only defined efficacy or rational determinations. Such advancement is often associated with ideals of being conceived based on basic or clinical research, new or refined technology, and imagination to develop ground-breaking and life-saving techniques. Often forgotten are social, economic, marketing, engineering materials, relationships to specialty, and regulatory contexts, as well as whether there is confirmation of efficacy.

Percutaneous vertebroplasty (VP) became one of the fastest emerging techniques in spine surgery over the last decades. VP progressed from a virtually unknown procedure to one that is performed on hundreds of thousands of patients annually. The invention of VP provides a historically exciting case study into a rapidly adopted procedure, which had a significant impact on the direction of spinal surgery and became an often cited example for comparative-effectiveness research. VP was the synthesis of information gained from spinal biopsy developments, the inception of biomaterials used in medicine, and the unique health care climate within France

Disclosure Statement: The authors have nothing to disclose.
[a] Department of Radiology, Moffitt Cancer Center, 12902 USF Magnolia Drive, Tampa, FL 33612, USA;
[b] Department of Radiology, Johns Hopkins Hospital, North Caroline Street, Baltimore, MD 21287, USA;
[c] Einstein Healthcare Network, 5501 Old York Road, Philadelphia, PA 19141, USA; [d] Department of Radiology, Mercy Catholic Medical Center, 1500 Lansdowne Avenue, Darby, PA 19023, USA; [e] Department of Neurosurgery, Barrow Neurological Institute, St. Joseph's Hospital and Medical Center, 350 West Thomas Road, Phoenix, AZ 85013, USA
* Corresponding author.
E-mail address: kushchayev@gmail.com

Neuroimag Clin N Am 29 (2019) 481–494
https://doi.org/10.1016/j.nic.2019.07.011
1052-5149/19/© 2019 Elsevier Inc. All rights reserved.

during the 1980s. It was designed as a revolutionary technique that was determined to safely and effectively treat vertebral body fractures with minimal side effects experienced by the patient, and which was rapidly adopted and marketed in the United States. The impact of VP on spine surgery was profound.

Percutaneous Approach to Vertebral Bodies

Ball,[1–3] in 1934, published a method for percutaneous spinal biopsy via needle aspiration, and Ball and Robertson[3] used an radiography-assisted aspiratory biopsy method that ensured relative safety and accuracy and allowed for the precise pathology diagnosis. Valls and colleagues[4] suggested that each vertebral segment should not be considered equal and altered Ball and Robertson's methods, depending on the vertebral level of the lesion to ensure more accurate and safe aspiration. In 1949, Michele and Krueger[5] proposed 5 methods of direct approaches to the thoracic and lumbar vertebral bodies, including using a trephine passed through the pedicles into the vertebral body. The method was important not only for lesion access, which resided only within the vertebral body, but also their more direct approach to the vertebral body via the pedicles allowed supplemental procedures after the biopsy, such as injection medications and other materials into the vertebral body. From the late 1940s through the 1950s, various improvements to percutaneous biopsies were made. In 1955, Ottolenghi[6] reported a large series (1061 procedures) of orthopedic biopsies, including spinal procedures, with results positive in 84.3%. In 1956, Craig,[7] in an attempt to increase the success rate and decrease the impact of vertebral body biopsies on patients, developed a new set of needles, which became highly effective and achieved long-lasting use. Those early reports described methods of blind insertion of the needle. It seems that Rabinov and colleagues[8] in 1967 were the first to improve the spinal biopsy technique using intraoperative fluoroscopy during the procedure. In 1981, Adapon and colleagues[9] first described 22 patients who underwent a computed tomographic (CT)-guided percutaneous needle spinal biopsy that allowed safe and accurate biopsy at virtually all segments of the spine.

Bone Cement in Spinal Surgery

In the late nineteenth century, chemists began to synthesize methyl methacrylate from acrylic acid, and in 1877, German chemists, Fitting and Paul, successfully polymerized the monomer, creating polymethyl methacrylate (PMMA).[10] In 1934, another German chemist and pharmacist, Röhm, a pioneer in the field of plastics, developed a large number of acrylic and methacrylic compounds, including Plexiglas. By 1936, PMMA was generally marketed and widely used, such as in aircraft and military equipment, during World War II. PMMA was initially used in dental applications. PMMA began to be used with a growing interest in functional and cosmetic surgeries for veterans after World War II and replaced metallic cranioplasty implants because of "almost a social stigma to having 'a silver plate in the head.'"[11]

After a series of animal experiments that indicated usability of PMMA for cranial surgery, acrylic masses were introduced in neurosurgery.[12] In 1946, Elkins and Cameron[13] reported 70 clinical cases in which PMMA was used for cranioplasty, concluding that acrylic worked well to repair skull defects, and there were no significant surgical or postoperative complications. Based on the use of acrylics in cranioplasty, Hamby and Glaser[14] replaced intervertebral discs with PMMA in 1959. Within the same year, Knight[15] related using PMMA to cover vertebral segments in order to improve spine stabilization and alleviate issues associated with arthritis, spondylosis, and injury.

Until 1960, acrylics had been used for superficial repair or replacement of the bone or joint in entirety. In 1960, Charnley[16] demonstrated the use of "cold-curing" acrylic cement for the placement of femoral prostheses. The resin was not radiographically visible, and therefore, a small amount of barium sulfate by volume was added to the mixture. Using that experience from orthopedic surgery, in 1967, Scoville and colleagues[17] reported the use of acrylic inlays over individual and multiple vertebral elements to alleviate vertebral body collapse and instability (**Fig. 1**). These first reported cases of spinal deformities, aside from intervertebral disc replacement, were repaired through open surgery using acrylic inlays, which indicated positive patient recovery with no severe adverse side effects. In 1981, Harrington[18] reported complete replacement of the vertebral body using PMMA in vertebral metastases (**Fig. 2**). Since that time, vertebroplasty has been performed as an open procedure, mostly in combination with instrumentation. Moreover, applying PMMA demonstrated many advantages over bone autografts.

Percutaneous Vertebroplasty

Following World War II, France adopted a social security-based health care system operated and managed by state-sanctioned oversight committees composed mainly of union and corporate

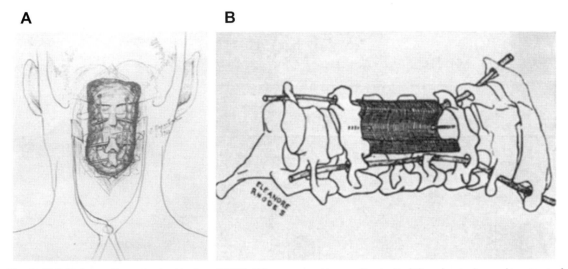

A   **B**

Fig. 1. PMMA for malignant spinal lesions (1967). Wires encased by acrylic plastic (*A*) and anterior replacement of cervical vertebral bodies by acrylic plastic (*B*). (*From* Scoville WB, Palmer AH, Samra K, Chong G: The use of acrylic plastic for vertebral replacement or fixation in metastatic disease of the spine. Technical note. Journal of Neurosurgery 27:274–279, 1967 with permission.)

representatives. Cost-saving measures had great appeal, although primary research within France that might lead to new medical breakthroughs or procedures, was not looked on favorably until the 1980s.

In 1984, neurosurgeon Galibert and the neuroradiologist Deramond at the University Hospital of Amiens in France, after a series of experiments on cadavers, developed a technique of percutaneous injection of bone cement to fill large vertebral cavities.[19,20] The first patient to receive the new VP procedure had severe cervical pain and a vertebral hemangioma encompassing the entire C2 vertebral body with extension into the epidural space. After performing a C2 laminectomy to excise the epidural component of the lesion, a 15-gauge needle was inserted percutaneously using the anterolateral approach into the C2 vertebral body for cement injection for structural reinforcement (**Fig. 3**). For augmentation, Galibert and colleagues[19] used "Simplex" (Stryker, Kalamazoo, MI, USA) bone cement that contained

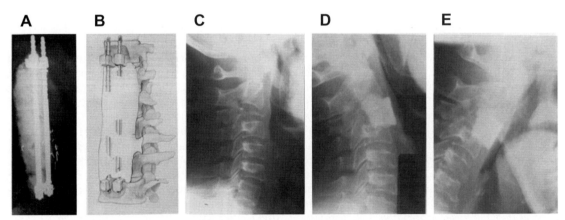

A   **B**   **C**   **D**   **E**

Fig. 2. Open vertebroplasty: the use of PMMA for vertebral-body replacement (1981). Postoperative radiograph (*A*) and sketch (*B*) of anterior stabilization from the T10-L4 using PMMA reinforced by Harrington rods. Preoperative (*C*) and postoperative (*D, E*) radiographs after anterior stabilization in the cervical spine using PMMA. Functional postoperative study demonstrates stability of the composite. (*From* Harrington KD. The use of methylmethacrylate for vertebral-body replacement and anterior stabilization of pathological fracture-dislocations of the spine due to metastatic malignant disease. J Bone Joint Surg Am 63:36–46, 1981; with permission.)

A

B

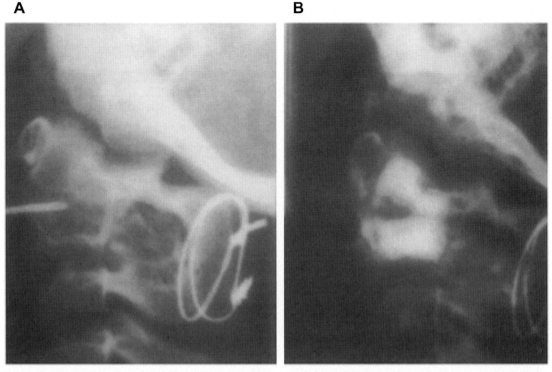

Fig. 3. The first VP. First intraoperative radiographs. (*A*) Lateral view of C2 with a cannula in place in the vertebral hemangioma cavity. (*B*) Lateral view of C2 after composite injection. (*From* Mathis J.M., Belkoff SM., Deramond H. History and Early Development of Percutaneous Vertebroplasty. In: Mathis J.M., Deramond H., Belkoff S.M. (eds) Percutaneous Vertebroplasty and Kyphoplasty. Springer, New York, NY, 2002 with permission.)

10% barium sulfate. Three milliliters of the composite was injected based on the calculations using transosseous venography. A skilled interventional radiologist and well-known arteriovenous malformation expert, Deramond injected the cement. After the surgery, the patient experienced complete relief of pain. By 1987, the investigators described 6 other patients with aggressive hemangiomas treated with VP and published their first paper entitled, "Note préliminaire sur le traitement des angiomes vertébraux par vertébro-plastie acrylique percutanée."

Inspired by the initial success of the VP, other teams of French neuroradiologists in Lyons, Paris, and Strasbourg introduced percutaneous augmentation in their hospitals. The early clinical experience was focused on the treatment of aggressive hemangiomas.[21,22] Dusquenel adapted the procedure to treat pain resulting from the compression fractures associated with osteoporosis and malignancy.[20]

For a long time, VP was performed only in France. It appears that this technique was virtually unknown in North America until 1993, perhaps because the first articles were published in French. However, there were 2 attempts to draw attention

to vertebroplasty in the United States. In 1989, Kaemmerlen and colleagues[23] from Lyon published a short letter to the editor in the *New England Journal of Medicine*, where the investigators stressed: "Our preliminary experience seems to demonstrate that this technique relieves the pain of metastatic bone diseases in vertebrae within 48 h and may be a good method of preventing vertebral-body collapse." Deramond and colleagues also presented a small abstract at the Radiological Society of North America meeting in November 1990, although these publications did not achieve notoriety.

Attention to the procedure was generated in 1993 when VP was presented at the American Society of Neuroradiology annual meeting by another French researcher, Depriester-Debussche.[22] Inspired by this report, Jensen and Dion[22] successfully implemented VP and treated the first patient in the United States in 1993, remarking, "In 1993 we attended the annual meeting of the ASNR [where vertebroplasty] sounded promising and ... we were asked to see a patient with a painful compression fracture caused by lung metastases."[22] Unlike Europeans, who preferred CT guidance, they adopted fluoroscopy for intraoperative navigation and introduced intraoperative venography to evaluate the vertebral body venous drainage pattern and prevent possible extravertebral cement leakage. In May 1997, Jensen and colleagues[22] reported the first case series of vertebroplasty for osteoporotic vertebral compression fractures in the United States. Shortly thereafter, the University of Virginia Medical Center became the major teaching center for this new percutaneous augmentation technique.

Biomechanical studies of VP initiated by Belkoff at the Johns Hopkins University Medical Center provided a strong research background for clinical use of vertebral body augmentation. The first 4 papers published in 1999 by Belkoff addressed the most critical clinical aspects, namely, temperature effect from PMMA polymerization, biomechanical properties of injected cement, comparative assessment of unipedicular versus bipedicular VP.[24] Such research on the biomechanics of augmentation provided a theoretic framework for understanding and optimizing the technology and created reliable fundamental guidance on how to achieve excellent results and predetermined the further success and widespread use of this technique. The first controlled trial of VP versus conservative therapy published in 2003 was an important message from a policy perspective. This study provided strong evidence that VP had an immediate effect on pain relief, increased functioning, and decreased analgesia use in patients with acute or subacute osteoporotic vertebral fractures.

Initial high success rates reported for pain relief with VP prompted the development of related surgical techniques and devices. Medical technology companies directed effort toward the development of a new generation of injectable bone composites and systems for delivery of the cement. At the time, the Food and Drug Administration reviewed only devices and materials; the safety and efficacy of the procedures themselves were not subject to regulation. As a result, procedures could be broadly disseminated before the development of rigorous evidence and were supported by early insurance coverage.[25] Thoracic and lumbar (but not cervical) vertebroplasty and associated imaging procedures were assigned unique Current Procedure Terminology (CPT) billing codes in 2001.[26] In 2005, the Centers for Medicare and Medicaid Services Coverage Advisory Committee reached no conclusions regarding vertebroplasty effectiveness and generated no national coverage decisions. Nevertheless, many state-level Medicare contractors and private insurers covered VP under various circumstances, since at least 2001.[26] In 2003, the Society of

Interventional Radiology introduced Standards of Practice for VP.[27] VP received appraisals of treatment patients in different countries around the world. The National Institute of Health and Care Excellence in the United Kingdom in 2003 published guidance stating: "Current evidence on the safety and efficacy of percutaneous vertebroplasty appears adequate to support the use of the procedure, provided that normal arrangements are in place for consent, audit and clinical governance."[28] Also, in 2003, the German Radiological Society released guidelines and recommendations.[29] In 2005, Australian Medical Services Advisory Committee approved VP for painful osteoporotic vertebral compression fractures not controlled by conservative medical therapy in patients with pain from metastatic deposits or multiple myeloma in a vertebral body.[30]

Kyphoplasty

Despite the increasing popularity of vertebroplasty, cement leakage and associated damage to the surrounding spinal cord and nerves remained the major drawback to the procedure. In 1994, Reiley, an orthopedic surgeon, Scholten, an engineer and inventor of surgical products, and Talmadge, a biochemist, attempting to mitigate extrusion and improve cement localization, percutaneously inserted an inflatable balloon tamped into a compressed vertebral body before injecting the PMMA cement to make VP safer, restore vertebral height, and reduce kyphotic deformity.[31] In essence, a balloon angioplasty technique had been developed to repair spinal fractures.[31] In 1996, the device was given 510k approval by the Food and Drug Administration as a "bone tamp."[32] In 1998, Reiley performed the first kyphoplasty (KP) for osteoporotic vertebral compression fracture. Kyphon held the patent for the height-restoration device.[33] Kyphon began selling its balloon device in 1999, and by the end of the year posted sales of $261,000, with sales increasing to more than $6 million in 2000, topping $36 million in 2001, $76.3 million in 2002, and more than $131 million in 2003.[31] About 50,000 patients worldwide underwent KP in 2004, a number that increased to 73,000 in 2005.[31] In 2006, Kyphon reported worldwide sales of approximately $408 million, with US sales of $324 million.[34] In 2006, KP received a specific CPT code. This growth reflected positive results from clinical studies, and corporate educational efforts made steady progress in convincing doctors to consider the new procedure and then received training to perform it. Mathis and Deramond were invited to be instructors at the Kyphon workshops. Interestingly, commercial promotions and advances by Kyphon facilitated widespread use not only of KP but also of VP, because to master KP, the physician should master VP first. The commercial success of Kyphon was impressive, and in 2007, Medtronic acquired Kyphon, reportedly for $3.9 billion, creating what was historically the most expensive medical technology acquisition.[35]

Vertebroplasty Versus Kyphoplasty

Height restoration and kyphosis reduction are thought to be potential advantages of KP over VP. However, the analysis was and is difficult, because many studies listed percent height resto-ration determined by comparison to the initial postfracture height.[33] Moreover, a 50% to 75% height gain appears impressive, but a close anal-ysis of many studies revealed that many investiga-tors mean only 3 mm of height recovery from an initial 4-mm height loss.[33] KP appeared to be more expensive than traditional vertebroplasty. The KP kit (without bone cement) costs approxi-mately $3,400, whereas a vertebroplasty kit (with bone cement) was less than $400.[32] KP was usu-ally performed in the operating room with general anesthesia, and therefore, the patients usually stayed overnight in the hospital for observation, whereas VP was usually performed with intrave-nous sedation with patients discharged home after the procedure. In 2006, Hulme and colleagues[36] summarized 69 clinical studies on VP and KP. They demonstrated that pain relief was achieved in 87% of patients after VP and 92% after KP, with cement leaks identified in 41% of VP and 9% KP procedures. They also showed that new fractures of adjacent vertebrae occurred after augmentation at rates approximately equivalent to the general osteoporotic population that had a previous vertebral fracture. Analysis of 72,693 pa-tients from the 2006 Medicare Provider Analysis and Review File database revealed that vertebral augmentation procedures were associated with more prolonged patient survival compared with nonoperative treatment, with KP having better as-sociation with survival than VP.[37] However, KP was more significantly likely to result in a subse-quent augmentation procedure than was VP (9.4% vs 7.9%, retrospectively).

VP and KP both became popular for the treat-ment of painful vertebral compression fractures. Most physicians agreed that both augmentation techniques VP and KP had a dramatic effect in reducing patient pain and improving functional outcomes by providing strong mechanical stabili-zation of fractured vertebral bodies.[33] Clinically significant complications associated with both

procedures are typically less than 1% for most op-erators dealing with osteoporotic fractures and slightly higher in pathologic fractures.[33]

Other than financial aspects, the division of percutaneous augmentations into the VP group and the KP group "wastes time and intellectual en-ergy."[38] Beyond these basics, the discussion around the augmentation techniques seems to be blurred by the jargon.[32] Manufacturers and champions of any device describe their individual advantages.[32] Regardless of which procedure is selected, safety depends on operator experience, imaging equipment, and adequate cement opaci-fication. The complications that occurred most often were the result of poor operator judgment and experience or inadequate anatomic and cement visualization but not the technique cho-sen.[39] New devices, including vertebral body stents and vertebral augmentation implants, have been developed and implemented into clinical practice. In 2016, 3 orthopedic conglomerates, DePuy Synthes, Medtronic, and Stryker, domi-nated the global market for vertebral fracture repair products in 2016.[40]

Vertebroplasty/Kyphoplasty: Do They Work or Not?

Since the 1990s, vertebroplasty has gained popu-larity. Initial reports from the late 1980s to the early 2000s indicated that VP provided an excellent outcome in 63% to 100% of patients.[41–45] Early studies of these procedures were neither random-ized nor blinded, because many of the patients chose VP rather than conservative treatment and also because the symptoms of compression frac-ture often abated over time. The lack of adequate controls made it impossible to determine whether clinical improvements that followed treatment would have occurred even without VP.[46] There were several attempts at double-blind randomized trials; however, accrual of patients proved to be extremely slow, and many of these efforts were abandoned for a variety of reasons.[47] Third-party payers were often content to have patients treated and rapidly improve rather than be on disability for protracted periods or requiring drugs, or even worse, be admitted for treatment to institutions; patients refused to participate in randomization, suggesting that this technique was highly effec-tive; and finally, the impressive clinical effect of VP was noted by many clinicians. US investigators launched a double-blind randomized study, and a similar study in Australia began recruiting patients in 2004. Finally, in 2009, results of these 2 studies were published in *The New England Journal of Medicine*. In 1 trial consisting of 131 participants with 1 or 2 painful osteoporotic vertebral fractures, vertebroplasty did not result in more significant improvement in overall pain, physical functioning, or quality of life assessed at 3 or 6 months after treatment.[48] Another trial involving 78 patients who underwent VP had improvements in pain and disability measures that were similar to those in patients who underwent a sham procedure.[49] Despite the long history of positive clinical outcomes research, both found no benefit to VP for compression fractures when compared with a sham procedure. The results of both studies conflicted with extensive clinical experience. The data surprised practitioners who performed VP every day and had believed the excellent results.[47]

Reaction from the medical society regarding these publications was sharp. A large number of responses, letters to editors, and articles written by physicians and professional societies, which performed and endorsed vertebroplasties criticizing these studies, were published immediately.[47,50–56] Titles of responses included: "Vertebroplasty: about sense and nonsense of uncontrolled 'controlled randomized prospective trials'"[54]; "The vertebroplasty affair: the mysterious case of the disappearing effect size"[56]; "The effects of randomized controlled trials on vertebroplasty and KP: a square PEG in a round hole"[55]; "Randomized vertebroplasty trials: bad news or sham news?"[52]

Most arguments against the NEMJ articles were strong, were professionally correct, and could not be ignored. Major pitfalls of these studies included improper study design, small numbers of patients, improper patient selection, the small amount of cement injected, the incomplete use of MR imaging or CT to confirm that the fracture was the likely source of pain, and the high rate of crossover from placebo to VP in one of the studies.[51,52,54,57] The inappropriately low quality of the 2 publications and the reputational damage that they caused led to the unusually emotional reaction to these publications: "I wonder whether the authors of these research studies … would proudly refuse vertebroplasty for themselves or their mothers in such a situation. If so, then let them find comfort in their own medicine. I am certain that their mothers would have a different opinion."[52]

The authors of these NEJM studies attempted to explain their unexpected results. Miller and Kallmes[58] suggested, "…the placebo reactivity of physicians may contribute to promoting positive placebo responses in patients. Clinicians' beliefs in the value of the treatments they recommend and administer are likely to help promote patients' expectations of therapeutic benefit, which in turn can enhance therapeutic responses." Later, Miller and colleagues[59] generated another hypothesis that observed results might be due to response bias, biased patient-reported outcomes. These 2 publications uncovered huge problems existing in medical research and the absence of responsibility for apparently low-quality publications in leading professional journals: "Sometimes, we cannot get rid of the impression that prestigious scientific journals occasionally tend to sell an ideology rather than to serve with objective science the sick human beings."[54]

Nevertheless, despite the loud protests from the professionals, in 2010 the American Academy of Orthopedic Surgeons (AAOS), based on results of these 2 publications, issued a "strong" recommendation against the use of VP in the treatment of patients with vertebral fractures.[60] In Canada, the Ontario Health Technology Advisory Committee ruled that VP should not be considered the standard treatment of osteoporotic vertebral fractures.[46] The most significant concern based on these studies was the possibility that insurance coverage could be withdrawn for VP and KP. In December 2009, Aetna sent a notice to its network clinicians that it planned to reclassify VP as "experimental" and thus rescind coverage for the procedure.[25] In late 2010, the Blue Cross Blue Shield Association's Medical Advisory Panel confirmed its decision that neither procedure met its criteria for established effectiveness. In 2010, Noridian Administrative Services, a Medicare intermediary for 11 Western states, issued a draft of a local noncoverage decision for percutaneous vertebral augmentation, proposing to deny reimbursement for these procedures for all indications.[25] The situation around VP uncovered serious problems about the policy mechanisms existing in the United States to interpret and act on negative research findings from studies of essential therapeutic techniques.[25]

Unfortunately, these 2 publications in NEJM affected tens of thousands of patients, who were denied a valuable procedure that the great bulk of studies to date had validated as a safe and effective therapy, and practitioners witnessed a considerable drop in referrals for vertebral augmentation in the United States and Europe.

In 2009, "Position statement on percutaneous vertebral augmentation: a consensus statement developed by the Society of Interventional Radiology (SIR), American Association of Neurological Surgeons (AANS) and the Congress of Neurologic Surgeons (CNS), American College of Radiology (ACR), American Society of Neuroradiology (ASNR), American Society of Spine Radiology (ASSR), Canadian Interventional Radiology Association (CIRA), and the Society of NeuroInterventional Surgery (SNIS)" was published. The statement supported and endorsed cement augmentation stating: "vertebral augmentation with vertebro-plasty or kyphoplasty is a medically appropriate therapy for the treatment of painful vertebral compression fractures refractory to medical ther-apy when performed for the medical indications outlined in the published standards. The Societies believe vertebral augmentation with vertebroplasty or kyphoplasty is established therapy and should be reimbursed by payors as a safe and effective treatment for painful compression fractures."[61] The North American Spine Society also released their concerns stating: "data from these two studies must be considered carefully and thoughtfully. As discussed above, the findings of these investiga-tions are not surprising and indeed not that dissim-ilar to previous data. The conclusions drawn by the authors, however, may not be as decisive as they appear. More practical conclusions should be made based on a thorough and systematic review of all the literature in order to better define the sub-group of patients for which vertebroplasty might be most appropriate."[50] Although publication of the tri-als and the AAOS guideline influenced the use of vertebroplasty and KP, results indicate that both procedures were at the time still widely used to treat patients with osteoporotic spinal fractures.

Results of 15 randomized clinical trials devoted to augmentation technique for osteoporotic compression fractures were published (**Table 1**). These studies used different methodology and techniques, and they show conflicting results. Eleven studies demonstrated positive outcomes, whereas the other 5 showed all negative results. Based on the published research, the role of VP in the treatment of acute osteoporotic vertebral compression fractures is unclear.

The Vertebroplasty Story: Mirror of Problems in Current "Bulk" Medical Research

Recent publications claim that physicians routinely prescribe medical treatments that are not based on sound science. Besides the vertebroplasty case, results of arthroscopic surgery for osteoar-thritis were found no better than those after a pla-cebo procedure[62]; percutaneous coronary intervention in stable angina in severe single-vessel coronary stenosis was not better than pla-cebo procedure,[63] and other studies questioned the value of spinal fusion or subacromial decom-pression.[64,65] Although every clinical problem raised requires a detailed and comprehensive analysis, there is 1 glaring problem. These studies were trying to evaluate procedures without the individualized analysis of patients included in the study. Instead of trying to identify the group of pa-tients who could benefit from the procedure, these

"all-in-one" studies aimed to find a "yes" or "no" answer. This "bulk" research failed to demonstrate real-world effectiveness of vertebroplasty and conflicted with results of individual operators, whose results are excellent. These results are based on an individual approach to patients on a case-by-case basis.

Placed at the top of the research hierarchy, ran-domized studies also are affected by many inherent significant limitations and weaknesses.[66] Often clinical studies have design-related prob-lems, have issues in the conduct and analysis re-sults, and fail to follow the rigorous methodology. To generate relevant research based on clinical practice, independent researchers who are leaders in the particular field must be actively involved and, importantly, supervise the clinical trial process. Most clinical drug research is spon-sored, organized, and supervised by the pharma-ceutical industry; however, in research devoted to procedures ("orphan research"), the supervision of clinical trials and an independent review of the research materials are not often performed or per-formed well. The increasing trend toward con-ducting clinical trials outside the United States is an aspect that may also be related to the defi-ciency of trials, besides cost savings and adminis-trative or initial regulatory avoidance.[66]

Economics of Augmentation Techniques

Percutaneous vertebral augmentation/consolida-tion techniques include VP, KP, and several methods involving percutaneous introduction of an implant (associated or not with cement injec-tion).[67] In most cases, these techniques are used for osteoporotic vertebral body fractures and ma-lignant lesions. The economics of VP and KP for benign (osteoporotic) fractures was investigated, whereas financial aspects of the application of these techniques for malignant cause were less evaluated. Vertebral compression fractures are responsible for almost 130,000 inpatient admis-sions and 133,500 emergency department visits annually, and the direct medical cost of osteopo-rotic fractures has been estimated at 10 to 22 billion dollars per year.[68,69] Earlier vertebral augmentation was linked to greater decreases in analgesic requirements, decreased costs of treat-ing vertebral fractures, decreased the indirect cost of treatment associated with morbidity, mortality as well as complications of bed rest and immo-bility.[70,71] In a Medicare population with malignant vertebral fractures, VP and KP predicted signifi-cantly reduced cost and length of hospital stay.[71,72] Therefore, Medicare and private insur-ance companies relatively quickly endorsed VP.

Table 1
Randomized clinical trials devoted to spinal augmentation techniques

	Author/Study, Reference, y	Number of Patients and Aims	Primary Outcome	Secondary Outcome	Clinical Follow-Up
1	Voormolen et al (VERTOS),[81] 2007	34; vertebroplasty vs nonoperative treatment	No	Yes	Yes
2	Wardlaw et al (FREE),[82] 2009	300; kyphoplasty vs nonoperative treatment	Yes	Yes	Yes
3	Kallmes et al (INVEST),[48,83] 2009	131; vertebroplasty vs sham intervention (blinded)	No	No	No
4	Buchbinder et al,[49] 2009	78; vertebroplasty vs sham intervention	No	No	No
5	Rousing et al,[84] 2010	49; vertebroplasty vs nonoperative treatment	No	Yes	Yes
6	Klazen et al (VERTOS II),[85] 2010	202; vertebroplasty vs nonoperative treatment	Yes	Yes	Yes
7	Farrokhi et al,[86] 2011	82; vertebroplasty vs nonoperative treatment	Yes	Yes	Yes
8	Blasco et al,[87] 2012	118; vertebroplasty vs nonoperative treatment	No	No	Yes
9	Chen et al,[88] 2014	96; vertebroplasty vs nonoperative treatment	Yes	Yes	Yes
10	Leali et al,[89] 2016	385; vertebroplasty vs nonoperative treatment	No	Yes	Yes
11	Yang et al,[90] 2016	130; vertebroplasty vs nonoperative treatment	Yes	Yes	Yes
12	Wang et al,[91] 2016	217; vertebroplasty vs nonoperative treatment	No	No	Yes
13	Clark et al (VAPOUR),[92] 2016	120; vertebroplasty vs sham intervention	Yes	Yes	Yes
14	Hansen et al (VOPE),[93] 2016	52; vertebroplasty vs sham intervention	Yes	Yes	Yes
15	Firanescu et al (VERTOS 4),[94] 2018	176; vertebroplasty vs sham intervention	No	Yes	Yes

Multiple publications demonstrated the financial benefits of vertebral augmentation techniques in osteoporotic vertebral fractures.[73] For example, analysis of 858,978 vertebral fractures taken from the Medicare database demonstrated that the cost per life-year gained for VP and KP patients ranged from $1863 to $6687 and $2452 to $13,543, respectively, compared with nonoperated patients.[74] However, in 2015, French researchers analyzed 21 publications devoted to the cost-effectiveness of augmentation techniques in order to assess the level of evidence.[75] Seemingly counterintuitively, the investigators concluded that the level of evidence used in economic evaluations of VP and KP is quite low, reflecting the quality of economic evaluations available for innovative medical devices.[75]

The economic impact of both VP and KP remains under careful analysis. According to the expert forecast, the North American KP market, including Canada, Mexico, and the United States, is expected to increase from $538.1 million in 2016 to around $1.1 billion by 2023, representing a compound annual growth rate of 11%.[40]

Vertebral Augmentation Rates and Specialties

In 2019, Rabei and colleagues[69] published a comprehensive analysis of the trends of vertebral augmentation in the elderly Medicare population. The study demonstrated that the most substantial spike in the utilization of augmentation techniques between 2005 and 2006 of 135% and the most significant decline in volume between 2008 and 2010 of 15.6%. Interestingly, overall, between 2006 and 2015, the annual volume of procedures declined by 11%.[69] According to this study, most procedures were performed by diagnostic radiologists controlling 71% of the procedural market share in 2005, and decreasing to 43% in 2015.[69] Orthopedic surgeons and neurosurgeons were the second and third largest providers in the Medicare population, performing 10% and 7% of procedures in 2005, with an increase to 22% and 17% in 2015. Anesthesia was the fourth major provider and demonstrated increasing market share from 7% in 2005 to 10% in 2015.[69] Overall, these 4 specialties performed about 92% of all augmentation procedures in the United States.

The majority, about 54% of procedures, were performed in the outpatient setting (58% for radiologists, 52% for orthopedic surgeons, 47% for neurosurgeons, and 35% for anesthesia). Almost 34% of procedures were done as inpatient procedures (radiology, 34%; orthopedic surgeons, 32%; neurosurgeons, 46%; and anesthesia, 7%). The minority, about 12% of all augmentations, were performed in office settings (7% radiology; 12% orthopedic surgery; 6% neurosurgery; 41% anesthesia).[69] Between 2005 and 2015, there was a significant increase in the volume of office-based KP among all providers.[69]

Cultural Aspects

Since 1984, VP was quickly adopted in different countries in Europe besides France. Initially, in Europe, augmentation techniques became popular to manage pain from tumor-related bone diseases, whereas VP and KP were mostly used for osteoporotic vertebral fractures. Although KP predominated in the United States, the VP technique was more popular in Europe.

VP is very popular in developing countries because of the high cost of materials for KP, which remains the major obstacle for their wide use.[76] Many practitioners in developing countries try to reduce the procedure cost and complexity. In Ukraine, a self-made metal injector using a Luer-lock syringe was developed and patented. This system allowed a significant reduction in procedure cost to around $70 (about $20 for the needle and $50 for bone cement)[77] (**Fig. 4**). Iranian investigators comparing the treatment of with VP and KP concluded that considering the high cost of materials for KP relative to VP, there was no reason to use KP in single-level refractory vertebral fractures in developing countries.[76] Chinese researchers suggested reuse of the balloon in KP and to perform single-balloon bilateral puncture for the treatment of nonneoplastic vertebral compression fractures in order to decrease the cost of the procedure.[78]

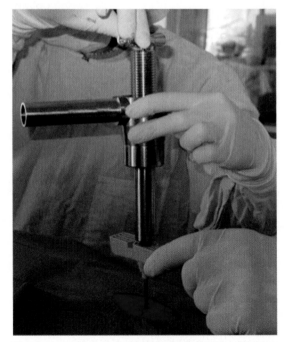

Fig. 4. A multiuse metal injector for a Luer-lock syringe for vertebroplasty.

Publications

Between 1994 and 2013, there was a rapid increase in the number of publications on VP and KP, with a more gradual increase in publications between 1994 and 2001, followed by an exponential increase by 2013, with a stable plateau afterward (Fig. 5). Since 2011, more than 300 papers per year have been published. Before 2001, articles consisted of descriptions of procedural technique, reports of adverse events, and small-uncontrolled case series, with the largest sample size of 47. Many articles published at that time had around 1000 citations. The hallmark 1987 article published in English by Galibert and colleagues,[19] "Preliminary note on the treatment of vertebral angioma by percutaneous acrylic vertebroplasty," has 2209 citations (accessed December 31, 2018).

Vertebroplasty-Based Techniques and Future of Vertebroplasty

VP and vertebroplasty-based modifications have tremendous potential to drastically decrease waiting times, health care costs, complication rates, and time to recovery and to increase patient satisfaction, both by replacing alternative surgical treatments and by offering treatments for diseases that were previously inoperable. Therefore, these image-guided spine vertebroplasty-based techniques continue to evolve and remain an intellectually active field for research.[38] Several additional variants of VP and KP have been developed. The fundamental aspect of these surgical techniques is to develop a cavity within the bone, contain the cement within a defined space, and achieve height restoration by using mechanical implants. A variety of new types of cement for augmentation, including biocompatible composites, are currently being developed, with the widespread introduction of high-viscosity material in order to decrease the risk of leak and restore the lost vertebral height.[79] Research and promotion of the procedure attempt to look beyond the simple augmentation procedure in order to enter the world of proper bone care and open a window to prophylactic bone augmentation in patients with diffuse osteoporosis.[38,80] For the treatment of malignant disease, the combination of VP with thermal ablation and intraoperative radiotherapy is being evaluated.

SUMMARY

Seized on as the gateway to relatively uncomplicated spine surgery by several medical specialties, VP provides a fascinating case history into what may be rational or irrational aspects of the adoption of a surgical procedure. Nevertheless, the development of VP stands at the vanguard of percutaneous spinal surgery procedures. The history of VP presents a unique study into the strength and influence of united medical specialties and societies upon procedures.

ACKNOWLEDGMENTS

This article was presented in part at the 2012 Annual Meeting of the American Association of Neurological Surgeons, where Dr Kushchayev received the Vesalius Prize in the History of Medicine from the AANS Section on History of Neurological Surgery. This study was supported in part by the Barrow Neurological Foundation and the Newsome Chair in Neurosurgery Research held by Dr M.C. Preul.

REFERENCES

1. Ball RP. Needle (aspiration) biopsy. J Am Med Assoc 1936;107:1381.
2. Ball RP. Needle (aspiration) biopsy. J Tenn Med Assoc 1934;27:203–6.
3. Robertson RC, Ball RP. Destructive spine lesions: diagnosis by needle biopsy. J Bone Joint Surg 1935;17:749–58.
4. Valls J, Ottolenghi CE, Schajowicz F. Aspiration biopsy in diagnosis of lesions of vertebral bodies. J Am Med Assoc 1948;136:376–82.
5. Michele AA, Krueger FJ. Surgical approach to the vertebral body. J Bone Joint Surg Am 1949;31:873–8.
6. Ottolenghi CE. Diagnosis of orthopaedic lesions by aspiration biopsy; results of 1,061 punctures. J Bone Joint Surg Am 1955;37-A:443–64.
7. Craig FS. Vertebral-body biopsy. J Bone Joint Surg Am 1956;38:93–102.

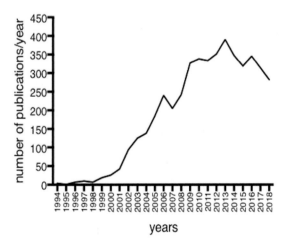

Fig. 5. Publication on vertebroplasty and KP (1994–2018) in PubMed per year.

8. Rabinov K, Goldman H, Rosbash H, et al. The role of aspiration biopsy of focal lesions in lung and bone by simple needle and fluoroscopy. Am J Roentgenol Radium Ther Nucl Med 1967;101:932–8.

9. Adapon BD, Legada BD Jr, Lim EV, et al. CT-guided closed biopsy of the spine. J Comput Assist Tomogr 1981;5:73–8.

10. Bauer W. Methacrylic acid and derivatives. Ullmann's Encyclopedia of Industrial Chemistry; 2000.

11. Spence WT. Form-fitting plastic cranioplasty. J Neurosurg 1954;11:219–25.

12. Mackay HJ. A method of cranioplasty using ready-made acrylic cranioprostheses. Surgery 1947;22:965–75.

13. Elkins CW, Cameron JE. Cranioplasty with acrylic plates. J Neurosurg 1946;3:199.

14. Hamby WB, Glaser HT. Replacement of spinal intervertebral discs with locally polymerizing methyl methacrylate: experimental study of effects upon tissues and report of a small clinical series. J Neurosurg 1959;16:311.

15. Knight G. Paraspinal acrylic inlays in the treatment of cervical and lumbar spondylosis and other conditions. Lancet 1959;274:147–9.

16. Charnley J. Anchorage of the femoral head prosthesis to the shaft of the femur. J Bone Joint Surg Br 1960;42-B:28–30.

17. Scoville WB, Palmer AH, Samra K, et al. The use of acrylic plastic for vertebral replacement or fixation in metastatic disease of the spine. Technical note. J Neurosurg 1967;27:274.

18. Harrington KD. The use of methylmethacrylate for vertebral-body replacement and anterior stabilization of pathological fracture-dislocations of the spine due to metastatic malignant disease. J Bone Joint Surg Am 1981;63(1):36–46.

19. Galibert P, Deramond H, Rosat P, et al. Preliminary note on the treatment of vertebral angioma by percutaneous acrylic vertebroplasty. Neurochirurgie 1987;33(2):166–8 [in French].

20. Mathis JM, Cho C. Percutaneous vertebroplasty. In: Mathis JM, Golovac S, editors. Image-guided spine interventions. New York: Springer New York; 2010. p. 249–78.

21. Cortet B, Cotten A, Deprez X, et al. Value of vertebroplasty combined with surgical decompression in the treatment of aggressive spinal angioma. Apropos of 3 cases. Rev Rhum Ed Fr 1994;61:16–22.

22. Jensen ME, Dion JE. Vertebroplasty relieves osteoporosis pain. Diagn Imaging (San Franc) 1997;19:68, 71-2.

23. Kaemmerlen P, Thiesse P, Jonas P, et al. Percutaneous injection of orthopedic cement in metastatic vertebral lesions. N Engl J Med 1989;321:121.

24. Jasper LE, Deramond H, Mathis JM, et al. The effect of monomer-to-powder ratio on the material properties of cranioplastic. Bone 1999;25:27S–9S.

25. Wulff KC, Miller FG, Pearson SD. Can coverage be rescinded when negative trial results threaten a popular procedure? The Ongoing Saga of Vertebroplasty. Health Aff 2011;30:2269–76.

26. Gray DT, Hollingworth W, Onwudiwe N, et al. Costs and state-specific rates of thoracic and lumbar vertebroplasty, 2001-2005. Spine 2008;33:1905–12.

27. McGraw JK, Cardella J, Barr JD, et al. Society of Interventional Radiology quality improvement guidelines for percutaneous vertebroplasty. J Vasc Interv Radiol 2003;14:S311–5.

28. Available at: https://www.nice.org.uk/guidance/ipg12/resources/percutaneous-vertebroplasty-pdf-52773974734021.

29. Helmberger T, Bohndorf K, Hierholzer J, et al. Guidelines of the German Radiological Society for percutaneous vertebroplasty. Radiologe 2003;43:703–8 [in German].

30. Available at: https://www.adelaide.edu.au/ahta/pubs/reportsmonographs/Vertebroplasty_reference_27_assessment_report_final_printready.pdf.

31. Available at: https://www.encyclopedia.com/books/politics-and-business-magazines/kyphon-inc.

32. Mathis JM, Ortiz AO, Zoarski GH. Vertebroplasty versus kyphoplasty: a comparison and contrast. AJNR Am J Neuroradiol 2004;25:840–5.

33. Mathis JM. Percutaneous vertebroplasty or kyphoplasty: which one do I choose? Skeletal Radiol 2006;35:629–31.

34. Available at: https://www.ftc.gov/sites/default/files/documents/cases/2007/10/071009analysis.pdf.

35. Available at: https://www.forbes.com/2007/07/27/medtronic-kyphon-kyphoplasty-biz-sci-cx_mh_0727kyphon.html - 7157e39c2831.

36. Hulme PA, Krebs J, Ferguson SJ, et al. Vertebroplasty and kyphoplasty: a systematic review of 69 clinical studies. Spine (Phila Pa 1976) 2006;31:1983–2001.

37. Chen AT, Cohen DB, Skolasky RL. Impact of nonoperative treatment, vertebroplasty, and kyphoplasty on survival and morbidity after vertebral compression fracture in the medicare population. J Bone Joint Surg Am 2013;95:1729–36.

38. Murphy KJ. Innovation in image-guided spine intervention. Semin Musculoskelet Radiol 2011;15:168–71.

39. Mathis JM, Deramond H. Complications associated with vertebroplasty and kyphoplasty. In: Mathis JM, Deramond H, Belkoff SM, editors. Percutaneous vertebroplasty and kyphoplasty. New York: Springer New York; 2006. p. 210–22.

40. Available at: https://www.globaldata.com/kyphoplasty-market-north-america-hit-1-1-billion-2023-says-globaldata/.

41. Gangi A, Kastler BA, Dietemann JL. Percutaneous vertebroplasty guided by a combination of CT and fluoroscopy. AJNR Am J Neuroradiol 1994;15(1):83–6.

42. Weill A, Chiras J, Simon JM, et al. Spinal metastases: indications for and results of percutaneous injection of acrylic surgical cement. Radiology 1996;199:241–7.

43. Barr JD, Barr MS, Lemley TJ, et al. Percutaneous vertebroplasty for pain relief and spinal stabilization. Spine (Phila Pa 1976) 2000;25:923–8.

44. Pedachenko EG, Kushchayev SV, Rogozhin VA, et al. Puncture vertebroplasty in aggressive hemangiomas of the vertebrae bodies. Zh Vopr Neirokhir Im N N Burdenko 2004;(1):16–20.

45. Murphy KJ, Deramond H. Percutaneous vertebroplasty in benign and malignant disease. Neuroimaging Clin N Am 2000;10:535–45.

46. Elshaug AG, Garber AM. How CER could pay for itself–insights from vertebral fracture treatments. N Engl J Med 2011;364:1390–3.

47. Munk PL. Vertebroplasty: where do we go from here? Skeletal Radiol 2011;40:371–3.

48. Kallmes DF, Comstock BA, Heagerty PJ, et al. A randomized trial of vertebroplasty for osteoporotic spinal fractures. N Engl J Med 2009;361:569–79.

49. Buchbinder R, Osborne RH, Ebeling PR, et al. A randomized trial of vertebroplasty for painful osteoporotic vertebral fractures. N Engl J Med 2009;361:557–68.

50. Bono CM, Heggeness M, Mick C, et al. North American Spine Society: newly released vertebroplasty randomized controlled trials: a tale of two trials. Spine J 2010;10:238–40.

51. Birkenmaier C, Wegener B, Bocker W, et al. Vertebroplasty–are osteoporotic vertebral fractures now excluded from vertebroplasty? Z Orthop Unfall 2010;148:12–4 [in German].

52. Noonan P. Randomized vertebroplasty trials: bad news or sham news? AJNR Am J Neuroradiol 2009;30:1808–9.

53. Gangi A, Clark WA. Have recent vertebroplasty trials changed the indications for vertebroplasty? Cardiovasc Intervent Radiol 2010;33:677–80.

54. Aebi M. Vertebroplasty: about sense and nonsense of uncontrolled "controlled randomized prospective trials". Eur Spine J 2009;18:1247–8.

55. Albers SL, Latchaw RE. The effects of randomized controlled trials on vertebroplasty and kyphoplasty: a square PEG in a round hole. Pain Physician 2013;16:E331–48.

56. Carragee EJ. The vertebroplasty affair: the mysterious case of the disappearing effect size. Spine J 2010;10:191–2.

57. Boszczyk B. Volume matters: a review of procedural details of two randomised controlled vertebroplasty trials of 2009. Eur Spine J 2010;19:1837–40.

58. Miller FG, Kallmes DF. The case of vertebroplasty trials: promoting a culture of evidence-based procedural medicine. Spine 2010;35:2023–6.

59. Miller FG, Kallmes DF, Buchbinder R. Vertebroplasty and the placebo response. Radiology 2011;259:621–5.

60. Available at: https://www.aaos.org/research/guidelines/SCFguideline.pdf.

61. Barr JD, Jensen ME, Hirsch JA, et al. Position statement on percutaneous vertebral augmentation: a consensus statement developed by the Society of Interventional Radiology (SIR), American Association of Neurological Surgeons (AANS) and the Congress of Neurological Surgeons (CNS), American College of Radiology (ACR), American Society of Neuroradiology (ASNR), American Society of Spine Radiology (ASSR), Canadian Interventional Radiology Association (CIRA), and the Society of NeuroInterventional Surgery (SNIS). J Vasc Interv Radiol 2014;25:171–81.

62. Moseley JB, O'Malley K, Petersen NJ, et al. A controlled trial of arthroscopic surgery for osteoarthritis of the knee. N Engl J Med 2002;347:81–8.

63. Al-Lamee R, Thompson D, Dehbi HM, et al. Percutaneous coronary intervention in stable angina (ORBITA): a double-blind, randomised controlled trial. Lancet 2018;391:31–40.

64. Mirza SK, Deyo RA. Systematic review of randomized trials comparing lumbar fusion surgery to nonoperative care for treatment of chronic back pain. Spine (Phila Pa 1976) 2007;32:816–23.

65. Beard DJ, Rees JL, Cook JA, et al. Arthroscopic subacromial decompression for subacromial shoulder pain (CSAW): a multicentre, pragmatic, parallel group, placebo-controlled, three-group, randomised surgical trial. Lancet 2018;391:329–38.

66. Naci H, Ioannidis JP. How good is "evidence" from clinical studies of drug effects and why might such evidence fail in the prediction of the clinical utility of drugs? Annu Rev Pharmacol Toxicol 2015;55:169–89.

67. Bousson V, Hamze B, Odri G, et al. Percutaneous vertebral augmentation techniques in osteoporotic and traumatic fractures. Semin Intervent Radiol 2018;35:309–23.

68. Goz V, Errico TJ, Weinreb JH, et al. Vertebroplasty and kyphoplasty: national outcomes and trends in utilization from 2005 through 2010. Spine J 2015; 15:959–65.

69. Rabei R, Patel K, Ginsburg M, et al. Percutaneous vertebral augmentation for vertebral compression fractures: national trends in the medicare population (2005-2015). Spine (Phila Pa 1976) 2019;44:123–33.

70. Teasell R, Dittmer DK. Complications of immobilization and bed rest. Part 2: other complications. Can Fam Physician 1993;39:1440–6.

71. Itagaki MW, Talenfeld AD, Kwan SW, et al. Percutaneous vertebroplasty and kyphoplasty for pathologic vertebral fractures in the Medicare population: safer and less expensive than open surgery. J Vasc Interv Radiol 2012;23:1423–9.

72. Trout AT, Gray LA, Kallmes DF. Vertebroplasty in the inpatient population. AJNR Am J Neuroradiol 2005; 26:1629–33.

73. Takura T, Yoshimatsu M, Sugimori H, et al. Cost-effectiveness analysis of percutaneous vertebroplasty for osteoporotic compression fractures. Clin Spine Surg 2017;30:E205–10.

74. Edidin AA, Ong KL, Lau E, et al. Cost-effectiveness analysis of treatments for vertebral compression fractures. Appl Health Econ Health Policy 2012;10: 273–84.

75. Martelli N, Devaux C, van den Brink H, et al. A systematic review of the level of evidence in economic evaluations of medical devices: the example of vertebroplasty and kyphoplasty. PLoS One 2015;10: e0144892.

76. Omidi-Kashani F, Samini F, Hasankhani EG, et al. Does percutaneous kyphoplasty have better functional outcome than vertebroplasty in single level osteoporotic compression fractures? A comparative prospective study. J Osteoporos 2013;2013:5.

77. Kushchayev S, Pedachenko E. Percutaneous vertebroplasty. Kiev (Ukraine): ASD; 2005.

78. Jing Z, Sun Q, Dong J, et al. Is it beneficial to reuse the balloon in percutaneous kyphoplasty for the treatment of non-neoplastic vertebral compression fractures? Med Sci Monit 2017;23:5907–15.

79. Hargunani R, Le Corroller T, Khashoggi K, et al. An overview of vertebroplasty: current status, controversies, and future directions. Can Assoc Radiol J 2012;63:S11–7.

80. Diel P, Freiburghaus L, Roder C, et al. Safety, effectiveness and predictors for early reoperation in therapeutic and prophylactic vertebroplasty: short-term results of a prospective case series of patients with osteoporotic vertebral fractures. Eur Spine J 2012;21(Suppl 6):S792–9.

81. Voormolen MH, Mali WP, Lohle PN, et al. Percutaneous vertebroplasty compared with optimal pain medication treatment: short-term clinical outcome of patients with subacute or chronic painful osteoporotic vertebral compression fractures. The VERTOS study. AJNR Am J Neuroradiol 2007;28:555–60.

82. Wardlaw D, Cummings SR, Van Meirhaeghe J, et al. Efficacy and safety of balloon kyphoplasty compared with non-surgical care for vertebral compression fracture (FREE): a randomised controlled trial. Lancet 2009;373:1016–24.

83. Comstock BA, Sitlani CM, Jarvik JG, et al. Investigational vertebroplasty safety and efficacy trial (INVEST): patient-reported outcomes through 1 year. Radiology 2013;269:224–31.

84. Rousing R, Hansen KL, Andersen MO, et al. Twelve-months follow-up in forty-nine patients with acute/semiacute osteoporotic vertebral fractures treated conservatively or with percutaneous vertebroplasty:

a clinical randomized study. Spine (Phila Pa 1976) 2010;35:478–82.

85. Klazen CA, Lohle PN, de Vries J, et al. Vertebroplasty versus conservative treatment in acute osteoporotic vertebral compression fractures (Vertos II): an open-label randomised trial. Lancet 2010;376: 1085–92.

86. Farrokhi MR, Alibai E, Maghami Z. Randomized controlled trial of percutaneous vertebroplasty versus optimal medical management for the relief of pain and disability in acute osteoporotic vertebral compression fractures. J Neurosurg Spine 2011;14: 561–9.

87. Blasco J, Martinez-Ferrer A, Macho J, et al. Effect of vertebroplasty on pain relief, quality of life, and the incidence of new vertebral fractures: a 12-month randomized follow-up, controlled trial. J Bone Miner Res 2012;27:1159–66.

88. Chen D, An ZQ, Song S, et al. Percutaneous vertebroplasty compared with conservative treatment in patients with chronic painful osteoporotic spinal fractures. J Clin Neurosci 2014;21:473–7.

89. Leali PT, Solla F, Maestretti G, et al. Safety and efficacy of vertebroplasty in the treatment of osteoporotic vertebral compression fractures: a prospective multicenter international randomized controlled study. Clin Cases Miner Bone Metab 2016;13:234–6.

90. Yang EZ, Xu JG, Huang GZ, et al. Percutaneous vertebroplasty versus conservative treatment in aged patients with acute osteoporotic vertebral compression fractures: a prospective randomized controlled clinical study. Spine (Phila Pa 1976) 2016;41: 653–60.

91. Wang B, Guo H, Yuan L, et al. A prospective randomized controlled study comparing the pain relief in patients with osteoporotic vertebral compression fractures with the use of vertebroplasty or facet blocking. Eur Spine J 2016;25:3486–94.

92. Clark W, Bird P, Gonski P, et al. Safety and efficacy of vertebroplasty for acute painful osteoporotic fractures (VAPOUR): a multicentre, randomised, double-blind, placebo-controlled trial. Lancet 2016; 388:1408–16.

93. Hansen EJ, Simony A, Rousing R, et al. Double blind placebo-controlled trial of percutaneous vertebroplasty (VOPE). Glob Spine J 2016;6. s-0036-1582763-s-1580036-1582763.

94. Firanescu CE, de Vries J, Lodder P, et al. Vertebroplasty versus sham procedure for painful acute osteoporotic vertebral compression fractures (VERTOS IV): randomised sham controlled clinical trial. BMJ 2018;361:k1551.

Percutaneous Vertebral Body Augmentations
The State of Art

Majid Khan, MBBS, MD[a],*, Sergiy V. Kushchayev, MD[b,c]

KEYWORDS

- Vertebral compression fracture • Balloon kyphoplasty (BK) • Percutaneous vertebroplasty (PV)
- Polymethyl methacrylate (PMMA) • Vertebral stent/implant (VI)

KEY POINTS

- Vertebral body augmentation techniques are minimally invasive procedures involving the image-guided injection of polymethyl methacrylate–based bone cements into compressed or fractured vertebral body.
- These techniques are effective means to provide mechanical support and symptomatic pain relief in patients with vertebral compression fractures from osteoporosis, malignant pathologic osseous involvement, and aggressive vertebral hemangiomas.
- These procedures are relatively easy to perform; however, successful results require understanding important concepts of spinal augmentation techniques and proper patient selection.

INTRODUCTION

Percutaneous vertebral augmentation techniques, including vertebroplasty and kyphoplasty, are minimally invasive interventional procedures in which bone cement, usually polymethyl methacrylate (PMMA), is injected via a percutaneous approach through a large-bore access needle under imaging guidance to restore the stiffness of the weakened vertebral body. French neurosurgeon Galibert and neuroradiologist Deramont[1] were the first to use percutaneous vertebroplasty (PV) for the treatment of aggressive vertebral hemangiomas of C2 vertebral body in 1987. In subsequent years, the procedure has been adopted for the treatment of acute symptomatic osteoporotic vertebral compression fractures and palliation of metastatic and myeloma osseous lesions.

Balloon kyphoplasty (BK) is a variant of vertebral augmentation using an inflatable balloon to create a cavity within the bone before injecting the PMMA cement within the created cavity within the vertebral body, resulting in increased cement deposition that also helps in restoring vertebral body height and reduces the incidence of cement leakage during injection. Vertebral body implants/stents have also been developed.[2] Vertebral augmentation procedures, including PV and BK, are both able to restore vertebral stiffness and load sharing toward near normal values, although it is thought that kyphoplasty (KP) is better at restoring vertebral body height.[3]

VERTEBRAL BODY BIOMECHANICS AND BACK PAIN

The vertebral body has high stiffness, which enables it to resist significant axial loading.[3] Osteoporosis or pathologic lesions owing to metastases or multiple myeloma lead to loss of

Disclosure Statement: M. Khan is Consultant for Stryker Medical Corporation and Medwaves Avecure Corporation. No conflict with the subject matter. S. Kushchayev has nothing to disclose.
[a] Division of Neuroradiology, Russell H. Morgan Department of Radiology, Johns Hopkins University Hospital, 7220, Bloomberg Building, 1800 Orleans Street, Baltimore, MD 21287, USA; [b] Department of Radiology, Johns Hopkins Hospital, North Caroline Street, Baltimore, MD 21287, USA; [c] Department of Radiology, Moffitt Cancer Center, 12902 USF Magnolia Drive, Tampa, FL 33612, USA
* Corresponding author.
E-mail address: mkhan9@jhmi.edu

Neuroimag Clin N Am 29 (2019) 495–513
https://doi.org/10.1016/j.nic.2019.07.002

normal bone stiffness, resulting in vertebra becoming more deformable and prone to development of compression fracture even without a traumatic inciting event. Osseous compression leads to altered disc pressure profile and decreased disc pressure during flexion with anterior load shift during flexion, resulting in increased stress on the anterior aspect of the adjacent disc, thereby increasing the risk for adjacent level fracture.[4] Most vertebral body fractures are painful, although "silent" vertebral compression fractures also occur, especially in patients with osteoporosis and myeloma.

Acute vertebral body fracture should be considered as a functionally unstable deformity: as when the patient stands up, the axial load increases with an increase in compression forces on vertebral body and endplates which leads to transitory anterior and lateral deformity of the vertebral body and local back pain. In supine or prone positions, the axial load decreases and the pain subsides. This acute axial (mechanical) back pain associated with a structural abnormality in the vertebral body occurs secondary the following mechanisms[5–7]:

1. Anterior and lateral deformity of the vertebral body with micromotion of the endplates and irritation of the periosteum nerve endings
2. Subperiosteal fractures
3. Endplate deformity and fractures
4. Intraosseus hematomas

Vertebral fracture also causes mechanical changes to the surrounding structures: abnormal adjacent disc biomechanics and loss of intradiscal pressure, laxity of intervertebral ligaments, and reduced bending and compressive mechanical changes of facet joints. All these elements may also contribute to the pain syndrome related to acute vertebral bony fracture and may cause symptoms in chronic deformities. Patients with pathologic vertebral fractures have the prolonged recovery period and may not experience the pain relief at all.

The main role of augmentation techniques is mechanical stabilization: restore the stiffness of fractured vertebral body toward prefracture levels with a resultant increase in adjacent discal pressure in order to reduce mechanical (axial) pain.

OSTEOPOROTIC COMPRESSION FRACTURES

Osteoporosis, defined as a clinical condition characterized by a "low bone mass and microarchitectural deterioration of bone tissue leading to decreased bone strength and an increased susceptibility to fractures" is a major global health problem.[8] Osteoporosis and low bone mass affect about 50 million people in the United States: every other person older than 50 years of age has low bone mass or osteoporosis.[9] Osteoporotic vertebral fractures are very common and represent a constant cause of morbidity and mortality. Utilization of augmentation techniques in the treatment of osteoporotic compression fractures has a long track record. Since the 1990s, vertebroplasty has gained popularity. Initial reports from late 1980s to early 2000s indicated that PV provided excellent outcome in 63% to 100% of patients.[10–14] Two clinical trials in 2009 brought conflicting opinions regarding the role of these procedures in the treatment of osteoporotic vertebral compression fractures.[9,15,16] Across the years, evidence has shown that patients subject to more rigorous selection, patients with severe pain secondary to acute vertebral body fracture in the setting of osteoporosis or pathologic compression with adequate corresponding imaging and local tenderness to palpation in the region of fractured vertebral body on clinical evaluation, should be considered for PV. Patient selection is the critical factor in achieving excellent results.

VERTEBRAL BODY METASTASIS AND MYELOMA

Treatment of spinal metastases requires a multidisciplinary approach. Percutaneous augmentation procedures are an effective palliative technique for pain management and consolidation of pathologic vertebral fractures and vertical vertebral instability owing to tumor infiltration.

The Spine Oncologic Study Group defined spine instability "as loss of spinal integrity as a result of a neoplastic process that is associated with movement-related pain, symptomatic or progressive deformity, and/or neural compromise under physiologic loads." This group established the Spine Instability Neoplastic Score to provide objective criteria to evaluate the stability of metastatic spinal lesions (**Fig. 1**). The risk of impending collapse in the thoracic spine is considered with 50% to 60% of destruction of the vertebral body without involvement of other structures, or 25% to 30% vertebral body and costovertebral joint destruction. In the lumbar spine, the risk is the highest with more than 35% to 40% vertebral body involvement, or 20% to 25% vertebral body involvement with posterior elements destruction.[17]

Augmentation of lytic lesions secondary to metastases and multiple myeloma is sometimes technically difficult and can be associated with relatively high risk of cement leakage. Destruction of the posterior wall of the vertebral body is not considered an absolute contraindication to

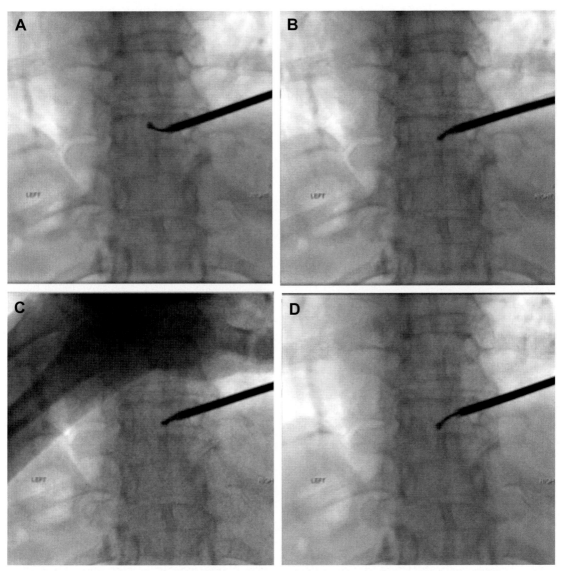

Fig. 1. Unipedicular approach percutaneous curette kyphoplasty used for bones with mixed density in which balloon expansion may not be achieved. (*A-D*) showing movement of the curette tip in the vertebra.

augmentation because now procedures can be safely performed in patients with advanced metastatic disease and pathologic fractures epidural involvement to alleviate back pain[18] by experienced users with utmost careful monitoring of needle access and cement delivery. Quality of life of patients with metastatic disease can be improved in many cases.[19]

Control of the tumor may be achieved with percutaneous radiofrequency ablation or cryoablation of the malignancy before injecting the cement (**Fig. 2**).

Combination therapy consisting of PV/KP and radiotherapy is often performed for malignant lesions. Often vertebral body augmentation is performed first to stabilize the involved vertebral body and control pain syndrome followed by radiation therapy to control the growth of osseous tumor burden. X-ray absorption value of cement containing about 30% barium is very high; therefore, dose distribution of an area containing bone cement calculated using the radiation treatment planning system may differ from actual dose distribution and needs to be individualized and adjusted.[20]

TRAUMATIC VERTEBRAL BODY FRACTURES

Recently, there has been increasing interest in minimally invasive augmentation techniques for

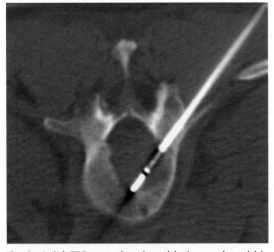

Fig. 2. Axial CT image showing ablation probe within the resection cavity in this patient with lytic breast Ca metastasis.

the management of acute traumatic vertebral fractures in order to avoid open surgery and extensive instrumentation. In 2004, Chen and Lee[21] published the first report on augmentation for 6 patients with traumatic burst fractures with excellent clinical outcome. Several other reports showed that augmentation can be successfully and safely used for patients with burst fractures without neurologic symptoms.[22–25] The primary goal is to create a cement bridge between the superior and inferior endplates to provide structural support for fractured vertebral bodies to heal and prevent development of osteonecrosis. The secondary aim of augmentation is to reduce kyphotic deformity, although it does not affect the clinical outcome.[25]

Patients with uncomplicated A1, and possibly A2 and A3 type (AOSpine classification) thoracolumbar fractures, without fracture lines extending to the posterior wall of the vertebral body may benefit from augmentations.[26] A lower amount of cement is required as compared with patients with osteoporotic fractures owing to normal volume intertrabecular spaces.[22] Ideally, the cement also should connect the displaced fragments of vertebral body and the rest of the vertebral body; therefore, attention should be given to place the needle tip away from the fracture lines to avoid cement leakage. KP in contrast to PV has a higher safety profile and allows improved restoration of posttraumatic kyphosis and endplate elevation and can theoretically reduce the risk of cement leakage.[25,27] Although the role of cement augmentation for acute traumatic vertebral body fractures has not been established yet, it definitely has a potentially valuable role in the treatment of certain patients with uncomplicated fractures.

BONE CEMENTS

The ideal filling materials for vertebral body augmentation require having good biocompatibility, biomechanical strength/stiffness, and radiodensity.[28] PMMA formulations are used almost universally. Because PMMA itself is radiolucent, radiodensity is achieved by adding contrast agent, usually barium sulfate. During PMMA polymerization, temperature can increase in excess of 90°C via exothermic reaction.[29] The exothermic reaction provides an analgesic effect because of the destruction of nerve endings and cytotoxic effect on malignant cells.[29] In addition, PMMA can suppress malignant cell proliferation, induce cell apoptosis, and inhibit cell cycle arrest.[30] However, if bone cement leaks into the spinal canal, the thermal effect may cause spinal cord and nerve injury.[31] New materials with different effects on the biomechanical properties of vertebral bodies (synthetic bone substitutes, eg, composite resin materials, calcium phosphate, or calcium sulfate cements) in addition to new PMMA formulations are now available for clinical use.[32,33]

CEMENT INJECTION, VOLUME, AND DISTRIBUTION

During the bone cement injection, displacement of the bone marrow particles causes migration of fat/bone marrow particles in the venous system. Research study on animals showed that this effect is associated with a temporary decrease in mean arterial pressure and an increase in pulmonary arterial pressure without changes in coagulation profile.[34–36] Apparently, similar changes occur in humans and virtually always remain unnoticeable. Consecutive augmentation of 4 vertebral bodies with PMMA induced a cumulative fat embolic event that gradually deteriorated baseline cardiovascular parameters.[34,35] To avoid this complication, not more than 3 augmentations in a single operation is recommended.[34,35]

In order to restore strength of the vertebral body, 2 to 3 mL of bone cement was found to be sufficient.[37] To restore the vertebral body stiffness, only 4 mL in thoracolumbar region and about 6 mL in lumbar region are required or to fill about 15% to 30% of the targeted vertebral body.[37,38] There is a positive association between cement volume and pain relief, but emphasis should be to achieve maximal safe filling of individual vertebral bodies, which usually translates to the above-mentioned volumes.[39,40]

Distribution of the filler material also plays an important role in the biomechanics of augmentation. The final position of the composite depends on the needle position and the property of the bone. During the procedure, the cement occupies the areas with scarce trabecular bone tissue, avoiding the areas of compacted bone. Therefore, the final position of the bone cement within the vertebral body is difficult to predict. Osteoporotic vertebral bodies where injected bone cement is noted closer to superior or inferior endplates is only up to 2 times stronger than nonaugmented vertebrae, whereas in vertebral bodies, where cement is bridging both endplates is found to be 1 to 8 times stiffer and 1 to 12 times stronger.[40,41] Unilateral distribution of composite within the vertebral body can promote single-sided load transfer, and toggle (medial-lateral bending motion), therefore, should be avoided as a biomechanically suboptimal distribution.[38–40] The unilateral approach is gaining popularity with the use of curved cement delivery coaxial nitinol needles.[42] In malignant lesions, it is important to achieve anchoring of the cement within the spongy vertebral body bone.

INDICATIONS AND PATIENT SELECTION

Vertebral body fractures may occur in the setting of either trauma or nontraumatic pathologic weakening of the bone owing to osteoporosis, multiple myeloma, and vertebral metastases or aggressive hemangiomas.

Careful patient selection and individual therapeutic strategy are the keys to successful and safe procedures. To be a candidate for vertebral augmentation, the patient should fulfill 3 criteria: compression vertebral body fracture or deformity, mechanical back pain from the fracture level, and failed initial conservative treatment.

The failure of medical therapy is defined as

A. Nonambulatory patients due to pain from a weakened/fractured vertebral body; pain persisting at a level that prevents ambulation despite 24 to 48 hours of potent analgesic therapy;
B. Patients with significant pain from a weakened/fractured vertebral body persisting at that level with no response to bed rest, bracing, analgesic therapy with no response to physical therapy;
C. Patients with a weakened/fractured vertebral body and unacceptable side effects due to the analgesic therapy necessary to reduce pain to a tolerable level.

The practice parameter paper defines 3 main indications for augmentation techniques[4]:

1. Painful osteoporotic vertebral fracture or fractures that are refractory to medical therapy;

2. Vertebral bodies weakened by neoplasm;
3. Symptomatic vertebral body microfracture (documented by MR imaging, nuclear imaging, and/or lytic lesion or lesions seen on computed tomography [CT] without obvious loss of vertebral body height).

Preprocedure assessment of patients is a key and should include comprehensive history, thorough neurologic examination for evidence of neural compression, and review of the most recent imaging. The patient should always be palpated and/or gently percussed in the region of fractured vertebral body in order to correlate symptoms with imaging findings.[43] It is essential to distinguish the pain caused by vertebral body fracture from numerous other causes of back pain.[44] Examining patients under fluoroscopy immediately before performing procedures, especially patients with multilevel disease who may have difficulty precisely localizing the level of pain, and in patients reporting diffuse pain and tenderness, can confirm this impression.[45,46]

Acute and subacute vertebral compression fractures should demonstrate marrow edema in the targeted vertebral body on short-tau inversion recovery (STIR) images. CT spine should be assessed in cases of traumatic vertebral fractures, and retropulsion, posterior cortical disruptions, and involvement of the posterior elements should be looked for.

The role of the diagnostic radiologist in patients with vertebral body pathology is 2-fold: to recognize imaging findings differentiating acute/subacute from chronic fractures and to identify contraindications on imaging; and to check for possible complications on follow-up studies.

Laboratory evaluation should include complete blood count, prothrombin time/partial thromboplastin time/international normalized ratio or activated clotting time, and platelet count. Blood urea nitrogen and creatinine levels were obtained in the past when intraoperative intraosseous venography was also performed by some before the injection of cement.[43,44]

CONTRAINDICATIONS

Absolute contraindications
1. Septicemia
2. Active osteomyelitis of the target vertebra or discitis of adjacent disc
3. Uncorrectable coagulopathy
4. Allergy to bone cement or opacification agent
Relative contraindications
1. Radiculopathy in excess of local vertebral pain, caused by a compressive syndrome

unrelated to vertebral collapse. Preoperative PV can be performed before a spinal decompressive procedure;

2. Retropulsion of a fracture fragment causing signs and symptoms of neurologic compromise;
3. Epidural tumor extension with significant encroachment on the spinal canal;
4. Ongoing systemic infection;
5. Patient improving on medical therapy;
6. Prophylaxis in osteoporotic patients (unless being performed as part of a research protocol);

Procedures are contraindicated when there is a clear disparity between the imaging findings and the clinical symptoms.[43] For patients with back pain of greater than 3 months' duration or without bone marrow edema in the targeted vertebral body on STIR images, augmentation can be performed, but it should be clearly explained to patients that the pain palliation may not be as good as if done for subacute fractures; at the same time, secondary benefit of arresting further compression at the fractured level with cement deposition can be achieved.

TECHNIQUE
Anesthesia and Patient Positioning

Procedures are usually performed using moderate sedation with administration of Midazolam, fentanyl, or other medications, with some patients with low pain threshold or patients who cannot lay prone having procedures performed under general anesthesia. Local anesthesia only, especially in elderly people with significant comorbidities, can be done.[47] Procedures under epidural anesthesia rarely can be performed.[48] A nurse is always present in the suite to monitor the patient, who is connected to an electrocardiograph, blood pressure cuff, and O_2 pulse oximeter.

The patient is positioned in the prone position, and rolled sheets under the chest and hips can be placed to cause lordosis, thereby facilitating reduction of the fracture responsible for the kyphotic deformity.[49]

Image Guidance

Most augmentation procedures are performed under fluoroscopic guidance, with CT used especially in patients with lytic pathologic lesions with posterior cortical disruption.

Technique

Augmentation procedures can be performed at all levels of the spine: cervical, thoracic, and lumbar.

Unilateral or bilateral transpedicular injection of cement can be performed. Both techniques are effective in the restoration of vertebral body strength and stiffness, especially now with the use of curved needle cement delivery systems.[42,50,51]

In the cervical and upper thoracic spine, both anterolateral and transpedicular approaches can be used (Fig. 3). In cervical levels, the transpedicular route can be difficult, and the right anterolateral approach is preferred with left anterior approach less favorable because of increased incidence of esophageal injury. In cervical and upper thoracic spine, smaller-gauge (13–15-gauge) access cannulas should be used. In mid/lower thoracic and lumbar regions, 10- or 11-gauge access cannulas should be used. In the thoracic spine, augmentation can be accomplished through transpedicular and parapedicular (transcostovertebral) approaches, whereas as the lumbar spine transpedicular approach is preferred, with the posterolateral approach sometimes used in select cases, especially in cases with lytic pedicular destruction.

The transpedicular approach is the technique of choice and is used overwhelmingly in most cases because it is the safest route to enter the vertebral body. After using the aseptic technique, 1% buffered lidocaine is used for skin, deep soft tissues, and periosteal injection for local anesthesia. After making a small skin incision, an access cannula is inserted under image guidance aiming for the lateral cortical margin of the pedicle at the 10:00 position on the left and the 2:00 position on the right (Fig. 4) for the unilateral transpedicular approach with barrel technique, using the center of the pedicle for bipedicular approach entry. Using a hammer, the needle is advanced through the pedicle with needle advancement done only using the anteroposterior (AP) projection (until the tip of needle enters the vertebral body), and the lateral plane used only to adjust the angle at which the cannula is entering the pedicle and the vertebral body.

The needle tip should always be positioned lateral to the medial border of the pedicle on the AP projection until it reaches the posterior margin of the vertebral body on the lateral projection to minimize the risk of breaching the medial cortex of the pedicle and entering the spinal canal. The bone needle can be advanced through the center of pedicle using so-called tunnel vision/barrel technique under the AP view and verification of needle trajectory at mid-pedicular level and posterior aspect of vertebral body on lateral view.[52,53]

If bone biopsy is needed, it can be easily done with special biopsy devices. For osteoporotic

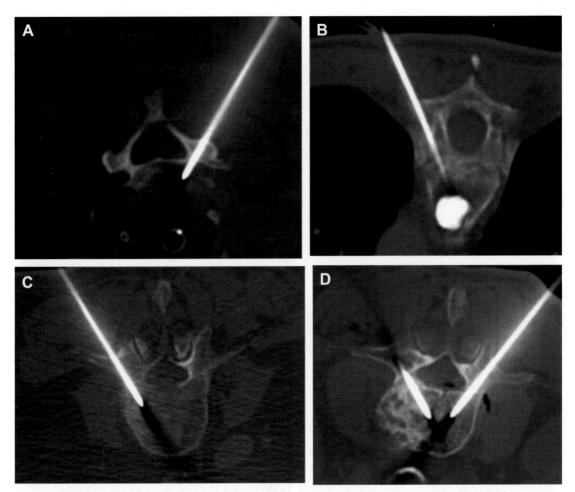

Fig. 3. Percutaneous approaches to spine. (*A*) Posterolateral approach to cervical vertebral body. (*B*) Costovertebral approach in thoracic vertebral body with CT balloon kyphoplasty. (*C*) Posterolateral approach for lumbar vertebra. (*D*) Bilateral posterolateral approach for lumbar vertebral body.

vertebral body fracture, the optimal position of the tip of the needle is a point approximately 1 to 1.5 cm posterior to the anterior vertebral body on the lateral view. For the unilateral approach vertebroplasty, the needle tip should be ideally be located at the base of the spinous process level for straight cannula vertebral injection, whereas for curved needle unilateral and bipedicular approach vertebroplasty, the needle tip should ideally be located in lateral one-third of the vertebra on AP view, with the coaxial curved needle crossing over to the other side of vertebra and the tip located adjacent to the contralateral pedicle.

For the bipedicular approach balloon kyphoplasty, ideal needle tip placement is the ipsilateral half of the vertebral body, with needle tips around the root of spinous processes on AP view and in the midanterior third of the vertebra on lateral view (**Fig. 5**).

For the unipedicular approach kyphoplasty using a curved balloon, the access cannula enters along the lateral edge of pedicle on AP view with final needle position in the lateral third of the vertebral body. The curved needle is introduced through the access needle crossing the midline with its tip close to the contralateral pedicle on AP view and anterior third of vertebra on lateral view (**Fig. 6**).

For patients with vertebral compression with mixed density vertebral stiffness, "curette kyphoplasty" can be used to create a cavity within such bone, because balloon inflation in such bones is hard to achieve with a high incidence of balloon rupture (see **Fig. 1**).

For kyphoplasty, the balloons are prepared to exclude the presence of air droplets, then are inserted through the access cannulas with the balloon tip in anterior third of vertebral body, and are then inflated using 100% iodinated contrast

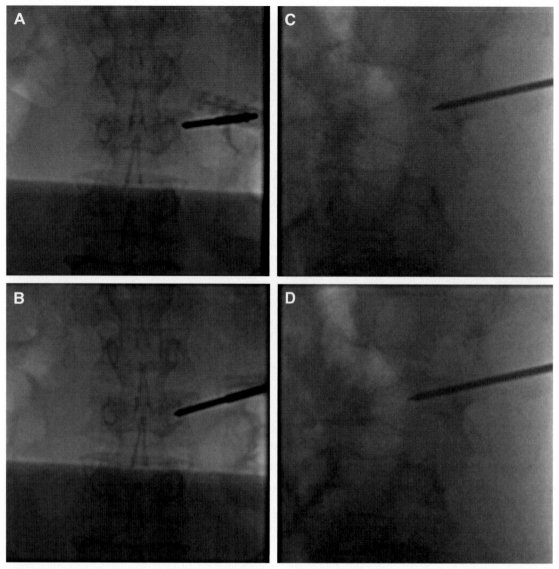

Fig. 4. The entry point of the needle for transpedicular approach. Lateral image used to ascertain correct angulation of the needle tip for entry into the vertebral body (*A*). AP view showing needle tip at 10:00 position (*B*) at the start of needle insertion into the pedicle with medial cortex of pedicle not breached until needle enters the body on lateral view (*C, D*).

for optimal visualization. After the desired height is reached and adequacy of balloon inflation is seen on both AP and lateral planes, the balloons are deflated completely before removal. The access cannulas are advanced with their tips around the anterior edge of the created cavity for optimal cement delivery (**Fig. 7**).

For vertebral stent implant kyphoplasty, access cannulas (10–11 gauge) are used for pedicle entry and then guide wire is introduced into the vertebral body. The pedicle size is measured in an axial plane on previously obtained CT for appropriate sized stent placement. Seven- to 8-gauge stent

introducer is pushed over the guide wire and manually drilled into the anterior third of the vertebra, and after confirming adequate position on both AP and lateral images, the vertebral stents are introduced into position. Then under careful image guidance, they are inflated with aim of raising the height of fractured endplate making sure that the stents ski's are as parallel as possible to the vertebral endplates during stent deployment. After optimal height restoration is achieved, the stent is disconnected from the delivery system and is ready to be injected with bone cement (**Fig. 8**).

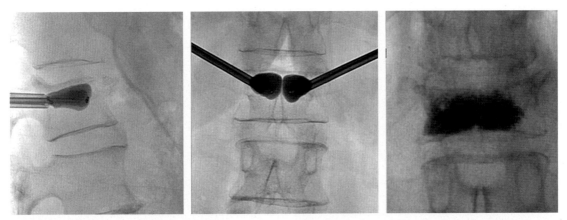

Fig. 5. Bipedicular approach kyphoplasty with balloons inflated with contrast on both AP and lateral images and final AP image with injected cement in place.

Cement Injection

The bone cement is prepared by mixing polymer powder with liquid monomer only after all needles are placed and are in adequate position for cement delivery. Cement is typically injected using commercial delivery systems under real-time x-ray or CT fluoroscopy. Toothpaste consistency of the composite is usually used for the injection. Administration of thick cement is considered safer than using a composite of liquid consistency.[47] During the procedure, injection pressure reaches 20 atm,[54] and thus, cement should be delivered slowly because this decreases the chance of cement leakage and also the patient feels less uncomfortable. Bone cement leaking outside the vertebral body is an indication to stop the injection. The leakage of the cement toward spinal canal requires the procedure be abandoned. If a small leak is noted in directions other than epidural space, cement delivery can be halted for 2 to 3 minutes to give extra time for the minimally leaked cement to solidify[55] and then resume cement deposition with careful continuous image guidance.

At the end of the procedure before the access cannula is removed, the trocar should be reinserted to prevent retrograde filling of the needle tract with cement. Ideally, the needles should be pulled back slowly, and once the needle tip is detached from the bone cement, they are pulled back into the pedicle and spot fluoroscopy is obtained to see that no cement is tracking along the tract into the pedicle. Once no extension of cement is confirmed, only then should the needles be removed completely, thus significantly minimizing accidental cement spillage. After the access cannulas have been removed, final postprocedure images should be obtained to confirm optimal cement positioning within the vertebral body before getting the patient off the table.

Postoperative Care

After the procedure, the patient is transferred to the recovery room and monitored for 2 to 3 hours, during which time hemodynamic and neurologic status can be assessed, the composite hardens, and also to ensure clearance and metabolic reversal of the sedation and anesthesia administered during the procedure. After the recovery from the medications, the patient can recline/sit in bed followed by standing up and ambulating before being discharged home.[56–63] Postprocedure CT of the operated level can sometimes be obtained to assess the efficacy of augmentation and detect cement leakage, especially in cases of persistent or new pain occurring postoperatively.

NEW ADJACENT VERTEBRAL BODY FRACTURES

The presence of a vertebral fracture increases the chance of fracture usually in the adjacent vertebra above the level of the fracture.[64] With systemic osteoporosis, all vertebral bodies lose their stiffness and become relatively "soft," allowing some degree of anterior and lateral deformity. In these setting, vertebral bodies work as a chain of shock absorbents, similar to intervertebral discs. A compression fracture changes this biomechanics because a fractured vertebral body has increased stiffness and is unable to deform as it used to do in the prefractured state.

Relative bone density also increases owing to compacted deformity and leads to proximal junctional kyphosis. In this setting, the vertebral body above the level of the fracture deforms more prominently against the rigid fractured vertebral body and thus absorbs more axial load. This changed biomechanics leads to increased fracture risk of the adjacent vertebra. Several studies demonstrated

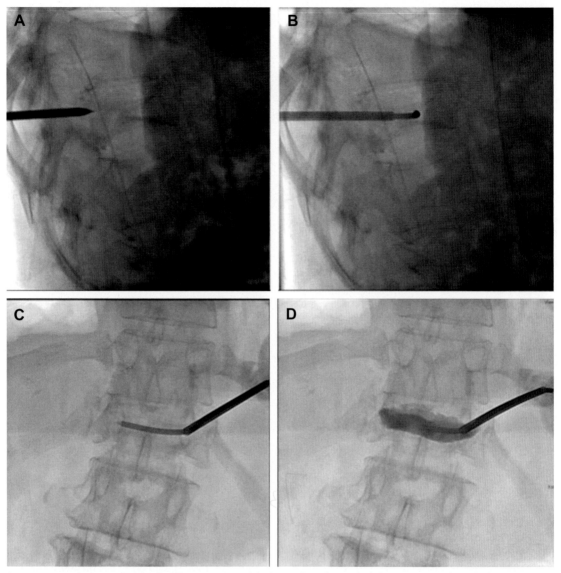

Fig. 6. Percutaneous unipedicular fluoroscopy-guided vertebroplasty showing access and curved needle entry into vertebral body (*A, B*) with needle seen crossing the midline on AP view (*C*) and uniform cement distribution (*D*).

increased risk of new adjacent vertebral body fractures in patients with osteoporosis with evidence of new factures incidence ranging between 8% and 52%. After vertebral augmentation, the incidence of adjacent level fracture decreases to 3% to 25% over the 3 years after augmentation, but usually new fractures occur during first 3 months after augmentation.[65–71] It is unclear whether the adjacent vertebral body fractures develop secondary to the compression fracture itself or because of increased stiffness related to augmentation. Interestingly, cement leakage, particularly into the disc, increases the risk of new fracture of adjacent vertebral body.[67,69]

EFFICIENCY AND SUCCESS RATES

Success of augmentation procedures is defined as achievement of significant pain relief, reduced disability, and/or improved quality of life.[5] Results should be measured by at least 1 of the relevant and validated measurement tools, such as the 10-point numerical pain rating scale score or a visual analogue scale score.[5] Expected success rates for neoplastic pathology are defined as 70% to 92% with threshold for the review of practice if the success rate is less than 60%, and 80% to 98% success rate for osteoporosis with less than 70% threshold for the review.[5]

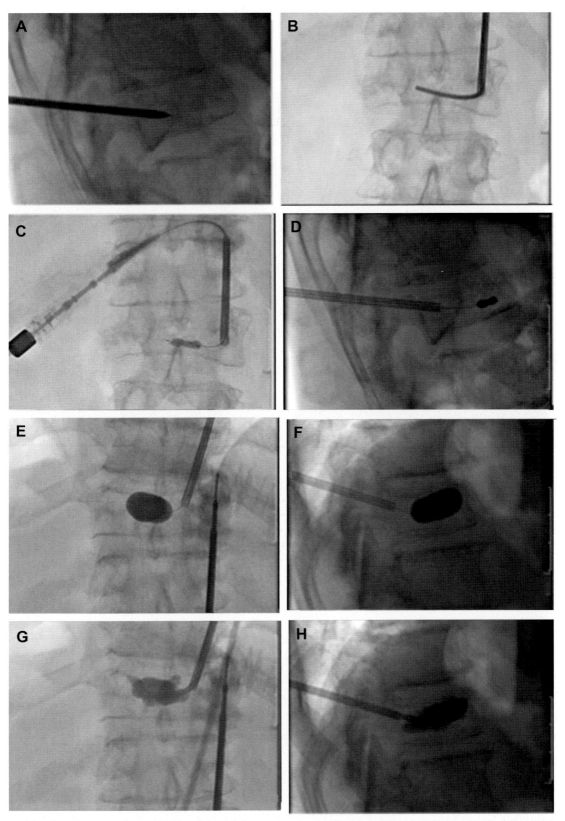

Fig. 7. Unipedicular approach balloon kyphoplasty. Access cannula entry into vertebral body (*A*) followed by curved balloon accessing anterior 3rd of vertebral body (*D*) and crossing over to the contralateral pedicle (*B*, *C*) with adequate balloon inflation with 100% iodinated contrast on AP/lateral images (*E*, *F*) followed by adequate cement fill (*G*, *H*).

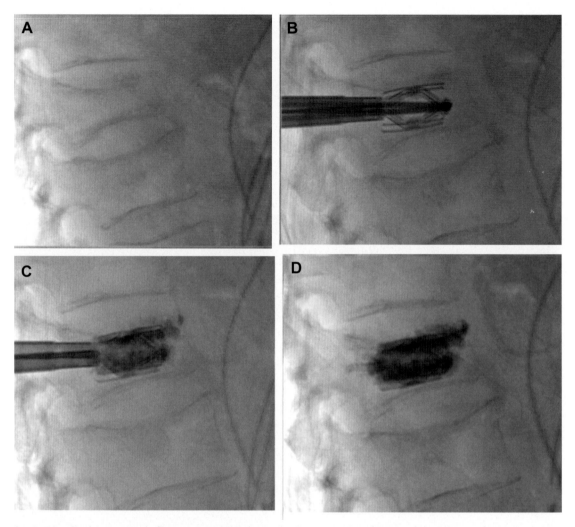

Fig. 8. Bipedicular approach fluoroscopy-guided vertebral compression fracture (*A*) and use of vertebral stent/implant (*B*) with adequate cement filling within (*C*) and around (*D*) the implant.

UNWANTED REACTIONS, INCIDENTS, AND COMPLICATIONS

All vertebral augmentation procedures are safe and associated with a very low risk of serious complications. Gangi and colleagues[72] outlined the most critical elements for successful augmentation procedures: proper patient selection, correct needle placement, good timing of cement administration, strict fluoroscopic control of injection, and operator's experience.

The overall procedure threshold for all complications resulting from vertebral augmentation performed for osteoporosis is 2%, and 10% when the procedures are performed for neoplastic pathology.[4] Published rates for individual types of complications and with threshold for the review of practice are detailed in **Table 1**. Complications should be separated from reversible unwanted reactions and incidents with reversible unwanted reactions developing during or after augmentation procedures and not related to procedure. An incident is an asymptomatic and clinically insignificant event usually related to minimal paravertebral or intradiscal cement leak.

Unwanted Reactions

Transient fever
The introduction of foreign material into the bone may result in transient inflammatory reactions with a fever up to 101°F.

Transient local pain
Local pain in the postoperative period at the site of puncture is a common event associated with

Table 1
Complications associated with vertebral augmentation and published rates and thresholds for review

Specific Complication	Published Rates, %	Thresholds for Review, %
Transient neurologic deficit (within 30 d of the procedure)		
Osteoporosis	1	>2
Neoplasm	10	>10
Permanent neurologic deficit (within 30 d of the procedure or requiring surgery)		
Osteoporosis	<1	>1
Neoplasm	2	>5
Fracture of rib, sternum, or vertebra	1	>2
Allergic or idiosyncratic reaction	<1	>1
Infection	<1	>0
Symptomatic pulmonary material embolus	<1	>0
Significant hemorrhage or vascular injury	<1	>0
Symptomatic hemothorax or pneumothorax	<1	>0
Death	<1	>0

trauma to soft tissue. The severity of these events is different: in many respects it depends on the level of the procedure, the number of puncture attempts, and the diameter of a puncture needle. Less often, pain developed during interventions on the thoracic spine; more often, pain developed on the lumbar spine owing to a large layer of muscle that the needle passes before reaching the targeted vertebra. Local pain syndrome is accompanied by muscular spasms. Typically, the pain resolves within 3 days of the procedure. Treatment includes prescription of anti-inflammatory medications or local injections.

Incidents

Paravertebral cement leakage
Paravertebral cement leakage is a fairly frequent event, and a minimal amount of leak can be seen in up to 60% patients with metastatic lesions and in patients with myeloma.[73] Cement leak can be classified into 3 types: those via the basivertebral vein (type B), those via the segmental vein (type S), and those through a cortical defect (type C)[74] and into the intervertebral disc (type D).

Type S leakage To prevent extravertebral leakage, the operator should place the tip of the needle in a proper location and inject the composite slowly under fluoroscopic control.[72] Although minimal paravertebral bone cement leaks almost always have no clinical significance, profound filling of paravertebral veins may lead to pulmonary cement embolism[72] (**Fig. 9A**). Paravertebral bone cement leakage into the paravertebral muscles followed by an exothermic reaction may lead to reactive myositis.[75] Fast injection of a large amount of cement into the vertebral body is associated with increasing intravertebral pressure, which may result in increased leakage. Keeping the needle in the bone detached from the cement for few minutes after injection is completed should be done to reduce the pressure and also to prevent retrograde filling of the tract (**Fig. 9B**).

Type D leakage The cement can extend into the intervertebral disc through the fractured end plates. A small amount of cement leakage in the intervertebral disc is quite common, is virtually always asymptomatic, but can be associated with delayed pain relief.[76] Intravertebral clefts and Schmorl nodes should be considered risk factors for intradiscal leakage.[77] Placing the needle tip far from the fractured endplate may decrease the risk.[78] It has been demonstrated that prominent intradiscal leakage changes spinal biomechanics and increases adjacent level fracture risk (**Fig. 9C**).[79]

Complications

Epidural leakage usually occurs in type B and S leaks.[74] These complications most often are the result of poor operator judgment and experience or inadequate anatomic and cement visualization.[80]

Epidural cement leakage
The main factors determining the development of this complication are the viscosity of the cement; vasculature at the site of cement administration; location of the distal end of the bone needle; integrity of posterior vertebral cortex; quality of intraoperative fluoroscopy; and diameter of the needle used.

Type C leakage
The leakage occurs as a result of the preexisting defect owing to malignant destruction of the posterior cortex and through a fracture involving the

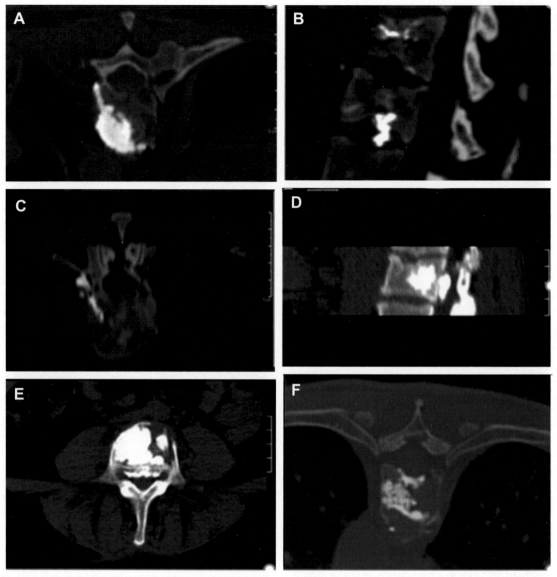

Fig. 9. Complications of augmentation techniques. (A) Paravertebral leakage. (B) Intradiscal leakage. (C) Retrograde filling of the tract. (D) Epidural cement leakage with spinal cord compression. (E) Epidural leakage due to osteolysis of the posterior wall of the vertebral body. (F) Epidural leakage due to filling the basivertebral vein.

posterior cortex in benign compression fractures as well as in iatrogenic injury.

Type C due to preexisting cortical defects In cases of malignant destruction of the posterior wall of the body, injection of the cement is associated with a high risk of epidural leakage. Thorough assessment of the integrity of the posterior wall of the vertebral body should always be made before the procedure to prevent this complication. For many years, this condition was considered a contraindication to augmentation procedures, particularly to PV, but recently this statement has been revised. KP with creation of a cavity and

then deposition of cement under low pressure can be the preferred way in view of posterior cortical wall destruction (**Fig. 9**D, E). Extreme care should be taken to make sure that cement stays in the anterior and middle third of the vertebra because posterior cement deposition/ extension in a case like this may at times cause retropulsion of the tumoral tissue into the epidural space.

Type B leakage
The vertebral venous system is a valveless collateral venous network that spans from the sacrum

to the foramen cranium and is divided into 3 inter-communicating parts:

1. Internal venous plexuses (epidural anterior and posterior plexuses).
2. The basivertebral veins, which are paired valve-less (intravertebral) veins that emerge in the anterior vertebral body and are directed poste-riorly draining venous blood directly into the anterior internal epidural plexus. The basiverte-bral veins communicate with the numerous venous channels within the vertebral body, and anteriorly, the basivertebral veins drain directly into the external vertebral venous plexus (**Fig. 9F**).
3. External vertebral venous plexuses (anterior and posterior) that communicate directly with the azygos venous system and the lumbar veins, and the superior and inferior vena cava.[81]

Radiculopathy

Radiculopathy after procedures may be related to fracture of the pedicle during the vertebral body access or in the setting of cement leak.

Fracture of the pedicle typically occurs when a large size needle is used for vertebral body access for patients with osteoporosis who have congeni-tally small pedicles or procedure performed in the upper thoracic spine with a large needle. If the patient presents with severe back or radicular pain during the pedicular access, fracture of the pedicle should be suspected.

Intraforaminal cement leak is more common in patients with metastatic lesions and may cause root irritation or radiculopathy. Root irritation is a temporary event that may resolve with local anes-thetic injections. Radiculopathy may develop as a result of a combination of thermal, toxic effects or root compression. Persistent compression radi-culopathy resistant to conservative therapy re-quires an open surgical decompression.

Embolism

Asymptomatic embolic events are common oc-currences, whereas embolic complications asso-ciated with embolic events are very rare but dangerous complications and may lead to death.

Fat embolism Fat embolism is an event character-ized by release of fat droplets into systemic circula-tion from the red bone marrow of the vertebral body as a result of the injection of the composite and "expulsion" of fat globules into the large venous collectors and dissemination of emboli through vascular system. Aebli and colleagues[34,35] demon-strated that cement during vertebral body augmen-tation leads to a transient sharp decrease in the heart rate, a drop in blood pressure, an increase

in central venous pressure, marked change in blood saturation, and an increase in CO_2 partial pressure. Rarely, fat embolism may lead to fat em-bolism syndrome, manifesting with respiratory distress, confusion, and chest pain and a charac-teristic petechial rash.[82]

Cement embolism Similarly, the cement displaced into venous system may migrate into the vena cava. Cement embolism can develop when the distal end of the needle is positioned in the imme-diate vicinity of a large venous collector. Patients with malignant compression fractures are at increased risk of such a complication.[83] Few cases of clinically significant cement-related pul-monary embolism were published.[84] Clinical symptoms of embolic syndrome are characterized by systemic hypotension, pulmonary hyperten-sion, and oxygen desaturation. In some cases, pulmonary infarct may develop.[55] Asymptomatic patients do not require treatment; however, clini-cally significant cases should be treated similarly to patients with thrombotic pulmonary embolisms with anticoagulation.[85–87] To reduce the risk of embolic syndromes, the number of augmented vertebrae during prophylactic multisegmental PV should be limited to 3 levels per session.[34,35] Cere-bral artery embolism as a paradoxic embolism may occur in patients with a patent foramen ovale through which emboli migrated into the systemic circulatory system.

Infection

The incidence of infection complications following augmentation procedures is rare and was reported in about 0.3% to 0.5%.[88–90] Infection may mani-fest after administration of the cement in preexis-tent spondylitis or spontaneously after an uncomplicated procedure. In pyogenic spondy-litis, the clinical presentation is more acute and oc-curs a few days after the procedure. Often spondylitis develops because of low virulence or-ganisms, such as coagulase-negative Staphylo-coccus, *Staphylococcus epidermis*, and Acinetobacter species so it takes a couple of weeks to several months to manifest.[90,91] Treat-ment of augmentation-related spondylitis is diffi-cult to treat and often requires vertebral corpectomy and debridement with instrumenta-tion. Patients always should be screened for sys-temic infection before procedures. Prophylactic intraprocedural intravenous antibiotics usually include of cefazolin 1 g; however, limited data are available to support or oppose their adminis-tration.[91] Augmentation-related spondylitis may develop even with parenteral preoperative antibiotics.[91]

Several cases of postvertebroplasty *Mycobacterium tuberculosis* spondylitis were also published.[92] Preexisting subtle tuberculous spondylitis was misdiagnosed as benign compression fractures in that case. Preoperative bone biopsy with microbiological evaluation of aspirate in any unclear cases is important to prevent this serious complication.

Miscellaneous complications

Bleeding Bleeding may develop in patients with underlying coagulopathy, usually in patients with multiple myeloma or malignant lesions who receive chemotherapy and therefore have a low platelet count. Mathis and Deramond[55] describe a case of retroperitoneal bleeding after a PV performed in a patient with myeloma. Undoubtedly, correction of the coagulation system parameters before the procedure is the key to preventing this complication.

Epidural hematoma Epidural hematoma following augmentation procedures may occur as a result of traumatization of the epidural venous plexus during the surgical procedure and iatrogenic fracture of the pedicle during needle advancement.[93]

Death A few procedure-related deaths were reported to have been attributed to anaphylactic reactions to the composited injected, pulmonary cement emboli, and fat emboli.[94]

REFERENCES

1. Galibert P, et al. Preliminary note on the treatment of vertebral angioma by percutaneous acrylic vertebroplasty. Neurochirurgie 1987;33:166–8 [in French].
2. Bousson V, et al. Percutaneous vertebral augmentation techniques in osteoporotic and traumatic fractures. Semin Intervent Radiol 2018;35(4):309–23.
3. Luo J, Adams MA, Dolan P. Vertebroplasty and kyphoplasty can restore normal spine mechanics following osteoporotic vertebral fracture. J Osteoporos 2010;2010:729257.
4. Tzermiadianos M, et al. Altered disc pressure profile after an osteoporotic vertebral fracture is a risk factor for adjacent vertebral body fracture. Eur Spine J 2008;17:1522–30.
5. Available at: https://www.acr.org/-/media/ACR/Files/Practice-Parameters/VerebralAug.pdf?la=en.
6. Dittmer DK, Teasell R. Complications of immobilization and bed rest. Part 1: musculoskeletal and cardiovascular complications. Can Fam Physician 1993;39:1428–37.
7. Teasell R, Dittmer DK. Complications of immobilization and bed rest. Part 2: other complications. Can Fam Physician 1993;39:1440–6.
8. Prevention and management of osteoporosis. World Health Organ Tech Rep Ser 2003;921:1–164. back cover.
9. Chandra RV, et al. Vertebroplasty and kyphoplasty for osteoporotic vertebral fractures: what are the latest data? AJNR Am J Neuroradiol 2018;39(5):798–806.
10. Pedachenko E, et al. Puncture vertebroplasty in aggressive hemangiomas of the vertebrae bodies. Zh Vopr Neirokhir Im N N Burdenko 2004;(1):16–20 [in Russian].
11. Gangi A, Kastler BA, Dietemann JL. Percutaneous vertebroplasty guided by a combination of CT and fluoroscopy. AJNR Am J Neuroradiol 1994;15(1):83–6.
12. Weill A, et al. Spinal metastases: indications for and results of percutaneous injection of acrylic surgical cement. Radiology 1996;199(1):241–7.
13. Barr JD, et al. Percutaneous vertebroplasty for pain relief and spinal stabilization. Spine (Phila Pa 1976) 2000;25(8):923–8.
14. Murphy KJ, Deramond H. Percutaneous vertebroplasty in benign and malignant disease. Neuroimaging Clin N Am 2000;10(3):535–45.
15. Kallmes DF, et al. A randomized trial of vertebroplasty for osteoporotic spinal fractures. N Engl J Med 2009;361(6):569–79.
16. Buchbinder R, et al. A randomized trial of vertebroplasty for painful osteoporotic vertebral fractures. N Engl J Med 2009;361(6):557–68.
17. Taneichi H, et al. Risk factors and probability of vertebral body collapse in metastases of the thoracic and lumbar spine. Spine (Phila Pa 1976) 1997;22(3):239–45.
18. Saliou G, et al. Percutaneous vertebroplasty for pain management in malignant fractures of the spine with epidural involvement. Radiology 2010;254(3):882–90.
19. Mohme M, et al. Circulating tumour cell release after cement augmentation of vertebral metastases. Sci Rep 2017;7(1):7196.
20. Komemushi A, et al. Does vertebroplasty affect radiation dose distribution?: comparison of spatial dose distributions in a cement-injected vertebra as calculated by treatment planning system and actual spatial dose distribution. Radiol Res Pract 2012;2012:571571.
21. Chen JF, Lee ST. Percutaneous vertebroplasty for treatment of thoracolumbar spine bursting fracture. Surg Neurol 2004;62(6):494–500 [discussion: 500].
22. Knavel EM, Thielen KR, Kallmes DF. Vertebroplasty for the treatment of traumatic nonosteoporotic compression fractures. AJNR Am J Neuroradiol 2009;30(2):323–7.
23. Kotil K, Ozyuvaci E. Fibrous dysplasia in axis treated with vertebroplasty. J Craniovertebr Junction Spine 2010;1(2):118–21.

24. Huwart L, et al. Vertebral split fractures: technical feasibility of percutaneous vertebroplasty. Eur J Radiol 2014;83(1):173–8.

25. Tsai PJ, et al. Is additional balloon kyphoplasty safe and effective for acute thoracolumbar burst fracture? BMC Musculoskelet Disord 2017;18(1):393.

26. Vaccaro AR, et al. AOSpine thoracolumbar spine injury classification system: fracture description, neurological status, and key modifiers. Spine (Phila Pa 1976) 2013;38(23):2028–37.

27. Zaryanov AV, et al. Cement augmentation in vertebral burst fractures. Neurosurg Focus 2014;37(1):E5.

28. Lai PL, et al. Chemical and physical properties of bone cement for vertebroplasty. Biomed J 2013;36(4):162–7.

29. Wegener B, et al. Heat distribution of polymerisation temperature of bone cement on the spinal canal during vertebroplasty. Int Orthop 2012;36(5):1025–30.

30. Fang J, et al. Cytotoxicity of polymethyl methacrylate cement on primary cultured metastatic spinal cells. Mol Cell Toxicol 2016;12(2):125–32.

31. Lai P-L, et al. Cement leakage causes potential thermal injury in vertebroplasty. BMC Musculoskelet Disord 2011;12:116.

32. Lieberman IH, Togawa D, Kayanja MM. Vertebroplasty and kyphoplasty: filler materials. Spine J 2005;5(6 Suppl):305S–16S.

33. Mauri G, et al. Safety and results of image-guided vertebroplasty with elastomeric polymer material (elastoplasty). Eur Radiol Exp 2018;2(1):31.

34. Aebli N, et al. Fat embolism and acute hypotension during vertebroplasty: an experimental study in sheep. Spine (Phila Pa 1976) 2002;27(5):460–6.

35. Aebli N, et al. Cardiovascular changes during multiple vertebroplasty with and without vent-hole: an experimental study in sheep. Spine (Phila Pa 1976) 2003;28(14):1504–11 [discussion: 1511–2].

36. Krebs J, et al. Influence of bone marrow fat embolism on coagulation activation in an ovine model of vertebroplasty. J Bone Joint Surg Am 2008;90(2):349–56.

37. Belkoff SM, et al. The biomechanics of vertebroplasty. The effect of cement volume on mechanical behavior. Spine (Phila Pa 1976) 2001;26(14):1537–41.

38. Liebschner MA, Rosenberg WS, Keaveny TM. Effects of bone cement volume and distribution on vertebral stiffness after vertebroplasty. Spine (Phila Pa 1976) 2001;26(14):1547–54.

39. Kaufmann TJ, Trout AT, Kallmes DF. The effects of cement volume on clinical outcomes of percutaneous vertebroplasty. AJNR Am J Neuroradiol 2006;27(9):1933–7.

40. Kim DJ, et al. The proper volume and distribution of cement augmentation on percutaneous vertebroplasty. J Korean Neurosurg Soc 2010;48(2):125–8.

41. Chevalier Y, et al. Cement distribution, volume, and compliance in vertebroplasty: some answers from an anatomy-based nonlinear finite element study. Spine (Phila Pa 1976) 2008;33(16):1722–30.

42. Papanastassiou ID, et al. Controversial issues in kyphoplasty and vertebroplasty in osteoporotic vertebral fractures. Biomed Res Int 2014;2014:12.

43. Nairn RJ, Binkhamis S, Sheikh A. Current perspectives on percutaneous vertebroplasty: current evidence/controversies, patient selection and assessment, and technique and complications. Radiol Res Pract 2011;2011:175079.

44. Stallmeyer MJB, Zoarski GH. Patient evaluation and selection. In: Mathis JM, Deramond H, Belkoff SM, editors. Percutaneous vertebroplasty and kyphoplasty. New York: Springer New York; 2006. p. 60–88.

45. Stallmeyer MJB, Zoarski GH, Obuchowski AM. Optimizing patient selection in percutaneous vertebroplasty. J Vasc Interv Radiol 2003;14(6):683–96.

46. Barr JD, Mathis JM. Extreme vertebroplasty: techniques for treating difficult lesions. In: Mathis JM, Deramond H, Belkoff SM, editors. Percutaneous vertebroplasty and kyphoplasty. New York: Springer New York; 2006. p. 185–96.

47. Mathis JM. Percutaneous vertebroplasty: procedure technique. In: Mathis JM, Deramond H, Belkoff SM, editors. Percutaneous vertebroplasty and kyphoplasty. New York: Springer New York; 2006. p. 112–33.

48. Jeon S-I, et al. Comparative clinical results of vertebroplasty using jamshidi® needle and bone void filler for acute vertebral compression fractures. Korean J Spine 2012;9(3):239–43.

49. Garnier L, et al. Kyphoplasty versus vertebroplasty in osteoporotic thoracolumbar spine fractures. Short-term retrospective review of a multicentre cohort of 127 consecutive patients. Orthop Traumatol Surg Res 2012;98(6 Suppl):S112–9.

50. Steinmann J, et al. Biomechanical comparison of unipedicular versus bipedicular kyphoplasty. Spine (Phila Pa 1976) 2005;30(2):201–5.

51. Tohmeh AG, et al. Biomechanical efficacy of unipedicular versus bipedicular vertebroplasty for the management of osteoporotic compression fractures. Spine (Phila Pa 1976) 1999;24(17):1772–6.

52. Kim DS, et al. Lumbar nerve root compression due to leakage of bone cement after vertebroplasty. Korean J Neurotrauma 2014;10(2):155–8.

53. Bernhard J, Heini PF, Villiger PM. Asymptomatic diffuse pulmonary embolism caused by acrylic cement: an unusual complication of percutaneous vertebroplasty. Ann Rheum Dis 2003;62(1):85–6.

54. Krebs J, et al. Clinical measurements of cement injection pressure during vertebroplasty. Spine (Phila Pa 1976) 2005;30(5):E118–22.

55. Mathis JM, Deramond H. Complications associated with vertebroplasty and kyphoplasty. In: Mathis JM,

Deramond H, Belkoff SM, editors. Percutaneous vertebroplasty and kyphoplasty. New York: Springer New York; 2006. p. 210–22.

56. Schmidt R, et al. Cement leakage during vertebroplasty: an underestimated problem? Eur Spine J 2005;14(5):466–73.

57. Gaudino S, et al. A systematic approach to vertebral hemangioma. Skeletal Radiol 2015;44(1):25–36.

58. Nabavizadeh SA, et al. Utility of fat-suppressed sequences in differentiation of aggressive vs typical asymptomatic haemangioma of the spine. Br J Radiol 2016;89(1057):20150557.

59. Jeromel M, Podobnik J. Magnetic resonance spectroscopy (MRS) of vertebral column—an additional tool for evaluation of aggressiveness of vertebral haemangioma like lesion. Radiol Oncol 2014;48(2): 137–41.

60. Kushchayev S, Pedachenko E. Percutaneous vertebroplasty. Kiev (Ukraine): ASD; 2005. p. 512.

61. Liu XW, et al. Vertebroplasty in the treatment of symptomatic vertebral haemangiomas without neurological deficit. Eur Radiol 2013;23(9):2575–81.

62. Premat K, et al. Long-term outcome of percutaneous alcohol embolization combined with percutaneous vertebroplasty in aggressive vertebral hemangiomas with epidural extension. Eur Radiol 2017; 27(7):2860–7.

63. Wang B, et al. Intraoperative vertebroplasty during surgical decompression and instrumentation for aggressive vertebral hemangiomas: a retrospective study of 39 patients and review of the literature. Spine J 2018;18(7):1128–35.

64. Klotzbuecher CM, et al. Patients with prior fractures have an increased risk of future fractures: a summary of the literature and statistical synthesis. J Bone Miner Res 2000;15(4):721–39.

65. Anselmetti GC, et al. Percutaneous vertebroplasty: multi-centric results from EVEREST experience in large cohort of patients. Eur J Radiol 2012;81(12): 4083–6.

66. Voormolen MH, et al. The risk of new osteoporotic vertebral compression fractures in the year after percutaneous vertebroplasty. J Vasc Interv Radiol 2006;17(1):71–6.

67. Lin EP, et al. Vertebroplasty: cement leakage into the disc increases the risk of new fracture of adjacent vertebral body. AJNR Am J Neuroradiol 2004; 25(2):175–80.

68. Borensztein M, et al. Analysis of risk factors for new vertebral fracture after percutaneous vertebroplasty. Global Spine J 2018;8(5):446–52.

69. Komemushi A, et al. Percutaneous vertebroplasty for osteoporotic compression fracture: multivariate study of predictors of new vertebral body fracture. Cardiovasc Intervent Radiol 2006;29(4):580–5.

70. Berton A, et al. A 3D finite element model of prophylactic vertebroplasty in the metastatic spine: vertebral stability and stress distribution on adjacent vertebrae. J Spinal Cord Med 2018;1–7. https://doi.org/10.1080/10790268.2018.1432309.

71. Kebaish KM, et al. Use of vertebroplasty to prevent proximal junctional fractures in adult deformity surgery: a biomechanical cadaveric study. Spine J 2013;13(12):1897–903.

72. Gangi A, et al. Percutaneous vertebroplasty: indications, technique, and results. Radiographics 2003; 23(2):e10.

73. Venmans A, et al. Postprocedural CT for perivertebral cement leakage in percutaneous vertebroplasty is not necessary–results from VERTOS II. Neuroradiology 2011;53(1):19–22.

74. Yeom JS, et al. Leakage of cement in percutaneous transpedicular vertebroplasty for painful osteoporotic compression fractures. J Bone Joint Surg Br 2003;85(1):83–9.

75. Maramattom B. Extraosseous cement leakage after vertebroplasty producing intractable low back pain. Neurol India 2017;65(2):375–6.

76. Churojana A, et al. Is intervertebral cement leakage a risk factor for new adjacent vertebral collapse? Interv Neuroradiol 2014;20(5):637–45.

77. Gao C, et al. Analysis of risk factors causing short-term cement leakages and long-term complications after percutaneous kyphoplasty for osteoporotic vertebral compression fractures. Acta Radiol 2018; 59(5):577–85.

78. Mirovsky Y, et al. Intradiscal cement leak following percutaneous vertebroplasty. Spine (Phila Pa 1976) 2006;31(10):1120–4.

79. Nouda S, et al. Adjacent vertebral body fracture following vertebroplasty with polymethylmethacrylate or calcium phosphate cement: biomechanical evaluation of the cadaveric spine. Spine (Phila Pa 1976) 2009;34(24):2613–8.

80. Mathis JM, Ortiz AO, Zoarski GH. Vertebroplasty versus kyphoplasty: a comparison and contrast. AJNR Am J Neuroradiol 2004;25(5):840–5.

81. Groen RJ, et al. Anatomical and pathological considerations in percutaneous vertebroplasty and kyphoplasty: a reappraisal of the vertebral venous system. Spine (Phila Pa 1976) 2004;29(13):1465–71.

82. Ahmadzai H, et al. Fat embolism syndrome following percutaneous vertebroplasty: a case report. Spine J 2014;14(4):e1–5.

83. Mansour A, et al. Cement pulmonary embolism as a complication of percutaneous vertebroplasty in cancer patients. Cancer Imaging 2018;18(1):5.

84. Habib N, et al. Cement pulmonary embolism after percutaneous vertebroplasty and kyphoplasty: an overview. Heart Lung 2012;41(5):509–11.

85. Krueger A, et al. Management of pulmonary cement embolism after percutaneous vertebroplasty and kyphoplasty: a systematic review of the literature. Eur Spine J 2009;18(9):1257–65.

86. Benneker LM, et al. Cardiovascular changes after PMMA vertebroplasty in sheep: the effect of bone marrow removal using pulsed jet-lavage. Eur Spine J 2010;19(11):1913–20.

87. Hershkovich O, et al. Bone marrow washout for multilevel vertebroplasty in multiple myeloma spinal involvement. Technical note. Eur Spine J 2019; 28(6):1455–60.

88. Park J-W, et al. Infection following percutaneous vertebral augmentation with polymethylmethacrylate. Arch Osteoporos 2018;13(1):47.

89. Abdelrahman H, et al. Infection after vertebroplasty or kyphoplasty. A series of nine cases and review of literature. Spine J 2013;13(12):1809–17.

90. Liao JC, et al. Surgical outcomes of infectious spondylitis after vertebroplasty, and comparisons between pyogenic and tuberculosis. BMC Infect Dis 2018;18(1):555.

91. Syed MI, et al. Vertebral osteomyelitis following vertebroplasty: is acne a potential contraindication and are prophylactic antibiotics mandatory prior to vertebroplasty? Pain Physician 2009;12(4):E285–90.

92. Kang JH, Kim H-S, Kim SW. Tuberculous spondylitis after percutaneous vertebroplasty: misdiagnosis or complication? Korean J Spine 2013;10(2):97–100.

93. Yaltirik CK, Ozdogan S, Atalay B. Thoracic epidural hematoma complicating vertebroplasty. Am J Case Rep 2017;18:1229–32.

94. Marden FA, Putman CM. Cement-embolic stroke associated with vertebroplasty. AJNR Am J Neuroradiol 2008;29(10):1986–8.

Sacral Fractures and Sacroplasty

Wende Nocton Gibbs, MD, MA[a],*, Amish Doshi, MD[b]

KEYWORDS

• Spine • Sacral insufficiency fracture • Osteoporosis • Sacroplasty • Ablation

KEY POINTS

- Traumatic and insufficiency fractures of the sacrum have traditionally been underrecognized, because they are poorly seen on radiographs.
- Increasing use of computed tomography in the trauma setting and MR imaging in the nonemergent setting is facilitating earlier diagnosis.
- Radiologists should have an understanding of, and create reports using the most current classification systems of the treatment team, to facilitate effective communication and optimal patient outcomes.
- Sacroplasty is a safe, minimally invasive treatment option for sacral fractures that provides fast and durable pain relief.
- Combined tumor ablation and sacroplasty can provide effective pain palliation for osseous sacral metastases.

Sacral fractures most commonly result from high impact trauma, or are pathologic fractures related to osteoporosis, radiation therapy, or malignancy. In the emergency setting, the increasing use of computed tomography (CT) has substantially increased the diagnosis of sacral fractures,[1] which are frequently occult on radiographs. Radiologists should be familiar with and create reports using the most current fracture classification systems, as this improves communication with the treatment team and optimizes patient care.

Sacral insufficiency fractures remain underdiagnosed due to nonspecific symptoms, poor visualization on screening radiographs, and underappreciation of the entity. This delay is increasingly problematic as osteoporosis is common in the aging population. Delayed diagnosis can result in substantial morbidity and poor quality of life. Once diagnosed, conservative treatment may facilitate eventual healing and pain relief. Alternatively, sacroplasty is a safe, minimally invasive procedure that can immediately and durably treat pain and help patients more rapidly return to normal activity. Sacroplasty can also treat the pain resulting from some types of traumatic fracture and pathologic fractures caused by benign and malignant tumors.[2] In patients with osseous metastatic disease, radiofrequency ablation performed before cement augmentation can alleviate pain, and in some cases provide local tumor control.

SACRAL FRACTURES: CAUSES AND CLASSIFICATION

Sacral fractures primarily occur in young patients in the setting trauma and in the elderly, who experience osteoporotic insufficiency fractures with minor trauma or no obvious inciting event. These fractures are increasingly diagnosed with the now near-routine use of CT in the emergency

Disclosure Statement: W.N. Gibbs: No relevant disclosures. A. Doshi: Merit Medical Speaker's Bureau.
a Neuroradiology Section, Department of Radiology, Mayo Clinic Arizona, 5777 East Mayo Boulevard, Phoenix, AZ 85054, USA; b Icahn School of Medicine at Mount Sinai, 1176 5th Avenue, MC Level, New York, NY 10029, USA
* Corresponding author.
E-mail address: Gibbs.Wende@Mayo.edu

Neuroimag Clin N Am 29 (2019) 515–527
https://doi.org/10.1016/j.nic.2019.07.003
1052-5149/19/© 2019 Elsevier Inc. All rights reserved.

neuroimaging.theclinics.com

setting, and more common use of CT and MR in the nonemergent setting for patients with back pain. Although relatively uncommon, these injuries can cause significant morbidity.

Traumatic Sacral Fractures

Traumatic sacral fractures typically occur in younger patients in high-speed or high-impact accidents. They are often associated with pelvic ring injuries and approximately 25% are associated with neurologic injuries. The presence of a neurologic deficit is the most important factor in predicting outcome.[1]

The Denis system has traditionally been used to categorize traumatic sacral fractures.[3] This classification divides the sacrum into 3 zones: zone I fractures are limited to the sacral ala and are occasionally associated with fifth lumbar nerve root injury (**Fig. 1**). These are the most common type, occurring in 50% of those with sacral fracture. Zone II fractures are the second most common type, approximately 34%. These fractures involve the sacral foramina and result in nerve injury in 28% of patients. Zone III fractures involve the spinal canal and sacral bodies. Fifty-seven percent of these fractures are associated with neurologic injury, often saddle anesthesia and loss of sphincter function (**Fig. 2**).

In 2016, the AOSpine Trauma Knowledge Forum devised a new traumatic sacral fracture classification to facilitate effective communication among members of the multidisciplinary treatment team and support development of optimal treatment algorithms. The rationale was that the existing sacral fracture classification systems, based on fracture morphology or inferred mechanism of injury, are too broad and simplistic, or too specific.[4] In the AOSpine classification, fractures are categorized by the effect on sacropelvic stability (**Table 1**). Type A fractures are lower sacrococcygeal injures with no impact on posterior pelvic or spinopelvic stability. Type B are posterior pelvic injuries that effect posterior pelvic stability, and type C, the most unstable, are spinopelvic injures. The type B injuries are a variation of the Denis system, although they are ranked by severity instead of location (type B1 is zone III, type B2 is zone I, and type B3 is zone II). The reader is referred to the AOSpine website for further description and figures.[5]

Sacral Insufficiency Fractures

Sacral insufficiency fractures are a significant source of debilitating low back pain in the older adult population. These fractures most commonly occur in individuals with osteoporosis, typically older women. Malignancy, prior radiation therapy for gynecologic or gastrointestinal cancer, rheumatoid arthritis, and metabolic bone disease are additional causes. These fractures can occur with little or no trauma. Pain from these fractures may gradually increase or present with acute pain exacerbated by weight bearing. Pain is most often in the sacral or buttock region, but may be referred to the hips or groin. Coexistent vertebral

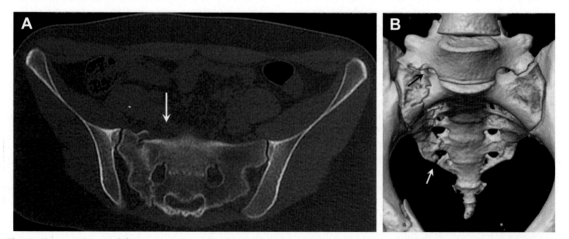

Fig. 1. Traumatic sacral fracture. A 22-year-old woman in a high-speed motor vehicle collision presented to the emergency room with severe back and pelvic pain and right leg radicular symptoms. The patient was taken immediately for a CT; no radiographs were obtained. An axial CT image (*A*) demonstrates a fracture through the right sacral ala involving the lateral aspect of the neural foramen. A small amount of presacral hemorrhage is present (*arrow*). A 3-dimensional CT reconstruction (*B*) clearly shows the fracture involving multiple right sacral foramina (*white arrow*), as well as the right L5 to S1 neural foramen (*black arrow*). This is a Denis zone II fracture type.

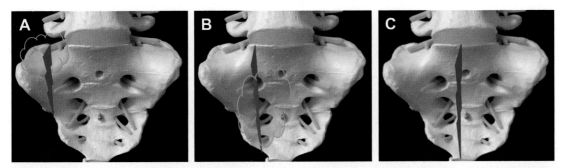

Fig. 2. Sacral fracture classification. The Denis classification of sacral fractures divides the sacrum into 3 zones. Zone I fractures (*A*) are lateral to the neural foramina. These fractures may rarely cause symptoms, most often related to injury of the exiting L5 nerve root. Zone II fractures (*B*) extend through the neural foramen and more frequently result in nerve injury. Zone III fractures (*C*) involve the spinal canal and lie medial the foramen. They also may involve a transversely oriented fracture component, typically below the S2 level. Zone III fractures are rare but often result in neurologic injury.

compression fractures may occur in osteoporotic patients: the radiologist should always check for spinal fractures when a sacral fracture is found, and vice versa.

Insufficiency fractures may involve multiple zones: transverse fractures commonly involve all 3 zones of the Denis classification system. The longitudinal component of the fracture may be unilateral or bilateral, and a transverse component is most commonly seen below the S2 vertebral body (**Fig. 3**).

Pathologic Fractures

Osseous metastases of the pelvis and sacrum can compromise structural weight-bearing integrity and precipitate pathologic fracture that can result in disabling mechanical pain. In addition, these patients may be further afflicted by superimposed pain related to their tumor, namely, pain owing to the stimulation of endosteal nociceptors and multiple chemical factors of the cancer microenvironment. Extension of the tumor into the neural foramina or epidural space can produce

Table 1
AOSpine classification of sacral fractures

Aospine	Type A	Type B	Type C
Injury type	Lower sacrococcygeal	Posterior pelvic	Spinopelvic
Significance	Does not cause posterior pelvic/spinopelvic instability	Posterior pelvic instability	Spinopelvic instability (with or without posterior pelvic instability)
Example	Injury below sacroiliac joint Avulsion fracture Compression fracture	Unilateral longitudinal sacral fracture	Sacral "U" fractures Bilateral longitudinal fractures
Neurologic injury	Higher grade subtypes may be associated with neurologic injury	As with Denis system, subtypes may cause neurologic injury based on location (likelihood increases from Denis zones I–III)	

INCREASING INSTABILITY

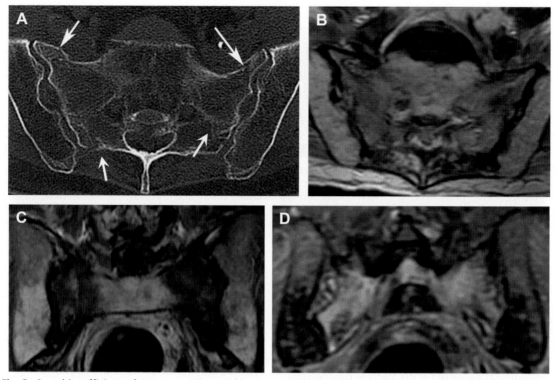

Fig. 3. Sacral insufficiency fracture. A 72-year-old woman with osteoporosis presents with severe back pain. The onset was sudden, without trauma. An axial CT scan (*A*) shows numerous longitudinal and transversely oriented fractures lines (*arrows*) within the osteoporotic bone. Axial T1 (*B*), coronal T1 (*C*), and coronal short T1 inversion recovery (*D*) images demonstrate T1 hypointense, short T1 inversion recovery hyperintense marrow edema within the fractured sacral ala.

radiculopathy, pain, and bowel and bladder incontinence. Primary malignant and benign tumors, such as hemangiomas, can also produce pain and result in pathologic fracture.

Radiation-Induced Fractures

Radiation therapy is an essential component of treatment for gynecologic and gastrointestinal malignancy. Large or locally advanced cervical cancers, postoperative or locally advanced endometrial cancers, and anal and rectal cancers are commonly treated with neoadjuvant external beam radiotherapy, which has shown benefit in local tumor control and patient survival. Adverse effects on the surrounding tissues are common. The sacrum is the most frequently involved osseous structure, given its location and large volume of red marrow. High loading forces and treatment-related or disease-related osteoporosis contribute to the risk of biomechanical failure. One study of pelvic insufficiency fractures after intensity-modulated radiation therapy for pelvic tumors found an overall incidence of 4.4% (20 fractures in 15 patients during

the 7-year study period). Of the 20 fractures, 13 involved the sacrum, 4 involved the superior pubic ramus, and 3 involved the inferior pubic ramus.[6] The development of sacral fractures after radiation, much like vertebral body fractures, is influenced by the presence of osteoporosis, age, weight, and medications, primarily corticosteroids.

Marrow reaction to radiation therapy can range from a transient osteitis to radiation necrosis. The range of insufficiency fracture incidence found in the literature is broad, at 1.7% to 89%, because of differences in length of follow-up, available imaging, and inclusion of asymptomatic patients in these studies.[7–10] Authors of a recent large study reported an incidence of 7.6% (31 of 410 patients).[11]

These osseous marrow reactions are T1 hypointense and T2 hyperintense on MR imaging in both symptomatic and asymptomatic patients. Meixel and colleagues[11] studied a group of 410 patients with pelvic malignancy treated with radiotherapy. Of these, 17.6% (72 patients) had new pathologic MR signal changes. Seventy-eight percent of patients (56/72) had eventual resolution of the

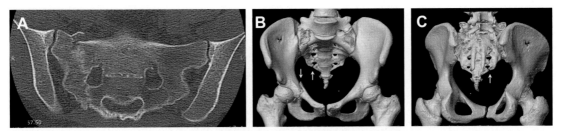

Fig. 4. The value of 3-dimensional CT reconstructed images. Axial CT image (*A*) from the 22-year-old woman described in **Fig. 1** do not fully capture the extent of her injuries. Anterior (*B*) and posterior (*C*) views from a 3-dimensional reconstruction show involvement of numerous right sided sacral foramina as well as a superior pubic ramus fracture (*arrows*).

treatment-related marrow edema, and 14% (10/72) had no recovery. Late insufficiency fractures were common 43% (31/72).

Imaging Evaluation

Plain films allow a rapid survey of the entire pelvis, but are limited by their low sensitivity (20%–38%) for sacral insufficiency fractures.[12] The identification of a fracture line or sclerosis along the fracture is rare. Osteopenia and overlying bowel gas contribute to obscuration of osseous structures. A 3-view series that includes inlet, outlet, and lateral views provides the highest sensitivity. Longitudinal fractures are best seen on inlet and outlet, because they provide orthogonal views of the sacrum. Lateral views are less useful, because there is often poor penetration owing to overlying pelvic anatomy, but these views may show angulated transverse fractures or displaced fractures. Transverse fractures show buckling or interruption of the sacral arcuate lines, which are the cortical reflections of the sacral foramen. Of note, fractures of the L5 transverse process or pubic rami are considered indirect evidence of a sacral fracture, prompting increased scrutiny or further evaluation with CT scanning or MR imaging.

CT scanning is now the mainstay for evaluation of suspected sacral and pelvic fractures in the trauma setting. Presacral edema or hematoma are highly suggestive of fracture. Three-dimensional reconstructions are useful for identifying fractures that may be subtle in the individual planes, finding additional injuries (**Figs. 4** and **5**). Three-dimensional volume-rendered images readily convey complicated spatial relationships and information, making them vital for surgical planning. The sensitivity of CT scans for sacral insufficiency fracture is 60% to 75%.[13] CT scanning is a useful adjunct to MR imaging to determine whether fractures involve the neural foramen and for surgical or sacroplasty planning.

MR imaging is the most useful modality for the identification of all types of sacral fracture. Fracture lines are T1 hypointense and the associated marrow edema is hyperintense on short T1 inversion recovery images. The fracture may enhance after contrast administration. In patients with a history of malignancy and concern for sacral metastasis, it may be difficult to differentiate an osteoporotic fracture from a pathologic fracture. Coronal oblique images nicely demonstrate vertically oriented fractures (**Fig. 6**). Sensitivity for acute and subacute fracture has been reported as high as 100%.[12]

Sacral insufficiency fractures often present with nonspecific low back pain, and lumbar spine MR imaging is often the initial imaging examination. The sagittal midline T1-weighted lumbar spine image should be carefully evaluated in older or osteopenic patients, because marrow edema

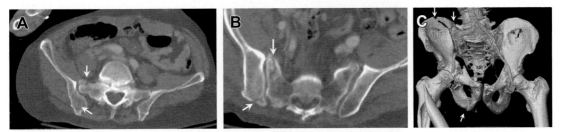

Fig. 5. A 3-dimensional reconstructed images best reveal full extent of injury. Axial CT images (*A*, *B*) from a 45-year-old man struck by an automobile. Several sacral fractures are seen (*arrows*). The 3-dimensional reconstruction (*C*) dramatically demonstrates the full extent of the injuries, including sacral, pelvic, and acetabular fractures (*arrows*), as well as a markedly displaced femoral fracture.

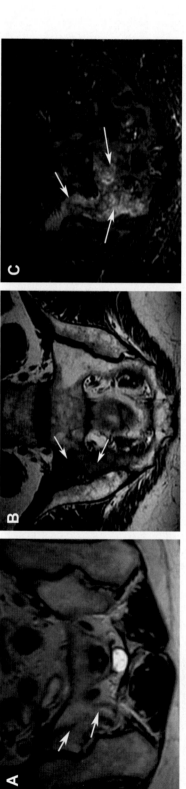
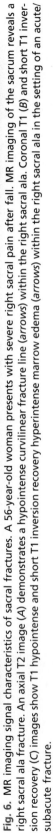

Fig. 6. MR imaging signal characteristics of sacral fractures. A 56-year-old woman presents with severe right sacral pain after fall. MR imaging of the sacrum reveals a right sacral ala fracture. An axial T2 image (A) demonstrates a hypointense curvilinear fracture line (*arrows*) within the right sacral ala. Coronal T1 (B) and short T1 inversion recovery (C) images show T1 hypointense and short T1 inversion recovery hyperintense marrow edema (*arrows*) within the right sacral ala in the setting of an acute/subacute fracture.

may be present and, if identified, can prompt dedicated imaging of the sacrum.

Technetium-99m methylene diphosphonate bone scintigraphy is highly sensitive: 96% for detection of sacral insufficiency fracture.[12] This test is valuable if MR imaging is contraindicated, as in the presence of a pacemaker or for a patient with claustrophobia. The posterior planar view is the most sensitive for fracture detection. A classic H-shaped distribution of radiotracer is considered by many to be pathognomonic for sacral insufficiency fracture, but other patterns of tracer uptake may be present.

SACROPLASTY
Treatment of Sacral Fractures

Traumatic sacral fractures may be treated with progressive weight bearing with an orthosis if the displacement is less than 1 cm and there are no neurologic deficits. If the fracture fragments are displaced by more than 1 cm, there is soft tissue compromise, there is instability, or there is persistent pain or displacement of the fracture with nonoperative treatment, surgical fixation is indicated. Neurologic injury requires prompt treatment with fixation and decompression.[14,15]

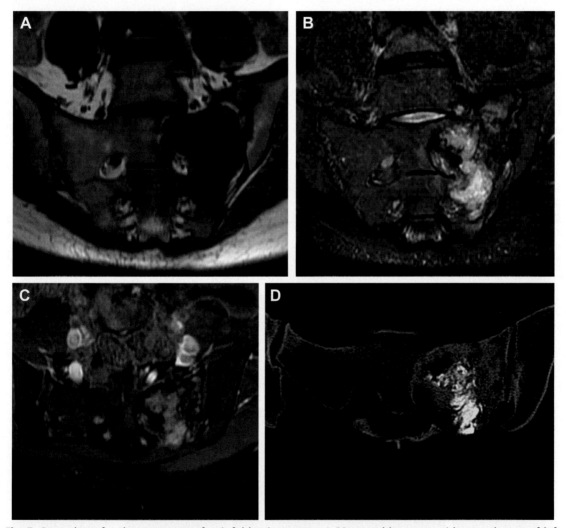

Fig. 7. Sacroplasty for the treatment of painful benign tumor. A 38-year-old woman with several years of left sacral pain presented with progressive worsening of symptoms. Coronal T1 (A), coronal short T1 inversion recovery (B), and axial postcontrast (C) images demonstrate an expansile, T1 hypointense, short T1 inversion recovery hyperintense, heterogeneously enhancing mass within the left sacral ala. Tissue sampling with CT-guided biopsy (images not shown) provided a diagnosis of sacral hemangioma. Cement augmentation was performed under CT guidance and the postprocedure CT axial image (D) shows PMMA cement filling the medial portion of the hemangioma. Upon completion of the procedure, the patient's pain improved significantly.

Similar options are available for the treatment of sacral insufficiency and pathologic fractures. Conservative treatment consists of pain medications, including opioids, bed rest, and physical therapy.[16,17] This course of treatment improves pain and functional disability in some patients; however, recovery can be lengthy, and patients have limited mobility with potential deleterious effects from bed rest including deep venous thrombosis, pulmonary emboli, progression of osteoporosis, decreased muscle strength, decubitus ulcers, and depression. Most patients experience some improvement in symptoms after 1 to 2 weeks and complete healing after 9 months.[18,19] Open surgical treatment has limited application in the elderly population, because the implantation and fixation of hardware in osteoporotic bone is technically challenging.

Sacroplasty, percutaneous injection of polymethyl methacrylate (PMMA) cement, with or without balloon assistance, is a safe, minimally invasive procedure analogous to spinal cement augmentation. In the pelvis, the injection of PMMA cement was originally described for the treatment of painful pathologic fractures resulting from metastases. After this, treating physicians began to use sacroplasty for insufficiency fractures, some types of minor traumatic fracture, and benign and malignant tumors (**Figs. 7** and **8**). In the case of insufficiency fractures, sacroplasty is typically limited to treatment of zone I fractures, lateral to the sacral foramina, owing to the greater risk of cement leakage into the foramina or canal in zone II and III fractures.[20]

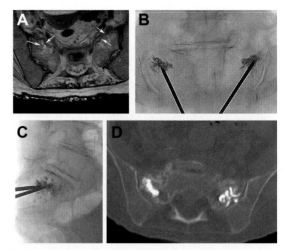

Fig. 9. Fluoroscopically guided sacroplasty. A 65-year-old man presented with severe back pain after a fall. He was found to have bilateral sacral fractures. The axial T2 image (*A*) shows linear T2 hypointense regions within the sacral ala consistent with fracture lines (*arrows*) surrounded by T2 hyperintensity representing edema. Fluoroscopic-guided sacroplasty was performed for pain control. Anteroposterior (*B*) and lateral (*C*) fluoroscopic images demonstrate needles and cement within the bilateral sacral ala. The postsacroplasty CT image (*D*) demonstrates shows PMMA cement stabilizing the sacral ala fractures.

Sacroplasty typically results in immediate and sustained pain relief[21–23] and improved, early patient mobility.[24] Compared with conservative treatment, including bedrest, medications, and

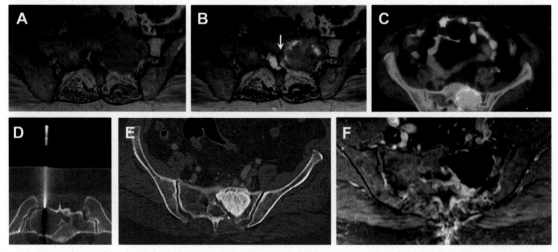

Fig. 8. Sacroplasty after partial sacrectomy. A 70-year-old woman presented to her doctor with progressive low back pain and left leg numbness. T1 (*A*) and T2 (*B*) images demonstrate a large left sacral mass. Note extension into the epidural space (*arrow*). An PET/CT scan with 18F-FDG-PET/CT (*C*) showed relatively intense FDG avidity. A percutaneous CT-guided biopsy facilitated the diagnosis of schwannoma. After tumor resection and partial sacrectomy, sacroplasty was used to stabilize the sacrum (*D*, *E*). Follow-up T1 postcontrast fat-saturated MR image (*F*) shows a large volume of hypodense cement in the surgical defect.

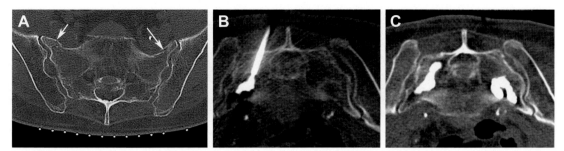

Fig. 10. CT-guided sacroplasty. A 72-year-old osteoporotic woman presented with severe sacral pain. She had no history of trauma. Sacroplasty planning CT scan (A) demonstrates diffuse demineralization of the sacrum with bilateral sacral ala fractures (arrows). An axial CT fluoroscopic image obtained during sacroplasty (B) demonstrates cement injection within the left sacral ala. Postsacroplasty axial CT scan (C) demonstrates cement filling the fractures of the sacral ala.

physical therapy, often for a protracted period of time, this procedure is cost effective and results in greater patient satisfaction.[24,25] Sacroplasty is safe, with few reported complications, and can be performed on an outpatient basis.

The technical aspects of the procedure vary by preference of the operator, but in general, PMMA cement is injected through bone biopsy needles into the fracture under CT, x-ray fluoroscopy, or CT fluoroscopic image guidance (Figs. 9 and 10). Preprocedure antibiotics are typically administered, and moderate sedation with fentanyl and midazolam (Versed) is adequate for procedural pain control. One difference between sacroplasty and cement augmentation of the spinal vertebral bodies is a lack of resistance during cement injection, owing to the large medullary cavity of the sacrum. For this reason, lower volumes of cement are used and close monitoring is required to avoid cement leakage. Leakage into the sacral foramina is the greatest potential risk, because this leaking may result in nerve compression. Breach of the anterior sacral cortex with leakage into the presacral space and leakage into the sacroiliac joint with potential for joint compromise are additional, although less substantial, concerns. Few cases of significant cement leakage have been reported.[20]

Several needle approaches are possible. The most common approaches are the long axis approach with placement of the needle in the caudad–cephalic direction along the ala, and the short axis approach, with needle entry in a posterior to anterior direction (Fig. 11). Proponents of

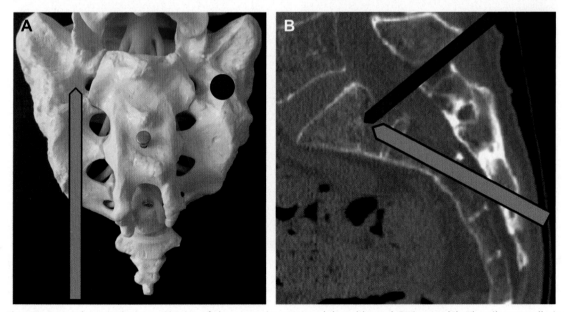

Fig. 11. Sacroplasty technique. Picture of the posterior sacrum (A) and lateral CT image (B). The silver needle in A and B shows the trajectory of the long axis approach. The dark gray needle (seen en face in A) shows the short axis approach.

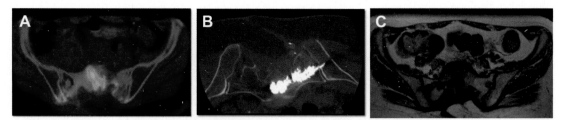

Fig. 12. A transiliac approach. A 54-year-old woman with history of chordoma treated with partial sacrectomy developed a painful pathologic fracture in the midline S1 body. (*A*) A 18F-FDG-PET/CT image shows increased avidity at the fracture site. Given the location, a transiliac approach (*B*) to cement augmentation was used for sacroplasty. (*C*) A T1-weighted image from a follow-up examination shows the T1 hypointense cement.

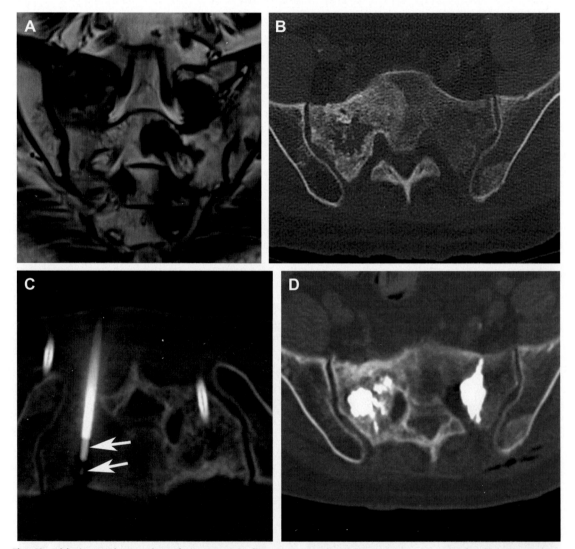

Fig. 13. Ablation and sacroplasty for metastatic disease. A 78-year-old man with a history of metastatic prostate cancer presented with severe low back and sacral pain. The coronal T1 image (*A*) shows multiple hypointense lesions throughout the sacrum reflecting metastases. The axial CT image (*B*) demonstrates a mixed sclerotic and lytic mass within the right sacral ala. The patient underwent CT-guided radiofrequency ablation followed by cement augmentation. The CT fluoroscopic image (*C*) demonstrates a radiofrequency ablation probe (*arrow*) placed coaxially thought an introducer needle. The final CT image (*D*) after ablation of the tumor and cement deposition shows good cement filling within the bilateral sacral ala.

the long axis approach cite better filling of the entire longitudinal fracture line with cement, and less potential for breaching the sacral anterior cortex as benefits of this needle trajectory. Studies of both techniques have shown similar effectiveness in treating pain and safety in terms of cement extravasation.[17,20,26–29] The transiliac approach, in which the needle enters the iliac bone and traverse the sacroiliac joint, has been found useful to reach sacral body lesions (**Fig. 12**).

Sacroplasty has an excellent safety record in the literature.[25] Similar to spinal cement augmentation, venous intravasation and cement embolism, infection, and extension into the neural foramen are potential complications. Cement leakage is the most common complication of sacroplasty. A wide range of incidence is cited in the literature: 8% to 73%, with a lower incidence when balloon kyphoplasty is used.[30,31] Adverse reactions are similar to other spinal procedures, including complications related to needle insertion (infection, bleeding) or anesthesia.

The mechanism by which injected cement provides pain relief is mainly attributed to structural stabilization, with treatment of the painful fracture micromotion and restoration of sacral strength and stiffness. However, a study by Richards and colleagues[32] found that cement augmentation did not restore the original strength and stiffness of the sacrum after cement injection. Another theory posits that the neurotoxic effect and exothermic reaction of PMMA could cause periosteal denervation.[2,33] At this time, the mechanism of pain relief remains unknown.

Tumor Ablation

Up to 7% of spinal metastases occur in the sacrum.[34] Chemical factors associated with the tumor microenvironment, pathologic fracture with micromotion, and mass effect on nerve roots are the primary causes of local pain. Radiotherapy is standard of care, but 40% to 60% of patients do not experience complete pain relief[35,36] and radiation does not treat the mechanical pain of pathologic fracture.

Percutaneous ablation is now an accepted alternative method of treating osseous metastasis in some patients. The most common type of ablation, radiofrequency ablation, uses high-frequency

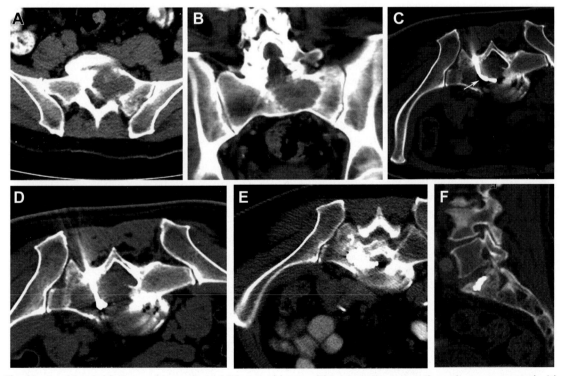

Fig. 14. Combined ablation and sacroplasty. A 54-year-old man with metastatic pancreatic carcinoma presented with severe left-sided back pain. Axial CT (*A*) and coronal CT (*B*) images show a lytic lesion within the left sacral ala extending toward midline. CT-guided radiofrequency ablation and sacroplasty was performed. Intraoperative CT scan (*C*) during radiofrequency ablation shows the tip of a curved ablation probe (*arrow*) within the central portion of the lytic lesion. After ablation, cement was injected into the lytic region (*D*). Follow-up axial (*E*) and sagittal CT (*F*) scans at 3 months demonstrates near-complete resolution of the lytic lesion postablation and sacroplasty.

alternating current to produce thermal injury and necrosis. The procedure is minimally invasive and may be performed in an outpatient setting. Ablation alone can treat pain, but given the risk of subsequent fracture, cement augmentation is frequently performed at the same time[2,37] (**Figs. 13** and **14**). Some authors believe that ablation and cement augmentation can provide pain palliation in a synergistic manner, greater than that of radiation therapy.[33,38] Multiple case series have shown decreased pain scores after radiofrequency ablation of painful osseous metastases with and without cementoplasty.[38] In a review of microwave ablation and cementoplasty performed for 69 patients with 102 painful spinal metastases, Khan and colleagues[36] found that 94% of patients had immediate pain reduction that was maintained for more than 6 months.

SUMMARY

Undiagnosed sacral fractures can lead to significant morbidity. Increased awareness and use of CT and MR imaging in the emergency and outpatient settings has facilitated diagnosis of this important injury. Fractures should be reported using the classification systems of the treatment team to ensure seamless communication and optimal patient care. Osteoporosis is an increasing problem as our population ages, and remains substantially undertreated. Sacral insufficiency fractures are often unsuspected, with vague symptoms and no history of injury. These patients often receive lumbar MR imaging for back pain before the sacrum is evaluated, and the radiologist should take care to carefully inspect the midline sagittal image for any signs of sacral marrow edema. Because patients with cancer are living longer with metastatic disease, sacral fractures from metastases or radiation treatment are also becoming more common. Percutaneous sacroplasty is a safe and effective procedure that rapidly and durably ameliorates the pain of sacral fracture. Radiofrequency ablation before cement augmentation is a useful option for palliating pain in patients with sacral metastatic disease.

REFERENCES

1. Bydon M, De la Garza-ramos R, Macki M, et al. Incidence of sacral fractures and in-hospital postoperative complications in the United States: an analysis of 2002-2011 data. Spine 2014;39(18):E1103–9.
2. Georgy BA. Percutaneous cement augmentations of malignant lesions of the sacrum and pelvis. AJNR Am J Neuroradiol 2009;30(7):1357–9.
3. Denis F, Davis S, Comfort T. Sacral fractures: an important problem. Retrospective analysis of 236 cases. Clin Orthop Relat Res 1988;227:67–81.
4. Schroeder GD, Kurd MF, Kepler CK, et al. The development of a universally accepted sacral fracture classification: a survey of AOSpine and AOTrauma members. Global Spine J 2016;6(7):686–94.
5. AOSpine. Available at: https://aospine.aofoundation. org/en/clinical-library-and-tools/aospine-injury-classification-system. Accessed January 31, 2019.
6. Bazire L, Xu H, Foy JP, et al. Pelvic insufficiency fracture (PIF) incidence in patients treated with intensity-modulated radiation therapy (IMRT) for gynaecological or anal cancer: single-institution experience and review of the literature. Br J Radiol 2017;90(1073):20160885.
7. Tokumaru S, Toita T, Oguchi M, et al. Insufficiency fractures after pelvic radiation therapy for uterine cervical cancer: an analysis of subjects in a prospective multi-institutional trial, and cooperative study of the Japan Radiation Oncology Group (JAROG) and Japanese Radiation Oncology Study Group (JROSG). Int J Radiat Oncol Biol Phys 2012;84(2):e195–200.
8. Blomlie V, Rofstad EK, Talle K, et al. Incidence of radiation-induced insufficiency fractures of the female pelvis: evaluation with MR imaging. AJR Am J Roentgenol 1996;167(5):1205–10.
9. Huh SJ, Kim B, Kang MK, et al. Pelvic insufficiency fracture after pelvic irradiation in uterine cervix cancer. Gynecol Oncol 2002;86(3):264–8.
10. Kwon JW, Huh SJ, Yoon YC, et al. Pelvic bone complications after radiation therapy of uterine cervical cancer: evaluation with MRI. AJR Am J Roentgenol 2008;191(4):987–94.
11. Meixel AJ, Hauswald H, Delorme S, et al. From radiation osteitis to osteoradionecrosis: incidence and MR morphology of radiation-induced sacral pathologies following pelvic radiotherapy. Eur Radiol 2018;28:3550–9.
12. Lyders EM, Whitlow CT, Baker MD, et al. Imaging and treatment of sacral insufficiency fractures. AJNR Am J Neuroradiol 2010;31:201–10.
13. Cabarrus MC, Ambekar A, Lu Y, et al. MRI and CT of insufficiency fractures of the pelvis and the proximal femur. AJR Am J Roentgenol 2008;191(4): 995–1001.
14. Rodrigues-Pinto R, Kurd MF, Schroeder GD, et al. Sacral fractures and associated injuries. Global Spine J 2017;7(7):609–16.
15. Mehta S, Auerbach JD, Born CT, et al. Sacral fractures. J Am Acad Orthop Surg 2006;14(12): 656–65.
16. Babayev M, Lachmann E, Nagler W. The controversy surrounding sacral insufficiency fractures: to ambulate or not to ambulate? Am J Phys Med Rehabil 2000;79(4):404–9.

17. Pommersheim W, Huang-hellinger F, Baker M, et al. Sacroplasty: a treatment for sacral insufficiency fractures. AJNR Am J Neuroradiol 2003;24(5):1003–7.

18. Lin JT, Lane JM. Sacral stress fractures. J Womens Health (Larchmt) 2003;12(9):879–88.

19. Sciubba DM, Wolinsky JP, Than KD, et al. CT fluoroscopically guided percutaneous placement of transiliosacral rod for sacral insufficiency fracture: case report and technique. AJNR Am J Neuroradiol 2007;28(8):1451–4.

20. Frey ME, Depalma MJ, Cifu DX, et al. Efficacy and safety of percutaneous sacroplasty for painful osteoporotic sacral insufficiency fractures: a prospective, multicenter trial. Spine 2007;32(15):1635–40.

21. Frey ME, Warner C, Thomas SM, et al. Sacroplasty: a ten-year analysis of prospective patients treated with percutaneous sacroplasty: literature review and technical considerations. Pain Physician 2017; 20(7):E1063–72.

22. Anselmetti GC, Marcia S, Saba L, et al. Percutaneous vertebroplasty: multi-centric results from EVEREST experience in large cohort of patients. Eur J Radiol 2012;81(12):4083–6.

23. Wang Z, Zhen Y, Wu C, et al. CT fluoroscopy-guided percutaneous osteoplasty for the treatment of osteolytic lung cancer bone metastases to the spine and pelvis. J Vasc Interv Radiol 2012;23(9):1135–42.

24. Talmadge J, Smith K, Dykes T, et al. Clinical impact of sacroplasty on patient mobility. J Vasc Interv Radiol 2014;25(6):911–5.

25. Gupta AC, Yoo AJ, Stone J, et al. Percutaneous sacroplasty. J Neurointerv Surg 2012;4(5):385–9.

26. Katsanos K, Sabharwal T, Adam A. Percutaneous cementoplasty. Semin Intervent Radiol 2010;27(2): 137–47.

27. Heron J, Connell DA, James SL. CT-guided sacroplasty for the treatment of sacral insufficiency fractures. Clin Radiol 2007;62(11):1094–100.

28. Wee B, Shimal A, Stirling AJ, et al. CT-guided sacroplasty in advanced sacral destruction secondary to tumor infiltration. Clin Radiol 2008;63(8):906–12.

29. Miller JW, Diani A, Docsa S, et al. Sacroplasty procedural extravasation with high viscosity bone cement: comparing the intraoperative long-axis versus short-axis techniques in osteoporotic cadavers. J Neurointerv Surg 2017;9(9):899–904.

30. Smith DK, Dix JE. Percutaneous sacroplasty: long-axis injection technique. AJR Am J Roentgenol 2006;186(5):1252–5.

31. Yang SC, Tsai TT, Chen HS, et al. Comparison of sacroplasty with or without balloon assistance for the treatment of sacral insufficiency fractures. J Orthop Surg (Hong Kong) 2018;26(2). 2309499018782575.

32. Richards AM, Mears SC, Knight TA, et al. Biomechanical analysis of sacroplasty: does volume or location of cement matter? AJNR Am J Neuroradiol 2009;30(2):315–7.

33. Kam NM, Maingard J, Kok HK, et al. Combined Vertebral Augmentation and Radiofrequency Ablation in the Management of Spinal Metastases: an Update. Curr Treat Options Oncol 2017;18(12):74.

34. Nader R, Rhines LD, Mendel E. Metastatic sacral tumors. Neurosurg Clin N Am 2004;15(4):453–7.

35. Agarawal JP, Swangsilpa T, Van der linden Y, et al. The role of external beam radiotherapy in the management of bone metastases. Clin Oncol 2006; 18(10):747–60.

36. Khan MA, Deib G, Deldar B, et al. Efficacy and Safety of Percutaneous Microwave Ablation and Cementoplasty in the Treatment of Painful Spinal Metastases and Myeloma. AJNR Am J Neuroradiol 2018;39(7):1376–83.

37. Lane MD, Le HB, Lee S, et al. Combination radiofrequency ablation and cementoplasty for palliative treatment of painful neoplastic bone metastasis: experience with 53 treated lesions in 36 patients. Skeletal Radiol 2011;40(1):25–32.

38. Madaelil TP, Wallace AN, Jennings JW. Radiofrequency ablation alone or in combination with cementoplasty for local control and pain palliation of sacral metastases: preliminary results in 11 patients. Skeletal Radiol 2016;45(9):1213–9.

Hot and Cold Spine Tumor Ablations

Anderanik Tomasian, MD[a], Jack W. Jennings, MD, PhD[b],*

KEYWORDS

- Minimally invasive thermal ablation • Spinal tumor • Pain palliation • Local tumor control

KEY POINTS

- The vertebral column is the most common site of osseous metastasis, and percutaneous minimally invasive thermal ablation is becoming an important contributor to multidisciplinary treatment algorithms.
- Continuously evolving minimally invasive image-guided percutaneous spine thermal ablation procedures have proven safe and effective in management of selected patients with spinal metastases to achieve pain palliation and/or local tumor control.
- Special attention to the details of procedure techniques including choice of ablation modality, thermo-protection, adequacy of treatment, and post-ablation imaging will translate into improved patient outcomes.

INTRODUCTION

Approximately 1.7 million patients are diagnosed with cancer in the United States annually, most of whom will develop metastases that in 40% of cases will involve the spine.[1,2]

The spinal column is the most common site of osseous metastasis due to the presence of vascular red marrow in adult vertebrae and communication of valveless vertebral venous plexuses with deep torso veins.[3] Approximately 90% of symptomatic patients with vertebral metastases present with pain due to pathologic fracture, biochemical stimulation of endosteal nociceptors due to tumor-produced cytokines, osteoclast-mediated osseous destruction, as well as spinal cord or nerve root compression, which occurs in 10% to 20% of patients and is most often due to tumor involvement of the posterior vertebral body or posterior elements.[4,5] Pain and neurologic deficits associated with spinal metastases often lead to impaired mobility, deficient functional independence, and overall diminished quality of life.[6] Management of metastatic spine disease requires multidisciplinary input.[7]

Radiation therapy is the current standard of care for local control and pain palliation of vertebral metastases, but when used alone has important limitations. First, particular tumors respond less favorably to radiation therapy, such as sarcoma, renal cell carcinoma, non–small-cell lung cancer, and melanoma.[8] Second, radiation therapy of vertebral metastases is limited by the cumulative tolerance of the spinal cord, which often precludes retreatment of recurrent tumor or progressive tumor at adjacent vertebrae.[9] Last, radiation therapy excludes patients from certain systemic chemotherapy clinical trials. Surgery (including stabilization, corpectomy, and gross tumor resection) is often of limited benefit in management of spinal metastases due to its morbidity and patients' often poor functional status and short expected life span, and is typically considered for patients with

Disclosure Statement: A. Tomasian: No disclosures. J.W. Jennings: Consulting Fee or Honorarium: Medtronic and Galil Medical.
a Department of Radiology, University of Southern California, 1500 San Pablo Street, Los Angeles, CA 90033, USA; b Mallinckrodt Institute of Radiology, 510 South Kingshighway Boulevard, St Louis, MO 63110, USA
* Corresponding author.
E-mail address: jackwjennings@wustl.edu

Neuroimag Clin N Am 29 (2019) 529–538
https://doi.org/10.1016/j.nic.2019.07.001
1052-5149/19/© 2019 Elsevier Inc. All rights reserved.

neurologic compromise or spinal instability. In addition, painful spinal metastases are often refractory to systemic therapies such as chemotherapy, hormonal therapy, radiopharmaceuticals, and bisphosphonates.[10] Pain palliation with systemic analgesics remains the only alternative option for many patients.[11]

Over the past few years, investigators have exploited minimally invasive percutaneous thermal ablation technologies, often combined with vertebral augmentation, for management of vertebral metastases, including radiofrequency ablation (RFA), cryoablation, and microwave ablation,[12–20] which may be performed in an outpatient setting under conscious sedation requiring minimal recovery, and do not hinder or compromise adjuvant radiation or chemotherapy. Percutaneous thermal ablation for vertebral metastases is performed to achieve pain palliation and/or local tumor control (often with vertebral augmentation for fracture stabilization or prevention) in patients who have not responded to or have contraindication to radiation therapy. In cases of osseous oligometastatic disease (fewer than 5 lesions), ablation may be performed with curative intent.

This review details the armamentarium available and the most recent advances in minimally invasive, percutaneous image-guided thermal ablation for management of vertebral metastases.

THERMAL ABLATION TECHNOLOGIES
Radiofrequency Ablation

In RFA, a generator delivers high-frequency, alternating current (375–600 kHz) to the target tissue through the exposed active tip of an electrode resulting in oscillation of charged tissue molecules within the ablation zone producing frictional heat. The thermal effect depends on the electrical-conducting properties of the target tissue and the characteristics of the electrode.[21] When local tissue temperature between 60 and 100°C is reached, protein denaturation and immediate coagulative necrosis occur.[21]

Several RFA electrode design technologies have been developed to achieve an improved ablation zone.[21] Unipolar systems use dispersing grounding pads placed on patient skin near the ablation site to serve as the receiving limb of the electrical circuit to prevent potential skin burn. Bipolar systems use built-in transmitting and receiving electrical elements within the electrode, which eliminate the need for grounding pads and the possibility of skin burn.[12,18,19] Internally cooled electrodes decrease tissue char (carbonization) by maintaining lower temperature surrounding the active electrode tip.[21]

Recently, navigational bipolar RFA electrodes with built-in thermocouples have become available that allow real-time intraprocedural monitoring of ablation zone size by measuring the temperatures along the periphery of the ablation zone based on predetermined manufacturer data.[12,18,19] The navigating tip of the electrode can be articulated in different orientations through the same entry site, which is beneficial for accessing lesions in challenging locations, particularly along the posterior vertebral body, and achieving larger ablation zones.[12,18,19]

Simultaneous bipedicular vertebral RFA is a novel technique that efficiently generates 2 confluent, coalescent, and overlapping ablation zones in close proximity that minimize the convective cooling effect (heat sink), and subsequently decrease the power required to conduct heat through tissue decreasing the risk of thermal injury and minimizing charring and impedance-related issues[19] (**Fig. 1**). This technique may result in a more thorough ablation of the vertebral body and pedicles, and support the stereotactic spine radiosurgery paradigm to treat the entire vertebral body volume and pedicles for improved local tumor control rates and more durable pain palliation.[19,22]

RFA is typically used for treatment of vertebral lesions with no or small extraosseous components. Specifically, navigational bipolar RFA electrodes are preferred for treatment of posterior vertebral body metastases that are not readily accessible with straight electrodes.[12,14,18,19] Built-in thermocouples along the navigational bipolar RFA electrodes allow real-time precise monitoring of ablation zone size and geometry beyond which tissues are safe from potential thermal injury.[12,14,18,19] Intact vertebral cortex is considered a boundary for undesired radiofrequency energy propagation.[23] RFA is mainly used for treatment of vertebral lesions that are primarily osteolytic, as the higher intrinsic impedance of osteoblastic lesions prevents the RF circuit from generating sufficiently high temperatures to ensure cell death and renders RFA ineffective.[24]

Limitations of RFA include nonvisualization of ablation zone boundary with computed tomography (CT), procedure-related pain, and, frequently, increased pain during the immediate postablation period.

In a retrospective multicenter study, investigators treated 128 vertebral metastases in 96 patients (vertebral augmentation in 92 patients) using bipolar navigational RFA electrodes implementing thermo-protective techniques and achieved pain palliation (improved visual analog scores and decreased opioid usage in most patients) in

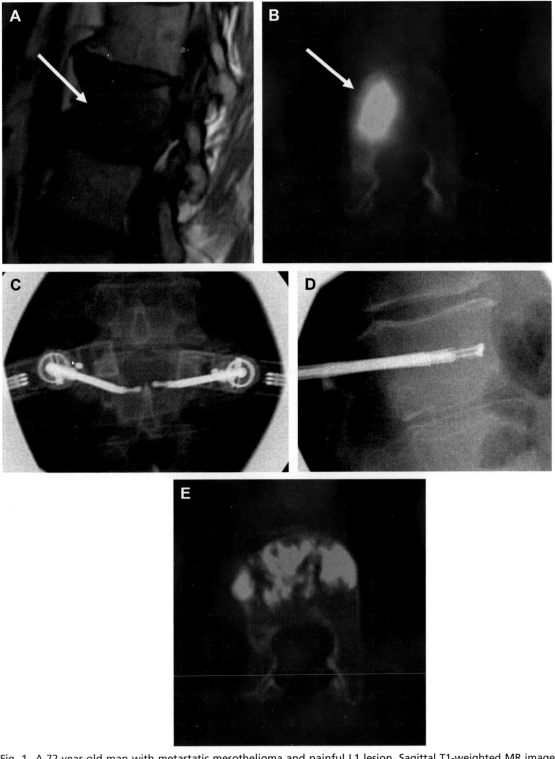

Fig. 1. A 72-year-old man with metastatic mesothelioma and painful L1 lesion. Sagittal T1-weighted MR image (*A*) and axial fludeoxyglucose (FDG)-PET/CT image (*B*) show a hypermetabolic bone marrow replacing lesion in the right aspect of L1 vertebral body with disruption of the inferior endplate and associated pathologic compression fracture (*A* and *B*, *arrow*).Simultaneous bipedicular RFA was performed to achieve local tumor control and pain palliation in alignment with the recent consensus recommendations by the international spine radiosurgery consortium to include the CTV. Prone anterior-posterior (*C*) and lateral (*D*) fluoroscopic images during

1-week, 1-month, and 6-month intervals following procedures with no major complication.[14]

In a retrospective study, combination of RFA (bipolar navigational electrodes) and vertebral augmentation was used to treat 55 patients with vertebral metastases. Local tumor control was achieved in 89%, 74%, and 70% of cases at 3-month, 6-month, and 1-year postprocedure time points (median follow-up of 34 weeks) with no major complications and no clinical evidence of metastatic spinal cord compression at treated levels.[12] In a multicenter prospective study, Bagla and colleagues[17] treated 50 patients with spinal metastases using RFA (69 ablations) and vertebral augmentation (96% of patients) and achieved significant reduction in pain and disability along with improvement in functional status and quality of life with no complications.

There has been a recent paradigm shift in stereotactic spine radiosurgery for management of vertebral metastases with specific consensus recommendations by the international spine radiosurgery consortium for definition of clinical target volume (CTV) versus gross tumor volume (GTV) to account for microscopic tumor spread and marginal radiation therapy failures.[22] The consensus recommendation defines CTV (to be treated by stereotactic spine radiosurgery) to include GTV plus surrounding abnormal bone marrow signal intensity on MR imaging to account for microscopic tumor invasion and adjacent normal osseous expansion to account for subclinical tumor spread in marrow space.[22] In support of this paradigm shift, Tomasian and colleagues[19] treated 33 tumors (27 patients) using simultaneous bipedicular RFA combined with vertebral augmentation and achieved local tumor control in 96% of cases with no complications and no clinical evidence of metastatic spinal cord compression at the treated levels (mean follow-up, 24.2 weeks).

Cryoablation

In closed percutaneous cryoablation systems, liquid argon is typically used to rapidly drop the temperature at the cryoprobe tip using the Joule-Thomson effect (pressurized gas, when allowed to expand, results in temperature drop). The rapid cooling is exchanged with adjacent tissues forming an enlarging ice ball with time followed by a "thawing" phase, resulting in osmotic gradient across the cell membrane.[21,25] Formation of extracellular ice results in relative imbalance of intracellular and extracellular electrolytes, and subsequently extracellular water shift by osmosis and cellular dehydration. The increase in intracellular electrolyte concentration results in damage to both the cellular enzymes and membrane.[21,25] Formation of intracellular ice crystals damages the cellular organelles. Both freezing and thawing lead to osmotic gradient and consequent cell membrane injury.[21,25] A temperature of -40°C or lower is necessary to ensure complete cell death.[26]

Currently, the cryoprobes of 2 major manufacturers are used in the pine with diameters ranging from 1.2 mm to 2.4 mm, generating predictable ablation zones, according to predetermined manufacturer data, using at least 1 freeze/active thaw/freeze cycle (typically 10 minutes/5 minutes/10 minutes).[13,16,27] Cryoablation is typically used for spinal metastases with large soft tissue components, or large lesions involving the posterior vertebral elements, and is preferred to RFA for management of osteoblastic lesions (**Fig. 2**).

Advantages of cryoablation include formation of a hypoattenuating ice ball in the soft tissues that is readily identified by CT, decreased intraprocedural and postprocedural pain compared with RFA or microwave ablation, and ability to use multiple cryoprobes in various orientations to achieve additive overlapping ablation zones. The intraosseous ice ball may not be visible on CT, particularly with osteoblastic lesions. An inter-cryoprobe distance of 1.0 to 1.5 cm is typically recommended with cryoprobe tips at bone-tumor or soft tissue-tumor interfaces.[13] The ice ball peripheral margin corresponds to 0°C, which is typically not sufficient for permanent tumor destruction. Reliable cell death is achieved at 3-mm margin from the peripheral edge, and therefore the ice ball should extend beyond tumor margins.[28] MR imaging–compatible cryoprobes offer an alternative approach, which may permit safe ablation of spinal lesions given the proximity of neural elements.[29] Advantages of MR imaging guidance include high tissue contrast resolution, lack of ionizing radiation, improved visualization of intraosseous ice ball, particularly in treatment of osteoblastic lesions, and possibility of real-time temperature mapping.

In a single-center retrospective study, Tomasian and colleagues[13] treated 31 vertebral metastases

simultaneous bipedicular RFA show transpedicular placement of bipolar navigational electrodes with medial articulation of the tips to achieve confluent coalescent ablation zones. Axial FDG-PET/CT performed 10 weeks after treatment (*E*) shows local tumor with no evidence of residual or recurrent tumor. Note cement augmentation performed immediately following RFA.

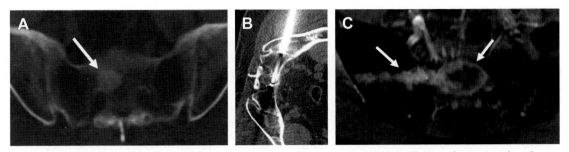

Fig. 2. A 51-year-old man prostate adenocarcinoma previously managed by radiation therapy and androgen deprivation therapy with Leuprolide (Lupron) for 2 years with new sacral metastatic lesion in radiation field. Cryoablation was performed for local tumor control. Axial CT image (*A*) shows an osteoblastic metastatic sacral lesion adjacent to the right S2 neuroforamen (*A, arrow*). Axial CT image with the patient in lateral decubitus position during cryoablation (*B*) shows positioning of a single cryoprobe within the target lesion with the tip at bone-tumor interface. Note that the ice ball is not clearly seen due to the osteoblastic nature of the lesion, which is a limitation of CT as compared with MR imaging for delineation of the cryoablation zone margins. Axial T1-weighted fat-saturated contrast-enhanced MR image (*C*) performed 8 weeks after cryoablation shows local tumor control with no evidence of residual or recurrent tumor. Note clear demarcation of the ablation zone and enhancing granulation tissue/vascular fibrosis along the ablation zone margin and needle tract (*C, arrows*).

in 14 patients with cryoablation implementing thermo-protective techniques and achieved 96.7% local tumor control and statistically significant pain palliation and decreased analgesics usage at 1-week, 1-month, and 3-month postprocedural time points with no major complications. Wallace and colleagues[27] treated 56 patients with musculoskeletal metastases using cryoablation, which included 16 patients with vertebral lesions. The investigators achieved statistically significant pain palliation at 1-day, 1-week, 1-month, and 3-month postprocedural time points as well as local tumor control at 3 months (90%), 6 months (86%), and 12 months (79%) after treatment with no major complications. However, the specific data regarding the vertebral lesions were not reported separately.

Microwave Ablation

Microwave ablation uses antennae to deliver electromagnetic microwaves (approximately 900 and 2450 MHz) to target tissue that results in agitation of ionic molecules, frictional heat, and tissue coagulative necrosis. It is postulated that microwave ablation is less influenced by variable tissue impedance and perfusion-mediated tissue cooling, potentially resulting in higher intratumoral temperatures, larger and more uniform ablation zones, and more efficient ablation using a single antenna, offering efficacy in management of osteoblastic lesions and obviating the need for grounding pads and thus diminished risk of skin burn.[15,20] Antenna shaft cooling systems implemented in the latest generations of microwave ablation equipment eliminate the risk of back-heating phenomena.

Rapid delivery of high amounts of power (up to 100 Watts) to large ablation zones might be a disadvantage when applied to spinal lesions, as surrounding overheating could potentially lead to neural injuries Although hypoattenuating ablated tissue is often identified on CT, margins of ablation zone are not well defined, which is a disadvantage of spinal microwave ablation.

In a retrospective single-center study, Khan and colleagues[20] successfully treated 102 vertebral lesions in 69 patients (multiple myeloma in 10 patients and metastases in 59 patients) and achieved statistically significant pain palliation at 2-week to 4-week and 20-week to 24-week postprocedural time points as well as local tumor control on post-treatment imaging at the 20-week to 24-week interval. The procedures were performed under general anesthesia with no thermal protection techniques, and the investigators reported complications in 2 patients (S1 nerve thermal injury and skin burn).

In a retrospective study, Kastler and colleagues[15] successfully treated 20 spinal metastases (17 patients) with microwave ablation (adjunct cementation in 9 cases) implementing thermoprotection in 4 cases. The investigators reported pain relief in 16 of 17 patients with significant pain reduction at 1-day, 1-week, 1-month, 3-month, and 6-month postablation time points with no major complications.

Patient Selection Algorithms

Treatment plans for patients with vertebral metastases should be determined by a multidisciplinary team of radiation and medical oncologists, interventional radiologists, and spinal oncologic surgeons. The metastatic spine disease multidisciplinary working group[7] declared in their algorithms that percutaneous spinal thermal ablation has no role in treatment of the following patient subsets: (1) asymptomatic spinal metastases in patients with poor performance status, life expectancy less than 6 months, or many visceral metastases; (2) unstable pathologic vertebral compression fracture; (3) metastatic epidural spinal cord compression (MESCC); and (4) stable pathologic vertebral compression fracture in patients with poor performance status, life expectancy less than 6 months, or many visceral metastases. Performance status is typically assessed by widely used and validated Karnofsky performance status.[7]

Vertebral metastases are ablated for pain palliation and/or local tumor control when there is persistent pain or imaging tumor progression despite maximum radiation therapy, radiation therapy is contraindicated, or there is inadequate response to systemic therapies and analgesics. Combination of radiation therapy and thermal ablation also is considered for radiation-insensitive tumors.[7] Vertebral augmentation is often performed following ablation for added pain relief or pathologic fracture prevention/stabilization.[12,14,19,30]

Spinal instability is a relative contraindication for percutaneous thermal ablation depending on severity. Spinal instability is determined using the spinal instability neoplastic score.[31] Scores range from 0 to 18, and higher scores indicate greater instability. Although there is no score cutoff to prompt surgery, surgical evaluation for potential tumor resection and/or stabilization is recommended for scores of 7 or higher.[32] At our institutions, we treat patients with spinal instability who are not surgical candidates with vertebral augmentation, which does not entirely restore stability but relieves pain related to motion at the fracture site. Surgery is the treatment of choice for spinal metastases complicated by central canal stenosis[33]; however, in the absence of spinal cord compression, thermal ablation may be considered as an alternative for patients who are not surgical candidates. CT and MR imaging are used to determine if central canal stenosis is due to tumor alone or in combination with retropulsion of fracture fragments, as ablation may arrest or cause retraction of epidural tumor but will not alleviate symptoms related to osseous central canal stenosis. Such patients are alternatively managed by epidural corticosteroid and long-acting anesthetic injections.[34]

Percutaneous spine thermal ablation is considered a valid option for the following patient subgroups: (1) asymptomatic spinal metastases in patients with life expectancy more than 6 months, good performance status, and few visceral metastases; (2) uncomplicated (lack of pathologic vertebral compression fracture and MESCC) painful spinal metastases; (3) stable pathologic vertebral compression fracture in patients with life expectancy more than 6 months, good performance status, and few visceral metastases.[7]

Thermal Ablation Planning: General Considerations, Preablation Imaging, and Procedure Guidelines

When multidisciplinary consensus is reached for a patient to undergo percutaneous minimally invasive therapy, pretreatment consultation with the patient is recommended and should include explanation of benefits, risks, potential complications, and alternative treatment options. Pretreatment consultation should include history and focused physical examination to reconfirm focal pain/tenderness at the tumor site and neurologic examination to assess for potential focal neurologic deficit. Laboratory tests are used to evaluate the coagulation status (platelet count more than 50,000/μL and international normalized ratio <1.5 are generally acceptable) and at times, possibility of systemic infection (complete blood count, erythrocyte sedimentation rate, C-reactive protein, and cultures, if clinically indicated). Thermal ablation of bone and soft tissue tumors is painful and requires moderate sedation or general anesthesia, particularly with technically challenging spinal ablations, to minimize patient movement and potential subsequent complications. General anesthesia is considered when motor/somatosensory-evoked potential monitoring is used to minimize potential neural thermal injury.

Percutaneous thermal ablation and vertebral augmentation may be performed with fluoroscopic or CT guidance. Cone-beam volume CT images may be acquired with some biplane flat-panel detector fluoroscopy units, using the strengths of both modalities.

RFA and vertebral augmentation are most commonly performed under fluoroscopic guidance, which is readily available, provides near real-time guidance, and affords efficient needle placement and immediate recognition of cement leakage. The main disadvantage of fluoroscopy is the often lack of visualization of the target lesion. Therefore, fluoroscopic images must be correlated with preprocedural cross-sectional imaging to confirm that the target lesion is ablated. Furthermore, preprocedural and intraprocedural vertebral segment counting is critical to account for potential anatomic variations, such as supernumerary ribs and transitional lumbosacral anatomy. The main advantage of CT guidance is detailed cross-sectional visualization of relevant anatomy, which affords accurate needle placement in the target lesion, and within epidural space or neuroforamina for thermal protection. When ablating tumor along the posterior vertebral body with bipolar navigational RFA electrodes, it is often easier to confirm with CT that the electrode is no closer than 10 mm from the posterior vertebral body cortex, the maximum short-axis radius of RFA volume.[14,18]

Cryoablation is typically performed under CT guidance, as the ablation zone is visualized as a hypoattenuating ice ball in soft tissues, confirming that paravertebral tumor is included in the cryoablated volume.[13] Although microwave ablation zone is largely CT occult, this procedure is generally performed under CT guidance because only straight microwave antennae are available, and accurate placement within the target lesion requires cross-sectional confirmation.[15,20] Conventional or cone-beam volume CT provides immediate cross-sectional localization of epidural or neuroforaminal cement leakage during vertebral augmentation.

Tumor location, size, and composition (osteolytic, osteoblastic, or mixed) are used to determine the choice of ablation modality. Anterior and posterolateral vertebral body lesions can be accessed using a transpedicular approach with traditional straight RF electrodes, cryoprobes, and microwave antennae, whereas central posterior vertebral body tumors may be accessed only from a transpedicular approach with navigational RF electrodes.[14,18,19] Osteoblastic lesions are better treated with cryoablation and microwave ablation, as RFA is rendered ineffective due to high impedance of sclerotic bone.[24] Cryoablation is also preferred for treatment of spinal tumors with an extraosseous soft tissue component as the cryoablated volume is identified on CT.

Preprocedure imaging includes dedicated weight-bearing spine radiographs, CT, and MR imaging. Radiographs are used to determine the presence and extent of vertebral compression fractures, spinal alignment, integrity of osseous central canal, and suitability of fluoroscopy as imaging guidance. CT accurately localizes the target tumor and provides information regarding the anatomy of the pedicles to ensure that the outer diameter of the introducing cannula can be accommodated. Otherwise, a partial lateral parapedicular approach may be considered, which is often necessary when accessing thoracic vertebrae, the pedicles of which are typically tall and narrow.[35] The main disadvantage of a parapedicular approach is the potential injury to the radicular arteries or the artery of Adamkiewicz, which may arise from either side of any vertebral level

between T8 and L3.[36] Cortical discontinuities caused by tumor or pathologic fracture clefts are readily identified with CT and may be a source of cement leakage during postablation augmentation. MR imaging is most accurate to determine tumor extent and provides guidance for procedure planning.

In general, we strive to ablate the entire volume of hyperintensity on fluid-sensitive sequences and enhancement on MR imaging, as well as an additional 3-mm margin to account for microscopic tumor spread.[37] In many cases, MR imaging affords detection of additional CT occult metastases in adjacent vertebrae potentially contributing to patients' pain. This is particularly important in the spine where the source of pain may be difficult to localize. In cases of RFA, we routinely perform simultaneous bipedicular ablations to include the entire CTV in alignment with the consensus recommendations by the international spine radiosurgery consortium resulting in more thorough ablation of the vertebral body and pedicles, for improved local tumor control rates and more durable pain palliation.[19,22]

The size and configuration of ablation zone for each specific applicator for a selected ablation modality is available based on validated manufacturer's data and is used to determine the number of applicators and ablation cycles required to achieve optimal treatment.[12-15,18-20]

Thermal Protection and Thermal Monitoring

Percutaneous thermal vertebral tumor ablation poses inherent risk of injury to the spinal cord and nerve roots due to proximity of ablation zone. Several parameters influence the extent and severity of neurologic thermal injury, including absolute temperature, duration of thermal effect, distance from margins of ablation zone, presence or absence of intact vertebral cortex, and type of nerve fiber.[29]

Current practice to minimize potential thermal injury during spine thermal ablation includes the use of thermal insulation, as well as temperature and neurophysiologic monitoring.[12,13,38,39] Thermal insulation may be achieved by hydrodissection and instillation of warm or cool liquid, which result in displacement of the structure at risk and modification of the temperature surrounding the structure at risk, respectively. Hydrodissection during RFA should be performed using nonionic solutions, such as 5% dextrose-in-water. Saline solutions should be avoided during RFA, as the electric conductivity may result in expansion of the ablation zone and creation of a plasma field.[12,29] Carbon dioxide injection of the epidural space and/or neuroforamina may be used to dissect and actively insulate the neural structures.[13,29] In addition to insulation, continuous real-time and precise temperature monitoring (passive thermal protection) may be undertaken by placing thermocouples close to the threatened structures, typically within the neuroforamina or epidural space.[38,39] In clinical practice, active thermoprotection is initiated once the temperature reaches 45°C (heat) and 10°C (cold).[38,39]

Neurophysiologic monitoring and nerve electrostimulation during spine thermal ablation have been performed using estimations of motor-evoked and somatosensory-evoked potential amplitudes.[13,38–40] Substantial reduction in amplitude and/or latency of evoked potential amplitudes afford early detection of impending neurologic injury, which should prompt active thermoprotection or modification during ablation.

Skin injury also is a potential complication of percutaneous thermal ablation. Accurate assessment of ablation zone boundaries minimizes the risk of skin injury. Active skin thermoprotection, such as surface application of warm saline in a glove or soaked gauze during cryoablation should be implemented to minimize skin injury. Furthermore, attention should be paid to prevent retraction of the outer cannula in cryoablation and unipolar RFA systems. Using a bipolar RFA system inherently obviates the risk of skin burn, and utilization of wider and more grounding pads with unipolar RFA systems decreases the risk of skin injury.

Posttreatment Imaging

Contrast-enhanced MR imaging is the modality of choice for posttreatment imaging of vertebral metastases. In our practice, we perform a baseline study 6 to 8 weeks after treatment to allow inflammation to subside, unless requested earlier by another physician. Subsequent imaging is performed when patients report new or increasing pain. Ablation typically generates a cavity of coagulation necrosis surrounded by an inner rim of hemorrhagic congestion and outer rim of granulation tissue.[41,42] Over time, the rim of granulation tissue evolves into vascular fibrosis.[43,44] On MR imaging, the ablated volume is identified by the lack of enhancement. The signal intensity of the ablated volume varies depending on relative combination of sclerotic bone, residual vascular and yellow marrow, and hemorrhagic products. The inner rim of hemorrhagic congestion contains hemosiderin and is T1 and T2 hypointense.[41] The outer rim of granulation tissue or vascular fibrosis is T1 hypointense and T2 hyperintense enhancing

tissue.[41,43,44] The marrow outside the ablated volume typically demonstrates no enhancement, as ablation frequently results in thrombosis of the vertebral vascular pedicle, particularly during ablation of posterior vertebral body lesions. Following vertebral augmentation, the cement produces hypointensity on all pulse sequences.

Widely used methods for evaluating treatment response, such as the Response Evaluation Criteria in Solid Tumors[45] and World Health Organization Handbook for Reporting Results of Cancer Treatment,[46] are not applicable to ablations because these methods are based on maximum dimensional measurements without considering tumor necrosis. Therefore, adequacy of treatment is determined by comparing the volume of the nonenhancing ablation cavity with tumor volume on pretreatment imaging. Residual or recurrent tumor is typically hyperintense tissue on fluid-sensitive MR sequences with nodular enhancement along the margin of the ablation cavity, most commonly in the posterior vertebral body and pedicles, where aggressive ablation may be precluded by the risk of potential nerve injury. Granulation tissue or vascular fibrosis may demonstrate identical MR imaging characteristics, and vascular fibrosis may evolve for years following ablation, mimicking tumor progression.[43,44] In such cases, PET/CT or PET/MR imaging may provide information on differentiating hypermetabolic tumor from fibrosis, which is not typically metabolically hyperactive. Ultimately, when clinical evaluations and imaging findings of tumor progression are discordant, tissue sampling should be performed before initiation of further radiation therapy, surgery, or change in systemic chemotherapy.

Complications

Thermal injury to the spinal cord and nerve roots is the most important potential complication of percutaneous spine thermal ablation, which may result in myelopathic and radicular symptoms, respectively. The vast majority of neural thermal injuries are transient and may be managed by transforaminal or epidural injection of steroids and long-acting anesthetics. Aseptic meningitis syndrome remains a potential complication as well. Following thermal ablation, there is potential bone weakening, and particularly in ablation of anterior vertebral body or pedicle lesions or tumors with large size, there is a potential risk of ablation-related fracture that may be minimized with cement augmentation. Cement leakage into the central canal/epidural space or neuroforamina may worsen pain related to central canal or neuroforaminal stenosis, or even result in spinal cord compression. Thermal spinal cord injury also may be caused by exothermic polymerization of extruded cement. In addition, cement pulmonary embolism caused by leakage into the caval or azygous venous systems should be recognized. There also remains a risk of thermal skin injury.

SUMMARY

Minimally invasive percutaneous spine thermal ablation has proved safe and effective in management of selected patients with vertebral metastases. These procedures have become a part of the treatment algorithm for a certain subgroup of patients with spinal metastases to achieve pain palliation and/or local tumor control. Special attention to the details of procedure techniques, including choice of ablation modality, thermoprotection, adequacy of treatment, and postablation imaging, will translate into improved patient outcomes.

REFERENCES

1. American Cancer Society. Cancer facts and figures 2018. Available at: https://www.cancer.org/content/dam/cancer-org/research/cancer-facts-and-statistics/annual-cancer-facts-and-figures/2018/cancer-facts-and-figures-2018.pdf. Accessed January 25, 2019.
2. Witham TF, Khavkin YA, Gallia GL, et al. Surgery insight: current management of epidural spinal cord compression from metastatic spine disease. Nat Clin Pract Neurol 2006;2:87–94.
3. Coleman RE. Clinical features of metastatic bone disease and risk of skeletal morbidity. Clin Cancer Res 2006;12:6243s–9s.
4. Bayley A, Milosevic M, Blend R, et al. A prospective study of factors predicting clinically occult spinal cord compression in patients with metastatic prostate carcinoma. Cancer 2001;92:303–10.
5. Klimo P Jr, Schmidt MH. Surgical management of spinal metastases. Oncologist 2004;9:188–96.
6. Kim JM, Losina E, Bono CM, et al. Clinical outcome of metastatic spinal cord compression treated with surgical excision ± radiation versus radiation therapy alone: a systematic review of literature. Spine 2012;37:78–84.
7. Wallace AN, Robinson CG, Meyer J, et al. The metastatic spine disease multidisciplinary working group algorithms. Oncologist 2015;20:1205–15.
8. Gerszten PC, Mendel E, Yamada Y. Radiotherapy and radiosurgery for metastatic spine disease: what are the options, indications, and outcomes? Spine 2009;34:S78–92.
9. Masucci GL, Yu E, Ma L, et al. Stereotactic body radiotherapy is an effective treatment in reirradiating spinal metastases: current status and practical considerations for safe practice. Expert Rev Anticancer Ther 2011;11:1923–33.
10. Rosenthal D, Callstrom MR. Critical review and state of the art in interventional oncology: benign and metastatic disease involving bone. Radiology 2012;262:765–80.
11. Hara S. Opioids for metastatic bone pain. Oncology 2008;74(suppl 1):52–4.
12. Wallace AN, Tomasian A, Vaswani D, et al. Radiographic local control of spinal metastases with percutaneous radiofrequency ablation and vertebral augmentation. AJNR Am J Neuroradiol 2016;37:759–65.
13. Tomasian A, Wallace A, Northrup B, et al. Spine cryoablation: pain palliation and local tumor control for vertebral metastases. AJNR Am J Neuroradiol 2016;37:189–95.
14. Anchala PR, Irving WD, Hillen TJ, et al. Treatment of metastatic spinal lesions with a navigational bipolar radiofrequency ablation device: a multicenter retrospective study. Pain Physician 2014;17:317–27.
15. Kastler A, Alnassan H, Aubry S, et al. Microwave thermal ablation of spinal metastatic bone tumors. J Vasc Interv Radiol 2014;25(9):1470–5.
16. Callstrom MR, Dupuy DE, Solomon SB, et al. Percutaneous image-guided cryoablation of painful metastases involving bone: multicenter trial. Cancer 2013;119:1033–41.
17. Bagla S, Sayed D, Smirniotopoulos J, et al. Multicenter prospective clinical series evaluating radiofrequency ablation in the treatment of painful spine metastases. Cardiovasc Intervent Radiol 2016;39:1289–97.
18. Hillen TJ, Anchala P, Friedman MV, et al. Treatment of metastatic posterior vertebral body osseous tumors by using a targeted bipolar radiofrequency ablation device: technical note. Radiology 2014;273:261–7.
19. Tomasian A, Hillen TJ, Chang RO, et al. Simultaneous bipedicular radiofrequency ablation combined with vertebral augmentation for local tumor control of spinal metastases. AJNR Am J Neuroradiol 2018;39(9):1768–73.
20. Khan MA, Deib G, Deldar B, et al. Efficacy and safety of percutaneous microwave ablation and cementoplasty in the treatment of painful spinal metastases and myeloma. AJNR Am J Neuroradiol 2018;39(7):1376–83.
21. Rybak L. Fire and ice: thermal ablation of musculoskeletal tumors. Radiol Clin North Am 2009;47:455–69.
22. Cox BW, Spratt DE, Lovelock M, et al. International Spine Radiosurgery Consortium consensus guidelines for target volume definition in spinal stereotactic radiosurgery. Int J Radiat Oncol Biol Phys 2012;83(5):e597–605.

23. Dupuy DE, Hong R, Oliver B, et al. Radiofrequency ablation of spinal tumors: temperature distribution in the central canal. Am J Roentgenol 2000;175(5): 1263–6.

24. Singh S, Saha S. Electrical properties of bone. A review. Clin Orthop Relat Res 1984;(186):249–71.

25. Gage AA, Baust JG. Cryosurgery for tumors. J Am Coll Surg 2007;205:342–56.

26. Weld KJ, Landman J. Comparison of cryoablation, radiofrequency ablation and high-intensity focused ultrasound for treating small renal cell tumors. BJU Int 2005;96(9):1224–9.

27. Wallace AN, McWilliams SR, Connolly SE, et al. Percutaneous image-guided cryoablation of musculoskeletal metastases: pain palliation and local tumor control. J Vasc Interv Radiol 2016;27(12): 1788–96.

28. Campbell SC, Krishnamurthi V, Chow G, et al. Renal cryosurgery: experimental evaluation of treatment parameters. Urology 1998;52(1):29–33.

29. Tsoumakidou G, Koch G, Caudrelier J, et al. Image-guided spinal ablation: a review. Cardiovasc Intervent Radiol 2016;39(9):1229–38.

30. Berenson J, Pflugmacher R, Jarzem P, et al. Balloon kyphoplasty versus non-surgical fracture management for treatment of painful vertebral body compression fractures in patients with cancer: a multicentre, randomised controlled trial. Lancet Oncol 2011;12:225–35.

31. Fisher CG, DiPaola CP, Ryken TC, et al. A novel classification system for spinal instability in neoplastic disease: an evidence-based approach and expert consensus from the Spine Oncology Study Group. Spine 2010;35:E1221–9.

32. Fourney DR, Frangou EM, Ryken TC, et al. Spinal instability neoplastic score: an analysis of reliability and validity from the Spine Oncology Study Group. J Clin Oncol 2011;29:3072–7.

33. Patchell RA, Tibbs PA, Regine WF, et al. Direct decompressive surgical resection in the treatment of spinal cord compression caused by metastatic cancer: a randomised trial. Lancet 2005;366:643–8.

34. Wallace AN, Greenwood TJ, Jennings JW. Use of imaging in the management of metastatic spine disease with percutaneous ablation and vertebral augmentation. Am J Roentgenol 2015;205(2): 434–41.

35. Mathis JM, Golovac S. Image-guided spine interventions. 2nd edition. New York: Springer; 2010. p. 2–5.

36. Charles YP, Barbe B, Beaujeux R, et al. Relevance of the anatomical location of the Adamkiewicz artery in spine surgery. Surg Radiol Anat 2011;33:3–9.

37. Lee YK, Bedford JL, McNair HA, et al. Comparison of deliverable IMRT and VMAT for spine metastases using a simultaneous integrated boost. Br J Radiol 2013;86:20120466.

38. Buy X, Tok CH, Szware D, et al. Thermal protection during percutaneous thermal ablation procedures: interest of carbon dioxide dissection and temperature monitoring. Cardiovasc Intervent Radiol 2009; 32:529–34.

39. Tsoumakidou G, Garnon J, Ramamurthy N, et al. Interest of electrostimulation of peripheral motor nerves during percutaneous thermal ablation. Cardiovasc Intervent Radiol 2013;36(6):1624–8.

40. Kurup AN, Morris JM, Boon AJ, et al. Motor evoked potential monitoring during cryoablation of musculoskeletal tumors. J Vasc Interv Radiol 2014;25: 1657–64.

41. Lee JM, Choi SH, Park HS, et al. Radiofrequency thermal ablation in canine femur: evaluation of coagulation necrosis reproducibility and MRI-histopathologic correlation. Am J Roentgenol 2005; 185:661–7.

42. Yoshimoto Y, Azuma K, Miya A, et al. A fundamental study of cryoablation on normal bone: diagnostic imaging and histopathology. Cryobiology 2014;69: 229–35.

43. Gervais DA, Arellano RS. Percutaneous tumor ablation for hepatocellular carcinoma. Am J Roentgenol 2011;197:789–94.

44. Sainani NI, Gervais DA, Mueller PR, et al. Imaging after percutaneous radiofrequency ablation of hepatic tumors. Part 1. Normal findings. Am J Roentgenol 2013;200:184–93.

45. Eisenhauer EA, Therasse P, Bogaerts J, et al. New response evaluation criteria in solid tumours: revised RECIST guideline (version 1.1). Eur J Cancer 2009; 45:228–47.

46. World Health Organization. WHO handbook for reporting results of cancer treatment. WHO offset publication no.48. Geneva (Switzerland): World Health Organization; 1979.

Conventional Image-Guided Procedures for Painful Spine

Miriam E. Peckham, MD, Troy A. Hutchins, MD, Lubdha M. Shah, MD*

KEYWORDS

• Epidural steroid injection • Facet joint injection • Sacroiliac joint injection • Synovial cyst rupture

KEY POINTS

- Image guidance is important for the accurate placement of medication at the affected spinal level and to avoid inadvertent intrathecal and intravascular injections.
- Scrutiny of the contrast spread pattern is imperative for site confirmation and avoiding intravascular injection.
- Different approaches can help avoid complications, such as nonparticulate steroids for transforaminal injections and the infraneural approach to avoid a radiculomedullary artery.
- Because facet and sacroiliac joint pain can be difficult to diagnose on imaging, as well as on clinical examination, diagnostic blocks can be helpful in pain generator localization.

INTRODUCTION

Painful degenerative conditions of the spine have multiple treatment options, ranging from medical management to surgical decompression.[1] Therapeutic steroid injections became a widely used treatment of spinal pain in the 1970s, with image guidance for these procedures introduced in the following decade.[2] In the following years, spinal injections have gained widespread popularity as a minimally invasive method for both diagnosis and treatment of spine pain generators,[2] with Medicare payments for these procedures increasing approximately 630% from 1994 to 2001.[3] Different imaging techniques, such as MR imaging and single-photon emission computed tomography (SPECT), allowed improved target specificity for pain generator diagnosis.[4,5] Also, for the interventionalist, image guidance provides more certainty of needle location. Having a detailed understanding of pathoanatomic correlations of spinal anatomy to the patient's symptoms, knowledge of different modalities for image-guidance, and awareness of the risks of spine interventions are imperative for not only targeting a site and delivering medication[6] but also for effectively treating the patient's low back pain (LBP).

MEDICATIONS

Anesthetics

Local anesthetics are often administered in conjunction with corticosteroids, both as a diagnostic tool and as therapeutic to provide the patient with immediate relief of symptoms. Local anesthetics inhibit nerve excitation and conduction, acting through inhibition of sodium-specific ion channels on neuronal cell membranes. There are 2 groups of local anesthetics: esters (eg, cocaine and procaine) and amides (eg, lidocaine, bupivacaine, ropivacaine). The ester preparations are associated with a risk of severe allergic reactions, whereas true allergic reactions are much less common with amide preparations. Increasing the dose of administered local anesthetic increases the degree of anesthesia and duration of

The authors have no commercial or financial conflicts of interest to disclose. The authors have no funding sources to disclose.
Department of Radiology, University of Utah, 30 North 1900 East, Room #1A71, Salt Lake City, UT 84132, USA
* Corresponding author.
E-mail address: Lubdha.Shah@hsc.utah.edu

action but does not change the time of onset of anesthesia.

There are excellent reviews providing an overview on the potencies of local anesthetics and corticosteroids used in spine interventions.[7] Lidocaine is typically administered to induce cutaneous analgesia at the time of a procedure. It has a quicker onset and a shorter duration of action than does bupivacaine. Bupivacaine is the most commonly administered local anesthetic in spine procedures because of its greater potency and longer duration of action compared with lidocaine. Typical doses of bupivacaine range from 0.5 to 2.0 mL in concentrations of 0.25% or 0.50%. Recommendations for maximum doses, although not evidence-based, are meant to prevent toxicity. The maximum safe dose of lidocaine is 300 mg and that for bupivacaine is approximately 150 mg (2 mg/kg).

Particulate Versus Nonparticulate

The steroids preparations may be particulate or nonparticulate, based on the solubility of the synthetic corticosteroids within water and on their aggregation characteristics. Particulate corticosteroids, such as triamcinolone acetonide, methylprednisolone acetate, and prednisolone acetate, are esters and can precipitate out of solution and crystallize within a hydrophilic environment. Most of the particles range in size between 0.5 and 100 μm.[8] Aggregation of the steroid into larger particles depends on the chemical ingredient (esters have larger particulate size), on the varying concentrations, on the drug vehicle, or on the drug mixtures with local anesthetics and/or contrast media prepared in situ for pain treatment.[7] These aggregates, particularly the larger particle sizes, have the potential to embolize with risk for occlusion of small vessels and subsequent neural ischemic injury.[9] Of the different steroids used for spine pain injections, particularly epidural steroid injections, dexamethasone sodium phosphate is considered safer because it is a nonparticulate steroid with a typical particle size of 0.5 μm,[7,9,10] approximately 10 times smaller than red blood cells. Furthermore, the particles do not aggregate, even in mixtures.[9,10] Given this pharmacokinetic profile, the multispecialty US Food and Drug Administration Safe Use Initiative expert working group has recommended dexamethasone as the first-line agent for lumbar transforaminal injections rather than particulate steroids,[11] which have been implicated in all cases of severe neurologic complications.

Particulate steroids have a delayed but sustained antiinflammatory effect, whereas nonparticulate steroids immediately dissolve.[12] Although it may be speculated that patients obtain longer lasting relief of symptoms after epidural injection of particulate steroids compared with nonparticulate steroids, the studies have shown mixed results.

Future: Platelet-Rich Plasma and Stem Cells

Platelet-rich plasma (PRP) is a novel therapeutic tool of autologous nature that has gained considerable attention as a treatment method for musculoskeletal conditions owing to its apparent safety and ability to potentially enhance soft tissue healing.[13,14] A centrifugation process separates the liquid and solid components of blood, and the resulting PRP has platelet concentrations above the physiologic baseline.

There are an increasing number of clinical studies that demonstrate overall good results when PRP injections are used for discogenic LBP.[14–19] A study of 10 subjects with LBP related to disc herniation treated with 5 mL autologous PRP via interlaminar lumbar epidural injection into area of affected nerve root showed improvements in their scores on these evaluation tools: visual analog scale, straight leg raising test, and Modified Oswestry Disability Questionnaire. Improvement was sustained during the 3-month study period and was not associated with any complications.[16] A major and notable advantage of PRP therapy is the safety; because autologous PRP is obtained from the patient's own blood, PRP therapy carries low risks of disease infection and allergic reaction.[20] In addition, it has been reported that PRP has antimicrobial properties.[21] For certain targets, such as the degenerated disc, the age of the target population needs to be considered as the number of functional cells in the intervertebral discs of older patients may hinder the efficacy of PRP injections. Future directions in PRP therapy include conducting more randomized, controlled, and unbiased clinical trials to provide higher quality evidence.

The use of stem cells to regenerate cells and increase disc matrix production is also currently being researched. Stem cell research with respect to healing degenerated intervertebral discs is focused on cell replacement and increase in the synthesis of proteoglycans and type II collagen. Although many cell lines have been considered, mesenchymal cells from either adipose tissue or bone marrow seem to hold the most promise. In vitro testing, animal models, and small pilot studies show success with matrix production. Several studies are currently underway, looking at the long-term benefits of intradiscal injection of stem cells, as well as the use of different stem cell lines, such as mesenchymal cells from adipose tissue or umbilical cord.[22]

IMAGE GUIDANCE

The modality for image guidance depends on operator preference and patient characteristics. Technical requirements to ensure safe and successful epidural steroid or anesthetic injection (ESI) include adequate institutional facilities, imaging and monitoring equipment, and support personnel.

No Image Guidance

Image guidance for all cervical and lumbar interlaminar injections is recommended to avoid inadvertent spinal cord penetration or intravascular or intrathecal placement.[11] Although ESIs have been performed without imaging guidance, there may be erroneous placement in up to 30% of injections in such cases.[23] In order to accurately place the medication at the affected level and to avoid the potential for intrathecal and intravascular injections, most interventionalists strongly recommend image guidance for spine interventions.

Fluoroscopy

Fluoroscopic guidance allows accurate needle placement when combined with contrast medium injection.[23-25] Lateral or oblique views are recommended to gauge the depth of needle insertion. Both C-arm and biplane fluoroscopy provide multiplanar imaging of the target anatomy, which can help reduce procedural time.[26]

Computed Tomography and Computed Tomography Fluoroscopy

Computed tomography (CT) guidance and CT-fluoroscopy (CTF) guidance allows for highly accurate needle guidance, with real-time cross-sectional visualization of needle placement into the epidural space to avoid neural and vascular structures, as well as impeding osseous structures.[27] In addition, CT and CTF enable the evaluation of spinal canal and paraspinal regions to permit diagnosis of synovial cysts, severe spinal stenosis, epidural scarring, and postoperative thecal sac deformity, which are potential causes of inaccurate needle placement or procedure failure.

The overall radiation dose from CTF is small compared with a diagnostic CT scan. Tube current selection for CTF procedures ideally balances the need for adequate anatomic visualization against the desire for individual patient dose reduction. Radiation dose to the patient and the interventionalist can be minimized with the use of intermittent fluoroscopy and a low milliamperage.[28-30]

Digital Subtraction Imaging Guidance

CT or CTF may have the theoretic disadvantage of lack of vessel opacification after contrast administration because the intravascularly injected contrast may be washed away by the time CT is performed or because the given vessel enters the cord at a different level and is therefore not imaged.[31] To reliably exclude inadvertent direct vessel puncture, some investigators have advocated real-time imaging with digital subtraction angiography when performed with fluoroscopy.[32-34]

Ultrasound

Ultrasonography can be used to accurately guide the spinal needle and has been shown to produce comparative treatment outcome as fluoroscopy.[35] The advantages of ultrasound guidance are no radiation and delineation of any vascular structures along the needle trajectory.[36] Patient body habitus and pathologic status, as well as operator skill, are important limitations.

EPIDURAL INJECTION
Indications

ESI is a technique used to treat LBP and radicular pain related to degenerative spinal etiologic factors after failure of more conservative treatments, such as oral pain medications and physical therapy.[1] Multifactorial degenerative changes, such as herniated disc, ligamentum flavum thickening, and osteophytic spurring along endplates and facet joints, are the leading cause of neck pain and LBP. A disc herniation may cause spinal nerve compression and inflammation, resulting in radicular pain.[37] Acquired degenerative spinal stenosis can cause neck pain or LBP, with radiation to the shoulders and arms in cases of cervical stenosis, or buttocks and lower extremities in cases of lumbar stenosis, by exerting pressure on adjacent nerves transiting or exiting the spinal canal. Pain characteristically worsens with activity and can be correlated to imaging findings of canal narrowing and/or nerve impingement.[38] The interlaminar ESI (ILESI) approach is used for central stenosis causing low back and radicular pain.[25] The transforaminal ESI (TFESI) approach is used in patients with a lateral disc bulge with primarily radicular or radiculopathic symptoms.[25]

Imaging Anatomy

Injections are targeted to the epidural space, an extradural fat-filled space surrounding the thecal sac within the osseous spinal canal and extending into the neural foramina through which course the exiting nerves. This space is seen subjacent to the spinolaminar line on fluoroscopy. On CT or CTF, the epidural space is identified by the fat attenuation surrounding the thecal sac. The extent of the epidural space allows 2 different routes for medication delivery to sites of stenosis: interlaminar, traversing the ligamentum flavum, and transforaminal, by way of the neural foramen.[25]

Technique

Interlaminar

In both the lumbar and cervical spine, the ILESI is performed by directing a needle (usually a blunt-tipped Touhy or Crawford needle between 17 and 22 gauge)[25] by a posterior paramedian approach to either the superior or inferior lamina when using posteroanterior (PA) fluoroscopy, or directly to the interlaminar space when using CT or CTF. While using PA fluoroscopy, aiming the needle at the adjacent laminae prevents inadvertent intrathecal puncture by providing an initial osseous barrier. Then a lateral or contralateral oblique view[39] can be used for depth assessment and further passage of the needle to the spinolaminar line.

When the needle tip has reached the firm-feeling ligamentum flavum at the spinolaminar line, a loss-of-resistance technique is used to access the epidural space. This technique can be performed by connecting a syringe filled with nonionic, myelographic-safe contrast or preservative-free saline. Forward pressure is placed on the syringe as the needle is advanced through the ligamentum flavum. When the ligamentum flavum is breached, there is loss of resistance, with free passage of contrast or saline into the epidural space. Dynamic fluoroscopic images are obtained to evaluate contrast spread within the epidural space. The contrast pattern appears blotchy and is often vacuolized (due to filling defects from epidural vessels) and asymmetric on the PA view; however, the contrast should appear as a uniform line just ventral to the spinolaminar line on the lateral or contralateral oblique view (**Figs. 1** and **2**).[6,25,39] There should be no evidence of intravascular or intrathecal spread.[6] By CTF, contrast should fill the posterior triangular epidural fat and can spread to surround the thecal sac posteriorly (see **Figs. 1** and **2**).

Transforaminal

The transforaminal approach is a target-specific approach allowing maximal delivery of medication to the relevant nerve root. A preganglionic TFESI (at the supraadjacent disc level) is preferred by some interventionalists instead of an ILESI injection when there is a lateralized lumbar disc herniation.[40,41] When there is a disc extrusion, a

ganglionic TFESI (at the exiting nerve root level) may be useful.[42]

Cervical In the cervical spine, a TFESI is performed by an anterolateral approach with the patient lying supine. An ipsilateral oblique view opening up the neural foramen is used for the trajectory on fluoroscopy (approximately 45°), with a 22-25–gauge Quincke needle directed to the posteroinferior aspect of the foramen. The AP view is used to determine needle depth, with optimal needle positioning along the outer third of the lateral mass and never beyond its midaspect.[42] Contrast is injected with real-time fluoroscopic imaging to ensure that there is no intravascular opacification due to the needle position, particularly the vertebral artery. Expected epidural contrast spread is often cephalad, with a variable degree of medial flow due to plica mediana dorsalis (**Fig. 3A, B**).[43] By CT or CTF, the needle is directed by an anterolateral approach to the posterior aspect of the epidural space, no deeper than the outer third of the lateral mass (**Fig. 3C**). Though this is a common approach, some interventionalists have used a posterior approach with similar efficacy.[44] The intraarticular facet steroid injection approach has been shown to deliver corticosteroids in the vicinity of the target spinal nerve root, and has been shown to be a viable alternative to the riskier transforaminal approach.[45–47]

Lumbar In the lumbar spine, an oblique so-called Scotty dog trajectory view is used. Both supraneural and infraneural needle positions are options for access to the lateral epidural space.

Supraneural In the supraneural approach, a 22-25–gauge Quincke or Chiba needle is aimed at the 6 o'clock position, directly beneath the pedicle on the oblique view. The needle is advanced with the PA view demonstrating optimal positioning below the midaspect of the pedicle and the lateral view demonstrating optimal positioning along the superior aspect of the neural foramen.[25] Contrast is injected to ensure positioning within the lateral epidural space, with a spread pattern of contrast contacting the medial aspect of the pedicle and extending craniocaudal in a thin line along the spinal canal by fluoroscopy (**Fig. 4A and B**).[6] By CT or CTF, contrast will fill the lateral epidural space and spread along the lateral margin of the spinal canal (**Fig. 4C**).

Infraneural In the infraneural approach, the needle is aimed along the lateral aspect of the superior articular process of the facet joint on the oblique view. The needle is advanced with the PA view, demonstrating optimal positioning below the

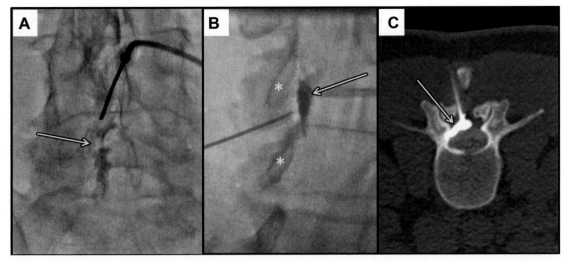

Fig. 1. Lumbar interlaminar epidural injection. (*A*) AP fluoroscopic image of lumbar interlaminar epidural injection shows expected irregular asymmetric contrast opacification with small amount of air, as well as venous filling defects in the epidural fat (*yellow arrow*). (*B*) Contralateral oblique fluoroscopic image from interlaminar lumbar epidural injection provides en face view of the lamina (*asterisks*) between which the needle is passing. Note expected linear epidural contrast (*yellow arrow*) just ventral to the spinolaminar line. (*C*) CTF axial image demonstrating contrast injected into the dorsal epidural space and extending along the periphery of the thecal sac (*yellow arrow*).

midaspect of the pedicle, and the lateral view, demonstrating optimal positioning along the inferior aspect of the neural foramen. The contrast spread pattern is at the level of the injection.

Complications

Image-guided ESIs have a high safety profile; however, complications can rarely occur. With an ILESI, inadvertent dural puncture can occur,

leading to an intrathecal injection of steroid or anesthetic, spinal cord or nerve injury, or cerebrospinal fluid leak. Intravascular injection can also occur, which extremely rarely can lead to spinal cord infarction, more commonly seen with TFESI and almost exclusively with usage of particulate steroids.[25,48–51] Because the radiculomedullary artery is most commonly located in the upper neural foramen, some investigators have

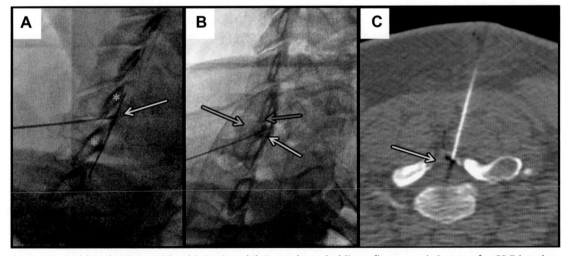

Fig. 2. Cervical interlaminar epidural injection. (*A*) Contralateral oblique fluoroscopic image of a C6-7 interlaminar epidural injection demonstrates expected thin linear contrast (*yellow arrow*) just ventral to the spinolaminar line. This view accurately shows the lamina en face (*blue asterisks*) and clearly depicts lower cervical anatomy often obscured by the shoulders on the straight lateral view. (*B*) Note interspinous contrast injected before entering the epidural space (*green arrow*). Ligamentum flavum appears as a clear space (*red arrow*) between interspinous and epidural contrast (*yellow arrow*). (*C*) CTF-guided epidural injection at C7-T1 using air to delineate the epidural space (*yellow arrow*) in a patient with an iodinated contrast allergy.

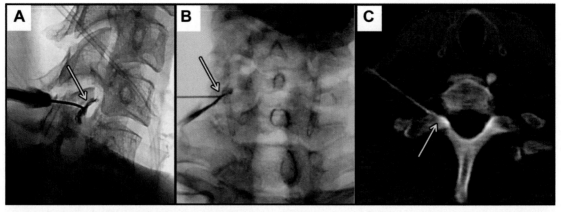

Fig. 3. Cervical transforaminal epidural steroid injection. (*A*) Foraminal oblique image from C6 selective nerve root block with expected needle position and contrast opacification in the posterior foramen (*arrow*). (*B*) AP fluoroscopic image of right C7 selective nerve root block shows expected contrast extending along the exiting nerve root sleeve (*arrow*). (*C*) CTF axial image demonstrating a C7 transforaminal epidural steroid injection from an anterolateral needle approach with contrast extending into the dorsolateral epidural space (*arrow*).

endorsed usage of the infraneural Kambin triangle approach in the lumbar spine to reduce the risk for vascular injury and infarction.[50,52] Though not a dangerous complication, one can inadvertently access the retrodural space of Okada during epidural injection, which will prevent the medication from getting to the targeted epidural space and potentially decrease treatment response.[53]

FACET JOINT INJECTION
Indications

Facetogenic pain is exacerbated by forward flexion and with twisting or rotary strain; there may or may not be associated radiation of pain.

In the lumbosacral spine, this pseudoradicular pain typically ends above the knee.[54] In the cervical spine, facet-related pain can radiate to the head, as well as the shoulders.[55]

Imaging Anatomy

Facet joints, also known as zygapophysial joints, are paired synovial joints formed by the joining of the inferior and superior articular processes from adjacent vertebrae. They are innervated by the medial branch nerve arising from the dorsal rami.[54,56] These joint spaces are approximately 1 to 2 mL in volume and are oriented along the anteriorly and laterally facing inferior articular process, and posteriorly and medially facing superior

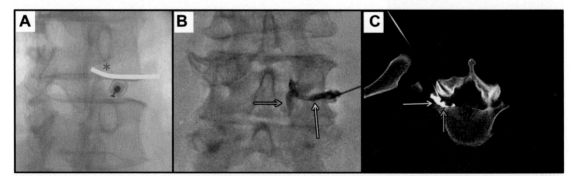

Fig. 4. Lumbar transforaminal epidural steroid injection. (*A*) Scotty dog oblique view demonstrating an infraneural trajectory for a transforaminal epidural steroid injection. The needle is lined up just lateral to the superior articular process of the facet (Scotty dog ear) placing it below the exiting nerve (*yellow line*). Though this imaging angle is not optimized for a supraneural approach, in a supraneural injection the needle would be lined up at approximately the 6 o'clock position of the pedicle above (*asterisk*). AP fluoroscopic (*B*) and CTF axial (*C*) images demonstrate lumbar transforaminal epidural injections that show expected contrast opacification along the exiting nerve root sleeve (*yellow arrows*), extending medially under the pedicle to the lateral epidural space (*blue arrows*).

articular process.[54,57] Although studies have shown no association of facet joint osteoarthritis on CT with clinical symptoms,[58] technetium-99m (^{99m}Tc) diphosphonate (bone) scintigraphy and SPECT fused with CT and MR imaging show great diagnostic promise. MR imaging can reveal soft tissue inflammatory changes[59,60] that can be seen with degenerative osteoarthritic processes. When combined with clinical provocation tests, facet joint effusion with or without edema on MR imaging can help detect a painful facet joint.[61] Because clinical and imaging findings can be unreliable for facet pain diagnosis, image-guided diagnostic blocks are considered the most reliable method for diagnosis.[62]

Technique

Techniques differ between the cervical, thoracic, and lumbar spine.

Cervical
In the cervical spine, both lateral and posterior approaches can be taken to access the facet joint.[63,64] Care is taken on the lateral projection to maintain the needle trajectory over the posterior elements to avoid vascular or subarachnoid puncture.[64] When contrast is injected, it should linearly fill the facet joint on both PA and lateral views (**Fig. 5**).[63] CT or CTF can also be used to target the cervical facet joint.

Lumbar
With fluoroscopy, an oblique view is used to best delineate the facet joint: the space between the ear of the lower Scotty dog sign and the leg of the upper Scotty dog sign. A 22-gauge spinal needle is then advanced from a posterior approach into the joint. Often, puncture through the capsule can be felt by the operator.[65] Nonionic contrast, used to confirm positioning, shows linear filling within the joint space with the potential of filling the inferior or superior joint recesses (**Fig. 6**).[65,66]

Thoracic
The thoracic spine approach is similar to the lumbar spine but often, because of the orientation of the joint space, the injection is more challenging and CT or CTF guidance must be used.[64]

In cases in which the facet joint cannot be easily accessed, prior studies have demonstrated no significant difference in pain relief between intraarticular and periarticular joint injections.[67] CT or CTF can be used for more precise targeting of the facet joint. Additionally, ultrasound guidance has also demonstrated similar efficacy for pain relief compared with CT.[68]

Complications

Most facet joint injections carry only minimal risk of allergy to contrast and bleeding. However, facet joint injections at higher cervical levels, particularly the C1-2 facet joint (**Fig. 7**), hold greater risk of arterial injury, potentially leading to stroke or injury of the spinal cord.[64,69]

SYNOVIAL CYST RUPTURE
Indications

Synovial cysts can arise from the degenerated facet joint, the ligamentum flavum, and

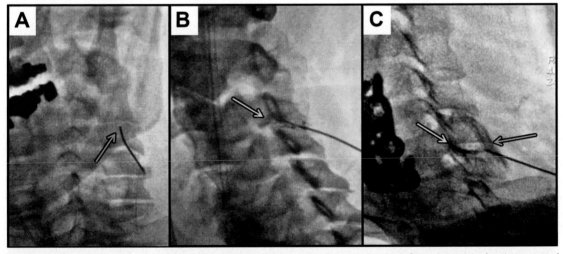

Fig. 5. Cervical facet injection. (*A*) AP fluoroscopic pillar view from right C3-4 facet injection (patient prone) shows needle tip (*blue arrow*) directed toward the joint space. (*B*) Oblique fluoroscopic image in same patient after contrast injection shows expected linear opacification of the joint space (*yellow arrow*). (*C*) Postcontrast oblique image in a different patient with contrast injected in the soft tissues (*green arrow*) before obtaining proper position within the joint space (*yellow arrow*).

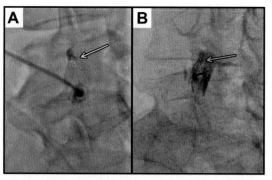

Fig. 6. Lumbar facet injection. (*A*) Ipsilateral oblique fluoroscopic images demonstrate a left lumbar nerve (L) 4-5 facet joint injection with needle tip in the inferior recess showing expected linear opacification of the joint with pooling in the superior recess (*yellow arrow*). (*B*) Attempted facet joint injection in another patient shows soft tissue opacification (*green arrow*) with no definite contrast within the joint.

interspinous bursa extending into the posterior epidural space, and can cause radicular symptoms from nerve compression or spinal stenosis.[70,71] Facet synovial cysts are far more common than epidural cysts and arise in the setting of degenerative arthropathy.[72–74] Image-guided rupture has been found to be a low-risk nonsurgical option for the treatment of cyst-related radiculopathy, leading to immediate symptom relief in up to 80% of patients, and up to half of patients not requiring subsequent surgical management.[71,74–78] Synovial cysts with internal T2 hyperintense and intermediate signal may be more amenable to percutaneous rupture.[79]

Imaging Anatomy

Symptomatic cysts have been found to arise from the anterior facet joint border and extend into the

neural foramen or spinal canal resulting in exiting or transiting nerve compression.[80] Because these cysts arise from the facet joint, they can be accessed indirectly through the posterior aspect of the joint, with some targeting the inferior recess.[74] Larger cysts can also be accessed through an interlaminar approach into the epidural space.[81] Dorsal epidural synovial cysts have been found to be associated with Baastrup disease, likely representing an interspinous bursa extending through a defect in the ligamentum flavum.[82,83] These can be accessed by a central interlaminar approach.

Technique

Both fluoroscopic and CT or CTF guidance can be used. Techniques vary between operators, patient body habitus and access to the synovial cyst. In general, an 18-22 gauge Quincke or Chiba needle is advanced to the facet joint space from a posterior approach. A 3 mL syringe is filled with different combinations of local anesthetic, steroid, saline, and nonionic contrast, and forcefully injected into the facet joint until the cyst is ruptured.[71,74,78] The patient often feels an acute escalation of pain and pressure during forceful inection.[71] Cyst rupture is confirmed by spread of contrast into the epidural space. In cases in which the cyst cannot be ruptured through the facet joint or the facet joint is inaccessible due to overgrowth, an interlaminar approach can be taken for direct fenestration (**Fig. 8**).[81,84]

Complications

Patients may experience increased radicular pain from forceful injection with nonrupture of the cyst.[71] Other complications include intrathecal puncture in procedures using an interlaminar approach.[84]

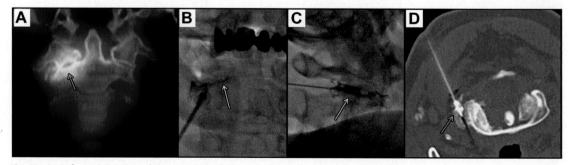

Fig. 7. C1-2 facet injection. (*A*) Bone SPECT demonstrates increased avidity (*blue arrow*) of the right C1-2 facet joint related to active inflammation. AP (*B*) and lateral (*C*) fluoroscopic images from left C1-2 facet injection (patient prone) demonstrate expected linear contrast filling the joint space (*yellow arrows*). (*D*) CTF image demonstrates a posterior needle approach (*blue arrow*) for C1-2 facet injection.

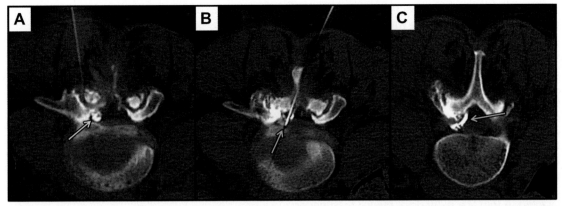

Fig. 8. Axial images from CT-guided left L4-5 synovial cyst rupture. (*A*) Needle tip first placed in the facet joint with expected contrast opacification of the joint and contiguous subarticular zone synovial cyst (*yellow arrow*). (*B*) After unsuccessful attempted rupture, the second needle tip is placed directly into cyst (*blue arrow*) from interlaminar approach. (*C*) Image after successful rupture shows linear epidural spread of contrast (*green arrow*) and collapse of the cyst.

SACROILIAC JOINT INJECTION
Indications

Patients with sacroiliac joint (SIJ) pain complain of buttock pain, localizing to the SIJ, with or without extension into the lower extremities.[56] Because of the complexity of the joint and surrounding ligaments, diagnostic localization can be challenging and is performed by a combination of history, imaging, physical examination, and diagnostic block.[85] Multitest physical maneuvers have shown to be promising for localization in many cases[86];

however, they have not received reliable consensus,[87] and the diagnostic standard remains pain reduction with intraarticular anesthetic injection.[88]

Imaging Anatomy

The SIJ is the largest axial joint and is composed of both fibrous portions in the upper two-thirds and a synovial portion in the lower third.[89–91] Due to the complex auricular shape of the joint, image guidance is necessary for joint injection.[92,93] The

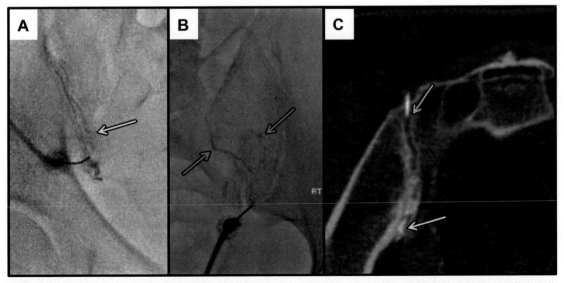

Fig. 9. SIJ injection. (*A*) Left anterior oblique fluoroscopic image (patient prone) of a left SIJ injection with needle tip in the SIJ inferior recess, which shows expected linear contrast opacification of the joint space extending cephalad (*yellow arrow*). (*B*) Right anterior oblique fluoroscopic image (patient prone) of a right SIJ injection in another patient shows abnormal curvilinear contrast opacification (*red arrows*) indicating a vascular injection. (*C*) Axial CTF image demonstrating the needle tip within the right SIJ (*blue arrow*) with contrast extending into the anterior portion of the joint (*yellow arrow*).

posteroinferior synovial aspect of the joint is targeted under image guidance with 25° to 35° obliquity to separate the posterior from the anterior part of the joint.[94]

Technique

With PA fluoroscopy, rotation of the C-arm or image intensifier between 25° to 35° is used to open the posteroinferior joint. A 22-25 gauge Quincke or Chiba needle is advanced from a posterior approach under image guidance into the joint space. A lateral view can be helpful to ensure adequate positioning.[91] When nonionic contrast is injected, a thin line extending inferior to superior along the contours of the joint space confirms intraarticular positioning (**Fig. 9A, B**).[91] In more challenging cases, a double-needle approach can be taken when the needle is not clearly within the joint.[95] Direct advancement of the needle into the SIJ can also be performed under CT or CTF (**Fig. 9C**).

Complications

Complications are primarily related to advancement of the needle too far anteriorly where there is increased potential of needle puncture to the bladder or bowel. A lateral view can be used to evaluate for depth to mitigate against these risks.[91]

SUMMARY

Image-guided therapeutic injections are low-risk treatment options in the setting of degenerative spine pain. Knowledge of the anatomic landmarks, understanding of pathoanatomic correlations of spinal anatomy to the patient's symptoms, and familiarity with the image-guidance modalities are essential for the spine interventionalist for precise targeting and effective treatment.

REFERENCES

1. Deer TR, Grider JS, Pope JE, et al. The MIST guidelines: the lumbar spinal stenosis consensus group guidelines for minimally invasive spine treatment. Pain Pract 2019;19(3):250–74.
2. Palmer WE. Spinal injections for pain management. Radiology 2016;281(3):669–88.
3. Friedly J, Chan L, Deyo R. Increases in lumbosacral injections in the Medicare population: 1994 to 2001. Spine 2007;32(16):1754–60.
4. el-Khoury GY, Ehara S, Weinstein JN, et al. Epidural steroid injection: a procedure ideally performed with fluoroscopic control. Radiology 1988;168(2):554–7.
5. Renfrew DL, Moore TE, Kathol MH, et al. Correct placement of epidural steroid injections: fluoroscopic guidance and contrast administration. AJNR Am J Neuroradiol 1991;12(5):1003–7.
6. Furman MB, Cuneo AA. Image and contrast flow pattern interpretation for attempted epidural steroid injections. Phys Med Rehabil Clin N Am 2018; 29(1):19–33.
7. MacMahon PJ, Eustace SJ, Kavanagh EC. Injectable corticosteroid and local anesthetic preparations: a review for radiologists. Radiology 2009; 252(3):647–61.
8. Benzon HT, Chew TL, McCarthy RJ, et al. Comparison of the particle sizes of different steroids and the effect of dilution: a review of the relative neurotoxicities of the steroids. Anesthesiology 2007;106(2):331–8.
9. MacMahon PJ, Shelly MJ, Scholz D, et al. Injectable corticosteroid preparations: an embolic risk assessment by static and dynamic microscopic analysis. AJNR Am J Neuroradiol 2011;32(10):1830–5.
10. Derby R, Lee SH, Date ES, et al. Size and aggregation of corticosteroids used for epidural injections. Pain Med 2008;9(2):227–34.
11. Rathmell JP, Benzon HT, Dreyfuss P, et al. Safeguards to prevent neurologic complications after epidural steroid injections: consensus opinions from a multidisciplinary working group and national organizations. Anesthesiology 2015;122(5):974–84.
12. MacMahon PJ, Huang AJ, Palmer WE. Spine injectables: what is the safest cocktail? AJR Am J Roentgenol 2016;207(3):526–33.
13. De La Mata J. Platelet rich plasma. A new treatment tool for the rheumatologist? Reumatol Clin 2013;9(3): 166–71.
14. Mohammed S, Yu J. Platelet-rich plasma injections: an emerging therapy for chronic discogenic low back pain. J Spine Surg 2018;4(1):115–22.
15. Akeda K, Ohishi K, Masuda K, et al. Intradiscal injection of autologous platelet-rich plasma releasate to treat discogenic low back pain: a preliminary clinical trial. Asian Spine J 2017;11(3):380–9.
16. Bhatia R, Chopra G. Efficacy of platelet rich plasma via lumbar epidural route in chronic prolapsed intervertebral disc patients-a pilot study. J Clin Diagn Res 2016;10(9):UC05–7.
17. Levi D, Horn S, Tyszko S, et al. Intradiscal platelet-rich plasma injection for chronic discogenic low back pain: preliminary results from a prospective trial. Pain Med 2016;17(6):1010–22.
18. Monfett M, Harrison J, Boachie-Adjei K, et al. Intradiscal platelet-rich plasma (PRP) injections for discogenic low back pain: an update. Int Orthop 2016;40(6):1321–8.
19. Tuakli-Wosornu YA, Terry A, Boachie-Adjei K, et al. Lumbar intradiskal platelet-rich plasma (PRP) injections: a prospective, double-blind, randomized controlled study. PM R 2016;8(1):1–10 [quiz: 10].
20. Nagae M, Ikeda T, Mikami Y, et al. Intervertebral disc regeneration using platelet-rich plasma and

biodegradable gelatin hydrogel microspheres. Tissue Eng 2007;13(1):147–58.

21. Fabbro MD, Bortolin M, Taschieri S, et al. Antimicrobial properties of platelet-rich preparations. A systematic review of the current pre-clinical evidence. Platelets 2016;27(4):276–85.

22. Knezevic NN, Mandalia S, Raasch J, et al. Treatment of chronic low back pain - new approaches on the horizon. J Pain Res 2017;10:1111–23.

23. White AH, Derby R, Wynne G. Epidural injections for the diagnosis and treatment of low-back pain. Spine 1980;5(1):78–86.

24. Johnson BA. Image-guided epidural injections. Neuroimaging Clin N Am 2000;10(3):479–91.

25. Watanabe AT, Nishimura E, Garris J. Image-guided epidural steroid injections. Tech Vasc Interv Radiol 2002;5(4):186–93.

26. Mathis JM. Epidural steroid injections. Neuroimaging Clin N Am 2010;20(2):193–202.

27. Wagner AL. CT fluoroscopy-guided epidural injections: technique and results. AJNR Am J Neuroradiol 2004;25(10):1821–3.

28. Paulson EK, Sheafor DH, Enterline DS, et al. CT fluoroscopy–guided interventional procedures: techniques and radiation dose to radiologists. Radiology 2001;220(1):161–7.

29. Fenster AJ, Fernandes K, Brook AL, et al. The safety of CT-guided epidural steroid injections in an older patient cohort. Pain Physician 2016;19(8):E1139–46.

30. Lazarus MS, Forman RB, Brook AL, et al. Radiation dose and procedure time for 994 CT-guided Spine pain control procedures. Pain Physician 2017; 20(4):E585–91.

31. Ryan TM, Kavanagh EC, MacMahon PJ. Is there a need for contrast administration prior to CT-guided cervical nerve root block? AJNR Am J Neuroradiol 2013;34(4):E45.

32. Hong JH, Kim SY, Huh B, et al. Analysis of inadvertent intradiscal and intravascular injection during lumbar transforaminal epidural steroid injections: a prospective study. Reg Anesth Pain Med 2013; 38(6):520–5.

33. Lee MH, Yang KS, Kim YH, et al. Accuracy of live fluoroscopy to detect intravascular injection during lumbar transforaminal epidural injections. Korean J Pain 2010;23(1):18–23.

34. McLean JP, Sigler JD, Plastaras CT, et al. The rate of detection of intravascular injection in cervical transforaminal epidural steroid injections with and without digital subtraction angiography. PM R 2009;1(7): 636–42.

35. Kao SC, Lin CS. Caudal epidural block: an updated review of anatomy and techniques. Biomed Res Int 2017;2017:9217145.

36. Jee H, Lee JH, Kim J, et al. Ultrasound-guided selective nerve root block versus fluoroscopy-guided transforaminal block for the treatment of radicular pain in the lower cervical spine: a randomized, blinded, controlled study. Skeletal Radiol 2013; 42(1):69–78.

37. Benyamin RM, Manchikanti L, Parr AT, et al. The effectiveness of lumbar interlaminar epidural injections in managing chronic low back and lower extremity pain. Pain Physician 2012;15(4):E363–404.

38. Mamisch N, Brumann M, Hodler J, et al. Radiologic criteria for the diagnosis of spinal stenosis: results of a Delphi survey. Radiology 2012;264(1):174–9.

39. Gill JS, Aner M, Nagda JV, et al. Contralateral oblique view is superior to lateral view for interlaminar cervical and cervicothoracic epidural access. Pain Med 2015;16(1):68–80.

40. Jeong HS, Lee JW, Kim SH, et al. Effectiveness of transforaminal epidural steroid injection by using a preganglionic approach: a prospective randomized controlled study. Radiology 2007;245(2):584–90.

41. Kamble PC, Sharma A, Singh V, et al. Outcome of single level disc prolapse treated with transforaminal steroid versus epidural steroid versus caudal steroids. Eur Spine J 2016;25(1):217–21.

42. Shim E, Lee JW, Lee E, et al. Fluoroscopically guided epidural injections of the cervical and lumbar spine. Radiographics 2017;37(2):537–61.

43. Demondion X, Lefebvre G, Fisch O, et al. Radiographic anatomy of the intervertebral cervical and lumbar foramina (vessels and variants). Diagn Interv Imaging 2012;93(9):690–7.

44. Wald JT, Maus TP, Geske JR, et al. Safety and efficacy of CT-guided transforaminal cervical epidural steroid injections using a posterior approach. AJNR Am J Neuroradiol 2012;33(3):415–9.

45. Bureau NJ, Moser T, Dagher JH, et al. Transforaminal versus intra-articular facet corticosteroid injections for the treatment of cervical radiculopathy: a randomized, double-blind, controlled study. AJNR Am J Neuroradiol 2014;35(8):1467–74.

46. Richarme D, Thevenin FS, Chevrot A, et al. Cervical radiculopathy: efficiency of CT-guided cervical facet joint corticosteroid injection. Chicago: Radiological Society of North America; 2008.

47. Kim KH, Choi SH, Kim TK, et al. Cervical facet joint injections in the neck and shoulder pain. J Korean Med Sci 2005;20(4):659–62.

48. Malhotra G, Abbasi A, Rhee M. Complications of transforaminal cervical epidural steroid injections. Spine 2009;34(7):731–9.

49. Diehn FE, Murthy NS, Maus TP. Science to practice: what causes arterial infarction in transforaminal epidural steroid injections, and which steroid is safest? Radiology 2016;279(3):657–9.

50. Gregg L, Sorte DE, Gailloud P. Intraforaminal location of thoracolumbar radicular arteries providing an anterior radiculomedullary artery using flat panel catheter angiotomography. AJNR Am J Neuroradiol 2017;38(5):1054–60.

51. Furman MB, Giovanniello MT, O'Brien EM. Incidence of intravascular penetration in transforaminal cervical epidural steroid injections. Spine 2003;28(1):21–5.

52. Park JW, Nam HS, Cho SK, et al. Kambin's triangle approach of lumbar transforaminal epidural injection with spinal stenosis. Ann Rehabil Med 2011;35(6):833–43.

53. Kranz PG, Joshi AB, Roy LA, et al. Inadvertent intra-facet injection during lumbar interlaminar epidural steroid injection: a comparison of CT fluoroscopic and conventional fluoroscopic guidance. AJNR Am J Neuroradiol 2017;38(2):398–402.

54. Perolat R, Kastler A, Nicot B, et al. Facet joint syndrome: from diagnosis to interventional management. Insights Imaging 2018;9(5):773–89.

55. van Eerd M, Patijn J, Lataster A, et al. 5. Cervical facet pain. Pain Pract 2010;10(2):113–23.

56. Kennedy DJ, Shokat M, Visco CJ. Sacroiliac joint and lumbar zygapophysial joint corticosteroid injections. Phys Med Rehabil Clin N Am 2010;21(4):835–42.

57. Datta S, Lee M, Falco FJ, et al. Systematic assessment of diagnostic accuracy and therapeutic utility of lumbar facet joint interventions. Pain Physician 2009;12(2):437–60.

58. Kalichman L, Li L, Kim DH, et al. Facet joint osteoarthritis and low back pain in the community-based population. Spine 2008;33(23):2560–5.

59. Weishaupt D, Zanetti M, Boos N, et al. MR imaging and CT in osteoarthritis of the lumbar facet joints. Skeletal Radiol 1999;28(4):215–9.

60. Carrino JA, Lurie JD, Tosteson AN, et al. Lumbar spine: reliability of MR imaging findings. Radiology 2009;250(1):161–70.

61. Mainka T, Lemburg SP, Heyer CM, et al. Association between clinical signs assessed by manual segmental examination and findings of the lumbar facet joints on magnetic resonance scans in subjects with and without current low back pain: a prospective, single-blind study. Pain 2013;154(9):1886–95.

62. Falco FJ, Manchikanti L, Datta S, et al. An update of the systematic assessment of the diagnostic accuracy of lumbar facet joint nerve blocks. Pain Physician 2012;15(6):E869–907.

63. Dussault RG, Nicolet VM. Cervical facet joint arthrography. J Can Assoc Radiol 1985;36(1):79–80.

64. Peh W. Image-guided facet joint injection. Biomed Imaging Interv J 2011;7(1):e4.

65. Dory MA. Arthrography of the lumbar facet joints. Radiology 1981;140(1):23–7.

66. Bykowski JL, Wong WH. Role of facet joints in spine pain and image-guided treatment: a review. AJNR Am J Neuroradiol 2012;33(8):1419–26.

67. Lilius G, Laasonen EM, Myllynen P, et al. Lumbar facet joint syndrome. A randomised clinical trial. J Bone Joint Surg Br 1989;71(4):681–4.

68. Wu T, Zhao WH, Dong Y, et al. Effectiveness of ultrasound-guided versus fluoroscopy or computed tomography scanning guidance in lumbar facet joint injections in adults with facet joint syndrome: a meta-analysis of controlled trials. Arch Phys Med Rehabil 2016;97(9):1558–63.

69. Tang E. Complications of C1-C2 facet injection. Anesthesiology 2011;114(1):222 [author reply: 224].

70. Pendleton B, Carl B, Pollay M. Spinal extradural benign synovial or ganglion cyst: case report and review of the literature. Neurosurgery 1983;13(3):322–6.

71. Kursumovic A, Bostelmann R, Gollwitzer M, et al. Intraspinal lumbar juxtaarticular cyst treatment through CT-guided percutaneus induced rupture results in a favorable patient outcome. Clin Pract 2016;6(4):866.

72. Kao CC, Uihlein A, Bickel WH, et al. Lumbar intraspinal extradural ganglion cyst. J Neurosurg 1968;29(2):168–72.

73. Abdullah AF, Chambers RW, Daut DP. Lumbar nerve root compression by synovial cysts of the ligamentum flavum. Report of four cases. J Neurosurg 1984;60(3):617–20.

74. Eshraghi Y, Desai V, Cajigal Cajigal C, et al. Outcome of percutaneous lumbar synovial cyst rupture in patients with lumbar radiculopathy. Pain Physician 2016;19(7):E1019–25.

75. Chazen JL, Leeman K, Singh JR, et al. Percutaneous CT-guided facet joint synovial cyst rupture: success with refractory cases and technical considerations. Clin Imaging 2018;49:7–11.

76. Haider SJ, Na NR, Eskey CJ, et al. Symptomatic lumbar facet synovial cysts: clinical outcomes following percutaneous CT-guided cyst rupture with intra-articular steroid injection. J Vasc Interv Radiol 2017;28(8):1083–9.

77. Huang AJ, Bos SA, Torriani M, et al. Long-term outcomes of percutaneous lumbar facet synovial cyst rupture. Skeletal Radiol 2017;46(1):75–80.

78. Lutz GE, Nicoletti MR, Cyril GE, et al. Percutaneous rupture of zygapophyseal joint synovial cysts: a prospective assessment of nonsurgical management. PM R 2018;10(3):245–53.

79. Cambron SC, McIntyre JJ, Guerin SJ, et al. Lumbar facet joint synovial cysts: does T2 signal intensity predict outcomes after percutaneous rupture? AJNR Am J Neuroradiol 2013;34(8):1661–4.

80. Janssen SJ, Ogink PT, Schwab JH. The prevalence of incidental and symptomatic lumbar synovial facet cysts. Clin Spine Surg 2018;31(5):E296–301.

81. Malik AS, Cairns KD. Percutaneous rupture of a symptomatic facet joint synovial cyst using 2-needle distention. Reg Anesth Pain Med 2015;40(5):635–8.

82. Hatgis J, Granville M, Jacobson RE. Baastrup's disease, interspinal bursitis, and dorsal epidural cysts:

radiologic evaluation and impact on treatment options. Cureus 2017;9(7):e1449.

83. Chen CK, Yeh L, Resnick D, et al. Intraspinal posterior epidural cysts associated with Baastrup's disease: report of 10 patients. AJR Am J Roentgenol 2004;182(1):191–4.

84. Ortiz AO, Tekchandani L. Improved outcomes with direct percutaneous CT guided lumbar synovial cyst treatment: advanced approaches and techniques. J Neurointerv Surg 2014;6(10):790–4.

85. Ko GD, Mindra S, Lawson GE, et al. Case series of ultrasound-guided platelet-rich plasma injections for sacroiliac joint dysfunction. J Back Musculoskelet Rehabil 2017;30(2):363–70.

86. Laslett M, Aprill CN, McDonald B, et al. Diagnosis of sacroiliac joint pain: validity of individual provocation tests and composites of tests. Man Ther 2005;10(3):207–18.

87. Thawrani DP, Agabegi SS, Asghar F. Diagnosing sacroiliac joint pain. J Am Acad Orthop Surg 2019;27(3):85–93.

88. Dreyfuss P, Michaelsen M, Pauza K, et al. The value of medical history and physical examination in diagnosing sacroiliac joint pain. Spine 1996;21(22):2594–602.

89. Egund N, Jurik AG. Anatomy and histology of the sacroiliac joints. Semin Musculoskelet Radiol 2014;18(3):332–9.

90. Puhakka KB, Melsen F, Jurik AG, et al. MR imaging of the normal sacroiliac joint with correlation to histology. Skeletal Radiol 2004;33(1):15–28.

91. Kasliwal PJ, Kasliwal S. Fluoroscopy-guided sacroiliac joint injection: description of a modified technique. Pain Physician 2016;19(2):E329–38.

92. Hansen HC. Is fluoroscopy necessary for sacroiliac joint injections? Pain Physician 2003;6(2):155–8.

93. Rosenberg JM, Quint TJ, de Rosayro AM. Computerized tomographic localization of clinically-guided sacroiliac joint injections. Clin J Pain 2000;16(1):18–21.

94. Chauhan G, Hehar P, Loomba V, et al. A randomized controlled trial of fluoroscopically-guided sacroiliac joint injections: a comparison of the posteroanterior and classical oblique techniques. Neurospine 2019;16(2):317–24.

95. Gupta S. Double needle technique: an alternative method for performing difficult sacroiliac joint injections. Pain Physician 2011;14(3):281–4.

Advanced Image-Guided Procedures for Painful Spine

Yian Chen, MD[a], Teresa Tang, MD[a], Michael Anthony Erdek, MD, MA[b],*

KEYWORDS

- Spine pain • Spinal stenosis • Neuromodulation • Failed back surgery syndrome
- High-frequency stimulation • Discography • Lumbar decompression
- Percutaneous lumbar decompression

KEY POINTS

- Spine pain is a prevalent and expensive condition worldwide.
- It manifests as several syndromes, including facetogenic pain, disc pain, failed back surgery syndrome, and degenerative spondylosis.
- Advanced procedures can be used to benefit patients with spine pain.
- Neuromodulation can be beneficial for patients who continue to have symptoms after spine surgery and multiple other interventions. Different frequencies have been studied in different painful conditions.
- For facet-mediated pain, radiofrequency thermoablation has been used to reduce arthropathic pain along the axial spine.

INTRODUCTION

Spine pain is significantly disabling and has a worldwide prevalence of 54% to 80%,[1] and its economic burden is similarly enormous, with back and neck problems accounting for $86 billion in US health expenditures in 2005.[2] The human spine is a complex structure with numerous possible pain generators, including the facet joints, discs, spinal nerve roots, and spinal cord itself. Conservative management and basic procedures, such as epidural steroid injections, are often paired with medications and physical modalities as mainstays of therapy for these conditions, but more advanced therapies can be used for patients who are recalcitrant to more basic therapies.

This article focuses on advanced techniques dedicated to the management of spine pain, including conventional spinal cord stimulation (neuromodulation), radiofrequency thermocoagulation for facet-mediated pain, and procedures for disc pain, as well as brief discussion of percutaneous minimally invasive lumbar decompression. These are more advanced procedures that can be completed under fluoroscopy or computerized tomography (CT) as image-guided techniques, thus expanding the repertoire of options available to patients. The article focuses on advanced therapeutic techniques that have been shown to be effective for syndromes associated with spine pain. In particular, it discusses spinal cord stimulation for failed back surgery syndrome and focally located lower back pain,

There are no disclosures for any of the authors.

[a] Department of Anesthesiology and Critical Care Medicine, Johns Hopkins School of Medicine, 550 North Broadway, Suite 301, Baltimore, MD 21205, USA; [b] Department of Anesthesiology and Critical Care Medicine, Johns Hopkins School of Medicine, Berman Institute of Bioethics, 550 North Broadway, Suite 301, Baltimore, MD 21205, USA

* Corresponding author.

E-mail address: merdek@jhmi.edu

Neuroimag Clin N Am 29 (2019) 553–561

https://doi.org/10.1016/j.nic.2019.07.005

and radiofrequency thermoablation for facet pain. Finally, it highlights discography and thermal ablation techniques for discogenic pain and minimally invasive lumbar decompression for lumbar spinal stenosis.

SPINAL CORD STIMULATION

Chronic spine pain that does not resolve from basic therapies can be successfully treated with more advanced modalities such as neuromodulation. Briefly, the use of electrical stimulation for treatment of pain has been present for centuries. One of the first documented uses was in 15 AD when Scribonius, a court physician to the Roman emperors, recommended torpedo fish treatment of pain after observing that gout pain was relieved by the electrical stimulation provided by the fish.[3] In 1965, the introduction of modulation as a potential treatment of pain accelerated with the gate theory by Melzack and Wall,[4] in which they proposed that pain perception involved a gate that can be opened or closed depending on the balance of large and small nerve fiber activity. Shortly after, in 1967, Norman Shealy, a neurosurgeon at Western Reserve Medical School, proposed the idea of stimulating large nerve fibers at the dorsal columns of the spinal cord, which, in turn, would alleviate pain; he demonstrated this principle in a patient with cancer.[3] It is now estimated that more than 40,000 new systems for spinal cord stimulators are implanted annually worldwide, with recent development of multiple forms of stimulation.[5]

From a technical standpoint, percutaneous or paddle leads composed of polyurethane and platinum are inserted or surgically placed into the posterior epidural space (Fig. 1). Cylindrical percutaneous leads generate a circumferential current; these are the primary device inserted percutaneously under image-assisted guidance. The leads are then connected to an implantable pulse generator. Patients most often undergo a trial of spinal cord stimulation that is completed under percutaneous guidance before the final surgical implant (which is also image-guided). Fluoroscopic guidance is used throughout the procedure and is essential for confirmation of the correct placement in the posterior epidural space.[6]

Tonic Stimulation

Different forms of spinal cord stimulation include conventional tonic stimulation, burst stimulation, and high-frequency stimulation. The first tonic stimulator was developed by Norman Shealy and Thomas Mortimer in 1967, and became

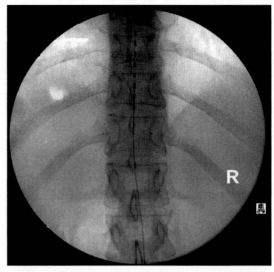

Fig. 1. A spinal cord stimulator lead advanced into the dorsal epidural space at midline, to the top of the thoracic nerve-10 vertebral body.

commercially available in 1968.[3] Tonic stimulation supplies a constant stimulation at frequencies between 40 to 60 Hz, with a pulse width between 150 to 500 microseconds, and at an amplitude that is adjusted for each patient to produce comfortable paresthesia in the painful area.[5] The mechanisms of spinal cord stimulation are multifold and continue to be clarified. Much of the basic science research has been in animal models of neuropathic pain, and there have been several proposed mechanisms. Spinal cord stimulation is thought to produce inhibition of dorsal horn wide dynamic range hyperexcitability, which induces release of gamma-aminobutyric acid. Additional studies have also demonstrated stimulation-induced release of adenosine, serotonin, noradrenalin, and acetylcholine, which contribute to descending inhibition resulting in pain reduction.[5] There have been randomized controlled trials on spinal cord stimulation for failed back surgery syndrome that showed significant improvement in pain and subject satisfaction in comparison with reoperation,[7] as well as significant improvement in pain, quality of life, and function in comparison with conventional medical management.[8]

Burst Stimulation

Burst spinal cord stimulation was introduced as a type of spinal cord stimulation that delivers 5 pulses of 500 Hz, each with 40 Hz frequency at a constant pulse width of 1 ms.[5] The groups of pulses are separated by pulse-free periods, which are supposed to resemble physiologic nervous activity. In addition, the amplitudes used are lower than those used in tonic stimulation, and approximately 17% of patients report paresthesia during burst stimulation.[9] The irregular bursts of firing of the stimulation are thought to be more similar to normal nerve activity and are thought to modulate both the lateral spinothalamic pathways, which are responsible for the discriminatory components of pain, as well as the medial spinothalamic pathway, which acts to modulate pain perception by influencing the affective components of pain.[5,10] There have been several randomized controlled trials comparing burst stimulation to tonic stimulation in subjects with both axial back and limb pain. In 2013, in a randomized placebo controlled trial in which 15 subjects with axial back pain and limb pain received tonic stimulation and burst spinal cord stimulation, as well as placebo, in a randomized fashion for a week each, De Ridder and colleagues[11] demonstrated that burst was superior to both tonic stimulation and placebo in decreasing visual analog scores (VAS) for axial back pain. In a similar trial design involving 20 subjects, Schu and colleagues[12] also demonstrated significant improvement in pain relief with burst stimulation. Most recently, Deer and colleagues[13] presented a randomized controlled trial in which 100 subjects with axial back pain and/or limb pain received tonic stimulation and burst stimulation in randomized sequence for 12 weeks at a time and demonstrated that burst stimulation was superior to tonic stimulation in decreasing VAS scores that were sustained through 1 year.

High-Frequency Stimulation

High-frequency stimulation provides frequencies up to 10,000 Hz (HF-10). Clinically, this is a paresthesia-free form of neuromodulation whereby patients do not sense stimulus. The definitive mechanisms of high-frequency spinal cord stimulation are not known. However, animal studies have demonstrated that administration of high-frequency stimulation has resulted in suppression of spontaneous activity and hyperpolarization of dorsal horn cells, decreasing the windup of these neurons.[5] Shechter and colleagues[14] (2013) showed that higher frequency stimulation at 1 kHz and 10 kHz reduced mechanical hypersensitivity in a spinal nerve ligation rat model at lower intensities. The first randomized controlled trial involving high-frequency spinal cord stimulation for back pain was published by Perruchoud and colleagues[15] in 2013, in which they demonstrated no significant difference in pain relief between subjects who had received high-frequency stimulation at 5 kHz and those who received placebo stimulation. In contrast,

Kapural and colleagues[16] published a randomized controlled study in which 198 subjects with both back and leg pain were randomized to either HF-10 or traditional low-frequency spinal cord stimulation. At 3 months and 12 months, more subjects with HF-10 stimulation had significant pain relief, defined as greater than 50% reduction in back pain, than the traditional stimulation group.[16] In a follow-up study, Kapural and colleagues[17] reported that effect was sustained at 24 months; in subjects receiving high-frequency HF-10 therapy, back pain was found to decrease more substantially (66.9%) than those receiving conventional spinal cord stimulation (41.1%).

Dorsal Root Ganglion Stimulation

Dorsal root ganglion stimulation has recently developed as an option for neuropathic and dermatomal-specific pain. From an anatomic standpoint, the paired dorsal root ganglia are located distal to the dorsal root in the lateral epidural space; they contain a variety of neural elements, including somatic and visceral sensory cell bodies, serving as a thoroughfare for sensorial information.[18] Dorsal root ganglionectomy involves open surgery for recalcitrant radicular pain,[19] although pulsed radiofrequency has been studied as a technique to change transcriptional activity and plasticity to contribute to pain relief.[20] Building off the observation that stimulation of dorsal root ganglion cell bodies reduces ectopic firing,[20,21] dorsal root ganglia have been directly stimulated via epidural leads directed through the intervertebral foramen and then in proximity to the dorsal root ganglion (**Fig. 2**). Liem and colleagues[22] reported significant benefit in a multicenter trial consisting of 32 subjects with complex regional pain syndrome, failed back surgery syndrome, radicular pain, and other conditions who proceeded to receive dorsal root ganglion stimulator implants. Through the course of this study, a total of 57.1%, 70%, and 88.9% of subjects reported greater than 50% improvement at 6 months of back, leg and foot pain, respectively.

RADIOFREQUENCY DENERVATION FOR FACET PAIN

It is estimated that facet-mediated pain is responsible for 15% to 45% of patients with low back pain and for 36% to 60% of patients with chronic neck pain.[23] Facet joints are true synovial joints composed of hyaline cartilage, which stabilize the entire length of the spine. In the lumbar spine, each facet joint is innervated by 2 medial branches of the dorsal rami: the medial branch from the same level and from the level above.[24] In the cervical spine, the innervation of the cervical facets

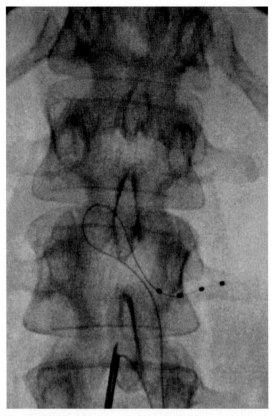

Fig. 2. A dorsal root ganglion stimulator 4-contact lead placed through intervertebral foramen and close to dorsal root ganglion.

is also from the same level and the level above, with the exception of the cervical nerve (C) 2-C3 and the atlantoaxial joint, which are more complex.[25] These medial branches can be targeted for radiofrequency ablation in those patients who have had a single medial branch block that resulted in greater than 50% improvement in pain. In the lumbar region, the active tip of the radiofrequency cannula is positioned at the junction of the transverse process and the superior articular process. In the cervical region, it is placed along the center of the articular pillars (Fig. 3). It is essential that the cannula lie parallel to the medial branches to create the optimal lesion size. Patients are then tested for the presence of sensory stimulation at 50 Hz at less than 0.5 V and for lack of motor contraction in the lower extremities with motor stimulation at 3 times the sensory threshold to ensure proper placement of the cannula before lesioning.[26]

To date, there have been 12 randomized controlled studies addressing lumbar medial branch ablation, with follow-up periods ranging from 3 to 6 months. The results from these studies are variable, given that some studies fail to select subjects appropriately through diagnostic blocks or fail to use optimal technique.[27] One such controversial study was the multicenter, non-blinded, randomized controlled trial on the effectiveness of Minimal Interventional Treatments for Participants with Chronic Low Back Pain (MINT)

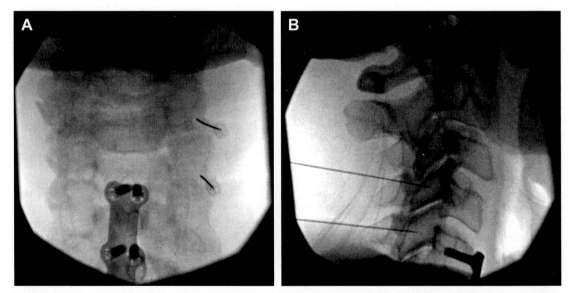

Fig. 3. (A) Anteroposterior view of cervical facet radiofrequency denervation; needles are directed toward the articular pillars. (B) Lateral view of cervical facet radiofrequency denervation, needle tips located at the center of the trapezoid of the articular pillar.

study published by Juch and colleagues.[28] This trial included 681 participants who had a diagnosis of chronic low back pain from the lumbar facet or sacroiliac joints, intervertebral disks, or any combination of those causes who were unresponsive to conservative care. These subjects were then randomized to receive a 3-month standardized exercise program or undergo radiofrequency denervation along with an exercise program. The conclusion of this study was that the radiofrequency denervation group showed no clinically significant improvement in the numeric rating scale (NRS) than the control group. There have been several criticisms of this study; specifically, that it is a pragmatic study as opposed to a clinical trial because the latter would be more rigorously designed to determine the efficacy of a treatment. In addition, the method of radiofrequency ablation was widely varied (monopolar, bipolar, cooled, and multielectrode radiofrequency ablation) and the approach of the needle, which was perpendicular to the medial branch as opposed to parallel, resulted in widely different lesion sizes and a much smaller likelihood of ablation of the medial branch.

In contrast, earlier studies by Lord and colleagues[29] and Stovner and colleagues[30] demonstrated the efficacy of cervical medial branch radiofrequency ablation in subjects with cervical facet arthropathy. Overall, there is favorable evidence for the use of radiofrequency ablation in patients with lumbar and cervical facet-mediated pain given that the patients are well selected and that proper techniques are used.[27]

Radiofrequency ablation has been investigated for its utility in treating cervicogenic headache at the C2-C3 joints and for arthropathy at the C1-C2 (atlantoaxial) joints, both conditions involving sites with complex anatomy. Lateral atlantoaxial injections have been used to successfully treatment arthropathy at this site but without significant duration of benefit. These can also be associated with adverse events. A case series reported from the Mayo Clinic indicated an adverse event rate of about 18.5% in such procedures.[31] For longer-lasting relief, conventional and pulsed radiofrequency have been used treat atlantoaxial pain. Halim and colleagues[32] reported successful pulsed radiofrequency (settings 45 V, 2 Hz, and 10 ms) of C1-C2 joint in a retrospective study of 86 subjects; in this group, 44.2% of subjects reported greater than or equal to 50% pain at 1 year. In this report, needles were placed toward the anteromedial aspect of the lateral atlantoaxial (C1-C2) joint. Studies have also examined the efficacy of radiofrequency denervation for lower cervical facet arthropathy. For example, Lord and colleagues[29] reported on a placebo-controlled trial in 24 subjects, comparing therapeutic lesioning at 80°C to sham lesioning at 37°C. The time to return of 50% of preprocedural pain was significantly higher (263 days) in the treatment group versus the sham group (8 days), P<.04, showing statistical significance.

DISCOGRAPHY AND BIACUPLASTY

Discogenic pain is responsible for about 40% of cases of lower back pain, particularly toward the later decades of life.[33] It is difficult to diagnose and has complex pathophysiology. The intervertebral disc is a complex structure comprising a tough annulus fibrosus encircling the soft nucleus propulsus.[34] Intervertebral discs can develop injuries such as fissures at a histopathological level but also exhibit cellular and molecular changes such as inflammation and neovascularization,[35,36] leading to the sensation of pain in patients.

Fluoroscopic imaging plays a role in both the diagnosis and therapy for discogenic pain. Although MR imaging can detect structural defects in intervertebral discs, provocative discography has been used to detect whether those lesions are symptomatic. In this procedure, the injection of contrast into the nucleus pulposus pressurizes the intervertebral disc; a positive result is noted if this causes pain.[37] Per the Spine Intervention Society guidelines, it is important that the pain resembles the patient's symptoms and that control disc pressurization at an adjacent level does not elicit pain. Discography is controversial and invasive, leading to possible complications such as infection, bleeding, and disc rupture; it is also associated with a high rate of false positives in some studies, although metaanalysis has revealed its utility in select populations.[33]

Discogenic pain has also been a target for therapeutic procedures aided with fluoroscopic visualization. Intradiscal electrothermal therapy (IDET) and intradiscal biacuplasty (IDB) are techniques that use electric current to generate heat, producing thermal lesions used to target innervation of the disc itself and the putative source of pain. The mechanism of action is suspected to involve either thermal modification of collagen fibers, other biochemical and cellular changes, or destruction of nociceptive nervous inputs in the disc itself. Because there is significant nerve intrusion into the annulus in disc degeneration, thermoablation of the posterior aspect of the annulus fibrosus has been a focus of some interventions.[38] Although these techniques have been a focus of research, reimbursement issues have limited their widespread use. For example, the Centers for

Medicare and Medicaid Services (CMS) issued a decision not to cover these services in 2008.[39]

IDET or annuloplasty is a minimally invasive technique that has been used in lieu of more invasive techniques such as spinal fusion. The technique was first reported by Saal and Saal[40] in 2000, whereby catheters were deployed through needles adjacent to the inner posterior disc annulus. A high success rate was reported in terms of percentage of patients endorsing improvement, and this improvement was also statistically significant. Multiple other studies have confirmed the successful application of IDET therapy in different study populations.[41,42] IDET has also been found to be effective in a significant number of 93 subjects in a recent retrospective study in which 86.52% of subjects who followed up showed improvement, verifying its utility in this clinical context.[43] This technique seems to have fallen out of favor recently due to difficulties with insurance recognition and reimbursement.

Biacuplasty involves a variation of thermotherapy in which radiofrequency probes (Baylis Medical Inc, Montreal, Canada) can be placed on the posterolateral sides of the annulus fibrosus, as first reported by Kapural and Mekhail[44] in 2007. In their case report, a patient endorsed improvement at 1 and 6 months. This technique was described to be less technically challenging than conventional IDET therapy. Kapural and colleagues[45] (2015) later described how 22 out of 27 subjects described improvement in symptoms at 6 and 12 months, further suggesting that this technique can be a useful procedure for discogenic pain. Desai and colleagues[46] (2016) performed an additional randomized multicenter trial, including 63 subjects, confirming a statistically significant difference in reduced VAS in subjects receiving IDB therapy versus conservative management for lumbar discogenic pain. At 6 months, subjects receiving IDB reported a mean 2.4 score decrease in pain, whereas those receiving conservative therapy reported a mean 0.56 score change. At 12 months, the investigators reported continued benefit in the interventional group.[47]

PERCUTANEOUS IMAGE-GUIDED LUMBAR DECOMPRESSION

Lumbar spinal stenosis is a common cause of lower back and lower extremity pain, and results from narrowing of the spinal canal. Anatomically, stenosis can result from degeneration, lipomatosis, ligamentum flavum hypertrophy, infection, or even cancer, whereas the symptoms, most notably neurogenic claudication, may result from ischemia or increased pressure.[48–50] This condition is progressive and can be challenging to treat with either conservative or interventional means. Percutaneous image-guided lumbar decompression is defined by the CMS as a technique completed under image guidance to debulk lamina and ligamentum flavum noninvasively. These techniques for treating lumbar spinal stenosis (Vertiflex, Vertos Medical, Aliso Viejo, CA, USA) can permit a less invasive removal of interlaminar bone, therefore permitting patients who may not be candidates for traditional decompression or fusion to undergo procedural intervention. Several manufacturers (MILD, Vertos Medical, Aliso Viejo, CA, USA, and Totalis, Vertiflex Spine, Carlsbad, CA, USA) have produced devices that are used for percutaneous imaged-guided decompression. Under monitored anesthesia care, trocars can be inserted percutaneously and used to facilitate decompression of laminar bone. Afterward tissue sculpters can be used to remove ligamentum flavum, decompressing stenotic regions of spine and relieving pressure.[51]

Several studies have compared the results of percutaneous lumbar decompression to conservative management or injections. Two prospective randomized controlled trials compared MILD directly to lumbar epidural steroid injections. Benyamin and Staats[52] randomized 302 subjects with symptoms consistent with lumbar stenosis to epidural steroids or minimally invasive decompression. Of subjects who underwent treatment and followed up at 1 year, those who received percutaneous decompression reported a statistically significant, relatively higher decrease in the NRS (mean −2.8 vs 0.7) and the Oswetry Disability Index score (mean −16.2 vs −4.4), reflecting greater improvements in pain sensation and function. A smaller study confirmed that minimally invasive decompression was more beneficial compared with epidural steroid injections in subjects who had failed conservative therapy.[53] In that study, of 38 subjects initially randomized, subjects were separated into groups receiving decompression or epidural steroid injection. Subjects receiving decompression reported a mean VAS score of 3.8 (compared with 6.3 at baseline) at 6 weeks versus achieving 6.3 from a baseline of 6.4 for subjects receiving epidural steroid injections.

Based on these trials, as well as prospective observational and retrospective studies, the Minimally Invasive Spine Treatment (MIST) guidelines have been developed to identify patients who are appropriate candidates for this procedure.[54] These guidelines have been published to determine appropriateness for minimally invasive spinal therapy for lumbar spinal stenosis. Published in

Table 1
Treatment of specific syndromes of spine pain

Spine Pain Syndrome	Technique
Failed back surgery syndrome Chronic low back pain secondary to facet arthropathy or lumbar radiculopathy not responsive to more conservative management	Spinal cord stimulation • Tonic • Burst • High-frequency
Lumbar facet arthropathy	Lumbar medial branch radiofrequency ablation
Cervical facet arthropathy	Cervical medial branch radiofrequency ablation
Discogenic pain	IDET IDB
Lumbar stenosis	Percutaneous image-guided lumbar decompression

2018, the MIST guidelines notably stated that there was level 1 evidence for percutaneous lumbar decompression as superior to epidural steroid injections and suggested MR imaging interpretation by the proceduralist and that reactivity is monitored to minimize any risks of injury.

SUMMARY

Spine pain is a symptom of a wide range of etiologic factors, ranging from discogenic pain to epidural scarring in patients who have undergone surgery. Interventional approaches for spine pain, including epidural steroid injections and facet denervation, have complemented conservative management such as medications and physical therapy. This article has highlighted more advanced approaches for specific disease states such as spinal cord stimulation, facet denervation, disc thermocoagulation, and percutaneous lumbar decompression, focusing on the role that these have in treatment of specific syndromes of spine pain **(Table 1)**. This is a rapidly emerging field, and new methodologies for image-guided minimally invasive therapy are on the horizon.

REFERENCES

1. Manchikanti L, Singh V, Datta S, et al, American Society of Interventional Pain Physicians. Comprehensive review of epidemiology, scope, and impact of spinal pain. Pain Physician 2009;12:E35–70.
2. Martin BI, Deyo RA, Mirza SK, et al. Expenditures and health status among adults with back and neck problems. JAMA 2008;299:656–64.
3. Gildenberg PL. History of electrical neuromodulation for chronic pain. Pain Med 2006;7:S7–13.
4. Melzack R, Wall PD. Pain mechanisms: a new theory. Science 1965;150:971–9.
5. Linderoth B, Foreman RD. Conventional and novel spinal stimulation algorithms: hypothetical mechanisms of action and comments on outcomes. Neuromodulation 2017;20:525–33.
6. Kreis PG, Fishman S. Spinal cord stimulation: percutaneous implantation techniques. New York: Oxford University Press; 2009. p. 1–8.
7. North RB, Kidd DH, Farrokhi F, et al. Spinal cord stimulation versus repeated lumbosacral spine surgery for chronic pain: a randomized controlled trial. Neurosurgery 2005;56:98–107.
8. Kumar K, Taylor RS, Jacques L, et al. The effects of spinal cord stimulation in neuropathic pain are sustained: a 24-month follow-up of the prospective randomized controlled multicenter trial of the effectiveness of spinal cord stimulation. Neurosurgery 2008;63:762–70.
9. De Ridder D, Vanneste S, Plazier M, et al. Burst spinal cord stimulation: toward paresthesia-free pain suppression. Neurosurgery 2010;66:986–90.
10. De Ridder D, Vanneste S, Plazier M, et al. Mimicking the brain: evaluation of St Jude Medical's Prodigy chronic pain system with burst technology. Expert Rev Med Devices 2015;12:143–50.
11. De Ridder D, Plazier M, Lamerling N, et al. Burst spinal cord stimulation for limb and back pain. World Neurosurg 2013;80:642–9.
12. Schu S, Slotty PJ, Bara G, et al. A prospective, randomised, double-blind, placebo-controlled study to examine the effectiveness of burst spinal cord stimulation patterns for the treatment of failed back surgery syndrome. Neuromodulation 2014; 17:443–50.
13. Deer T, Slavin KV, Amirdelfan K, et al. Success using neuromodulation with BURST (SUNBURST) study: results from a prospective, randomized controlled trial using a novel burst waveform. Neuromodulation 2018;21:56–66.
14. Shechter R, Yang F, Xu Q, et al. Conventional and kilohertz-frequency spinal cord stimulation produces intensity and frequency dependent inhibition of mechanical hypersensitivity in a rat model of neuropathic pain. Anesthesiology 2013;119:422–32.

15. Perruchoud C, Eldabe S, Batterham AM, et al. Analgesic efficacy of high-frequency spinal cord stimulation: a randomized double-blind placebo-controlled study. Neuromodulation 2013;16:363–9.

16. Kapural L, Yu C, Doust MW, et al. Novel 10-kHz high-frequency therapy (HF10 therapy) is superior to traditional low-frequency spinal cord stimulation for the treatment of chronic back and leg pain. Anesthesiology 2015;123:851–60.

17. Kapural L, Yu C, Doust MW, et al. Comparison of 10-kHz high-frequency and traditional low-frequency spinal cord stimulation for the treatment of chronic back and leg pain: 24-month results from a multicenter, randomized, controlled pivotal trial. Neurosurgery 2016;79:667–77.

18. Pope JE, Deer TR, Kramer J. A systematic review: current and future directions of dorsal root ganglion therapeutics to treat chronic pain. Pain Med 2013; 14:1477–96.

19. North RB, Kidd DH, Campbell JN, et al. Dorsal root ganglionectomy for failed back surgery syndrome: a 5-year follow-up study. J Neurosurg 1991;74: 236–42.

20. Liem L, van Dongen E, Huygen FJ, et al. The dorsal root ganglion as a therapeutic target for chronic pain. Reg Anesth Pain Med 2016;41:511–9.

21. Van Buyten JP. Dorsal root ganglion stimulation. In: Benzon HT, Raja SN, Fishman SM, et al, editors. Essentials of pain medicine. 4th edition. Philadelphia: Elsevier; 2018. p. 683–92.e2.

22. Liem L, Russo M, Huygen FJ, et al. A multicenter, prospective trial to assess the safety and performance of the spinal modulation dorsal root ganglion neurostimulator system in the treatment of chronic pain. Neuromodulation 2013;16:471–82.

23. Boswell MV, Colson JD, Sehgal N, et al. A systematic review of therapeutic facet joint interventions in chronic spinal pain. Pain Physician 2007;10:229–53.

24. Cohen SP, Raja SN. Pathogenesis, diagnosis, and treatment of lumbar zygapophysial (facet) joint pain. Anesthesiology 2007;106:591–614.

25. Bogduk N. The clinical anatomy of the cervical dorsal rami. Spine 1982;7:319–30.

26. Rathmell JP. Atlas of image-guided intervention in regional anesthesia and pain medicine. Philadelphia: Wolters Kluwer/Lippincott Williams & Wilkins Health; 2012.

27. Huang-Lionnet JH, Brummett C, Cohen SP. Facet syndrome. In: Benzon HT, Raja SN, Fishman SM, et al, editors. Essentials of pain medicine. 4th edition. Philadelphia: Elsevier; 2018. p. 591–600.e2.

28. Juch JNS, Maas ET, Ostelo RWJG, et al. Effect of radiofrequency denervation on pain intensity among patients with chronic low back pain. JAMA 2017; 318:68–81.

29. Lord SM, Barnsley L, Wallis BJ, et al. Percutaneous radiofrequency neurotomy for chronic cervical zygapophyseal joint pain. N Engl J Med 1996;335: 1721–6.

30. Stovner L, Kolstad F, Helde G. Radiofrequency denervation of facet joints C2-C6 in cervicogenic headache: a randomized, double-blind, sham-controlled Study. Cephalalgia 2004;24:821–30.

31. Aiudi CM, Hooten WM, Sanders RA, et al. Outcomes of C1-2 joint injections. J Pain Res 2017;10: 2263–9.

32. Halim W, Chua NHL, Vissers KC. Long-term pain relief in patients with cervicogenic headaches after pulsed radiofrequency application into the lateral atlantoaxial (C1-2) joint using an anterolateral approach. Pain Pract 2010;10:267–71.

33. Cohen SP. Discography. In: Benzon HT, Raja SN, Fishman SM, et al, editors. Essentials of pain medicine. 4th edition. Philadelphia: Elsevier; 2018. p. 627–38.e2.

34. Raj PP. Intervertebral disc: anatomy-physiology-pathophysiology-treatment. Pain Pract 2008;8: 18–44.

35. Garcia-Cosamalon J, del Valle ME, Calavia MG, et al. Intervertebral disc, sensory nerves and neurotrophins: who is who in discogenic pain? J Anat 2010;217:1–15.

36. Peng B, Wu W, Hou S, et al. The pathogenesis of discogenic low back pain. J Bone Joint Surg Br 2005; 87:62–7.

37. Gruver C, Guthmiller KB. Provocative discography. State pearls [Internet]. Treasure Island (FL): Stat Pearls Publishing; 2018.

38. Wetzel TF, McNally TA, Phillips FM. Intradiscal electrothermal therapy used to manage chronic discogenic low back pain: new directions and interventions. Spine (Phila Pa 1976) 2002;15: 2621–6.

39. Phurrough S, Salive ME, O'Connor D, et al. Decision memo for thermal intradiscal procedures (CAG-00387N) 2008. Available at: https://www.cms.gov/medicare-coverage-database/details/nca-decision memo.aspx?NCAId=215&bc=AAAAAAAAACAA&. Accessed January 26, 2019.

40. Saal JS, Saal JA. Management of chronic discogenic low back pain with a thermal intradiscal catheter: a preliminary report. Spine 2000;25:382–8.

41. Pauza KJ, Howell S, Dreyfuss P, et al. A randomized, placebo-controlled trial of intradiscal electrothermal therapy for the treatment of discogenic low back pain. Spine J 2004;4:27–35.

42. Freedman BA, Cohen SP, Kuklo TR, et al. Intradiscal electrothermal therapy (IDET) for chronic low back pain in active-duty soldiers: 2-year follow-up. Spine J 2003;3:502–9.

43. Tsou H, Chao S, Kao T, et al. Intradiscal electrothermal therapy in the treatment of chronic low back pain: experience with 93 patients. Surg Neurol Int 2010;1:37.

44. Kapural L, Mekhail N. Novel intradiscal biacuplasty (IDB) for the treatment of lumbar discogenic pain. Pain Pract 2007;7:130–4.

45. Kapural L, Vrooman B, Sarwar S, et al. Radiofrequency intradiscal biacuplasty for treatment of discogenic lower back pain: a 12-month follow-up. Pain Med 2015;16:425–31.

46. Desai MJ, Kapural L, Petersohn JD, et al. A prospective, randomized, multicenter, open-label clinical trial comparing intradiscal biacuplasty to conventional medical management for discogenic lumbar back pain. Spine (Phila Pa 1976) 2016;41: 1065–74.

47. Desai MJ, Kapural L, Petersohn JD, et al. Twelve-month follow-up of a randomized clinical trial comparing intradiscal biacuplasty to conventional medical management for discogenic lumbar back pain. Pain Med 2017;18:751–63.

48. Siebert E, Pruss H, Klingebiel R, et al. Lumbar spinal stenosis: syndrome, diagnostics and treatment. Nat Rev Neurol 2009;5:392–403.

49. Yoshiiwa T, Miyazaki M, Notani N, et al. Analysis of the relationship between ligamentum flavum thickening and lumbar segmental instability, disc degeneration, and facet joint osteoarthritis in lumbar spinal stenosis. Asian Spine J 2016;10:1132–40.

50. Kosaka H, Sairyo K, Biyani A, et al. Pathomechanism of loss of elasticity and hypertrophy of lumbar ligamentum flavum in elderly patients with lumbar spinal canal stenosis. Spine (Phila Pa 1976) 2007;32: 2805–11.

51. Lawrence MM, Hayek SM. Minimally invasive lumbar decompression: a treatment for lumbar spinal stenosis. Curr Opin Anaesthesiol 2013;26: 573–9.

52. Benyamin RM, Staats PS, for the MiDAS ENCORE Investigators. MILD® is an effective treatment for lumbar spinal stenosis with neurogenic claudication: MiDAS ENCORE randomized controlled trial. Pain Physician 2016;19:229–42.

53. Brown LL. A double blind, randomized, prospective study of epidural steroid injection vs. the mild® procedure in patients with symptomatic lumbar spinal stenosis. Pain Pract 2012;12:333–41.

54. Deer TR, Grider JS, Pope JE, et al. The MIST Guidelines: the Lumbar Spinal Stenosis Consensus Group guidelines for minimally invasive spine treatment. Pain Pract 2019;19(3):250–74.

Image-Guided Percutaneous Treatment of Lumbar Stenosis and Disc Degeneration

Stefano Marcia, MD[a],*, Chiara Zini, MD, PhD[b], Matteo Bellini, MD[c]

KEYWORDS

• Lumbar stenosis • Disc degeneration • Low back pain • Image-guided procedures

KEY POINTS

- Spinal stenosis has been defined as narrowing of the lumbar spinal canal, lateral nerve roots, and/or intervertebral neural foramina clinically related to neurogenic intermittent claudication.
- Pain caused by nerve root compression (so-called sciatica) is associated with numbness and paresthesia localized to the affected dermatome.
- Patients with spinal pain are initially managed conservatively with medical therapies and physical therapy, although the efficacy of steroid injection is controversial.
- The percutaneous minimally invasive approach in discogenic and radicular pain is designed to reduce the volume of the nucleus pulposus using chemical, thermal, or mechanical sources in patients with failure of medical therapy.
- Interspinous process devices decrease facet join overload, reducing the intradiscal pressure with segmental enlargement of the spinal canal, as shown in cadaveric studies.

INTRODUCTION

Low back pain (LBP) and lumbar spinal stenosis (LSS) are the most common of all chronic pain disorders leading to pain, disability, fall risk, and depression, in addition to the enormous related economic costs, societal impairment, and health impact.[1]

A recent meta-analysis showed a total of 266 million people (3.63%) worldwide with degenerative spine disease annually.[2]

The lifetime prevalence of spinal pain has been reported as 54% to 80%, with a recurrence rate ranging from 24% to 80%; currently, up to 50% of the population more than 65 years of age experiences LBP, so the incidence of spinal pain is projected to continue to grow as the population ages.[3–5]

The estimated cost of spinal pain in the United States has been calculated to range from $560 billion to $630 billion per year but it could also be higher because the incidence of spinal pain is increasing with the cost of spine-related care.[5,6]

Spinal stenosis has been defined as narrowing of the lumbar spinal canal, lateral nerve roots,

Disclosure: S. Marcia, Techlamed consultant; C. Zini, nothing to disclose; M. Bellini, nothing to disclose.
[a] Ahead Diagnostic and Interventional Radiology Unit, Hospital "Santissima Trinità", ATS Sardegna ASSL, Cagliari, Italy; [b] UOC Neuroimmagini e Neurointerventistica, Dipartimento di Scienze Neurologiche e Motorie, Azienda Ospedaliera Universitaria Senese, via Bracci 16, 53100 Siena, Italy; [c] UOC Neuroimmagini e Neurointerventistica, Dipartimento di Scienze Neurologiche e Motorie, Azienda Ospedaliera Universitaria Senese, via Bracci 16, 53100 Siena, Italy
* Corresponding author. Unità di Radiologia, Ospedale Santissima Trinità, ATS Sardegna ASSL, Via Is Mirrionis, 92, Cagliari 09121, Italy.
E-mail address: stemarcia@gmail.com

and/or intervertebral neural foramina caused by progressive hypertrophy of any of the surrounding osseous, fibrous, and ligamentous elements and resulting in neural and/or vascular compression.[7]

Clinical symptoms are generally an expression of the spinal stenosis grading and level of compression, ranging from LBP, sometimes associated with stiffness, to lower extremity pain, relived by setting and flexion with or without stiffness, paresthesia/weakness, and/or cramping; so-called neurogenic intermittent claudication (NIC).[8]

Pain caused by nerve root chronic compression, so-called chronic sciatica, is associated with numbness and paresthesia and it is usually localized to the affected dermatome.[8]

Patients with spinal pain are initially managed conservatively with medical therapies and physical therapy.[7]

Because of surgery-related risks and the good results in terms of outcomes, nonresponding patients are frequently treated with percutaneous treatments[8–11]; decompressive surgery is suggested to improve outcomes in patients with moderate to severe symptoms of LSS.[12]

NORMAL ANATOMY AND IMAGING TECHNIQUE

The basic anatomic unit of the spine consists of the paired zygapophysial joints and the intervertebral disc, able to support and stabilize the spine and prevent injury by limiting motion in all planes of movement.[13]

Intervertebral disc dehydratation and subsequent narrowing of the disc space lead to initial relative instability and hypermobility of the spine, with an increase of the pressure between the lumbar zygapophysial (l-z) joint resulting in zygapophysial joint degeneration, particularly at the level of the superior articular process.[13,14]

This process leads to a reduction of the spinal canal dimensions and compression of the neural elements.[14]

Anatomically, spinal stenosis can be categorized as central and lateral forms (**Figs. 1 and 2**).

A

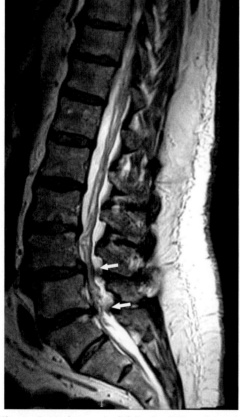

B

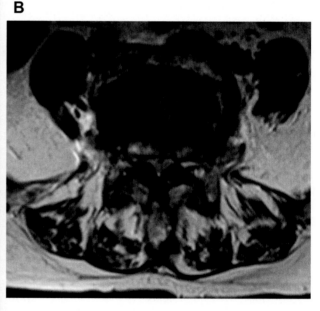

Fig. 1. Central stenosis. (*A*) Sagittal T2-weighted image shows a central canal stenosis with relevant compression of cauda equina caused by important disc bulging and facet joint degeneration (*arrows*). (*B*) Axial T2-weighted image shows spinal canal and foraminal degenerative stenosis with nerve root involvement.

A

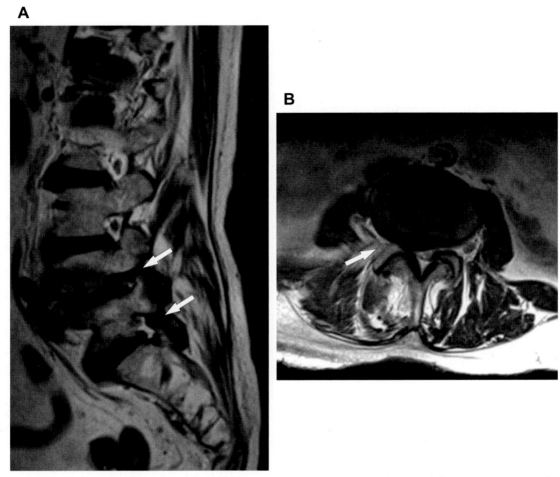

B

Fig. 2. Lateral stenosis. (*A*) Sagittal T2-weighted image shows relevant right foraminal degenerative stenosis (*arrows*). (*B*) Axial T2-weighted image shows nerve root involvement at the level of L4-L5 caused by foraminal stenosis and disc prolapse (*arrow*).

The central spinal stenosis is the result of the involvement of the area between the facet joints, occupied by the dura mater and its contents, frequently related to hypertrophy of the inferior facet articular process of cephalic vertebra[14,15]; it is clinically associated with NIC, resulting from the mechanical compression to the nerve root, the artery, and the vein surrounding the nerve root and leading to ischemic neuritis.[16]

In contrast, hypertrophy of the inferior facet articular process of caudal vertebrae leads to lateral stenosis.[15] Lateral recess stenosis could be related to the involvement of the lateral recess (also called Lee's entrance zone, anatomically described as being from the lateral border of the dura to the medial border of the pedicle), the foraminal area (the so-called Lee's midzone, occupied by the ganglion and the ventral motor root), and extraforaminal stenosis.[15]

Patients with lateral recess stenosis experienced pain with dermatomeric distribution, especially during rest and the nighttime but with more walking tolerance compared with patients with central stenosis.[14]

Spinal stenosis can be congenital or acquired; spinal acquired stenosis has been related to[14]:

- Degenerative disc disease
- Somatic osteophytosis
- Thickening and calcification of the ligament flavum
- Facet hypertrophy and osteophytosis

Accurate clinical history and physical examination are mandatory in the evaluation of patients with suspicious LSS and LBP (**Tables 1** and **2**).[17]

Plain radiographs are useful in evaluating alignment, loss of disc height, and osteophyte formation; however, they do not provide any

Table 1
Diagnostic criteria

Central stenosis (LSS is characterized by spinal canal narrowing)	• Lower extremity pain, relived by setting and flexion with or without stiffness, paresthesias/weakness, and/or cramping (NIC) • Usually bilateral • Pain distribution in the lower extremities depends on the area of stenosis • Stoop test can be positive
Lateral stenosis (LSS is characterized by chronic nerve root compression)	• Pain with dermatomeric distribution, especially during the rest and the nighttime but with more walking tolerance compared with the patients with central stenosis • Back pain • Straight leg raising and Lasègue tests may be positive

Table 2
Differential diagnosis

Central stenosis (LSS is characterized by spinal canal narrowing)	• Vascular claudication: pain usually in the calf and relieved by resting (flexing forward does not relieve pain); bicycling triggers claudication • Osteoarthritis of the hip and knee • Myelopathy as the cause of walking difficulties • Peripheral nerve entrapment involving a lower limb (meralgia paraesthetica, Morton neuralgia in foot pain) • Central disc herniation
Lateral stenosis (LSS is characterized by chronic nerve root compression)	• Back pain with a local cause and other factors • Muscle trigger points at the lumbar spine/buttock/lower limb • Other neurologic causes

information about the presence of anatomic narrowing of the spinal canal and/or the nerve root impingement.[14]

Magnetic resonance (MR) imaging is suggested as the most appropriate, noninvasive test to confirm the presence of anatomic narrowing of the spinal canal or the presence of nerve root impingement[12] (**Table 3**); in case of inconclusive or contraindicated MR imaging, computed tomography (CT) myelography results are comparable in the diagnosis of LSS.[18]

CT imaging (CTI) is the preferred test to confirm the presence of anatomic narrowing of the spinal canal and/or nerve root impingement for which MR imaging and CT myelography are contraindicated, inconclusive, or inappropriate.[12]

Normal spinal canal size has been defined as having a midsagittal diameter of more than 11.5 mm and an area more than 1.45 cm^2;[15] and a spinal stenosis is described as absolute stenosis, when the midsagittal diameter of the canal is less than 10 mm, or relative stenosis, when the midsagittal diameter of the canal is between 10 mm and 13 mm.[15,19]

Disk degeneration can be graded on MR imaging T2 spin-echo–weighted images using a grading system proposed by Pfirrmann and colleagues[20] and subsequently modified by Griffith and colleagues[21] (**Table 4**); herniation can be classified as contained, with intact outer fibers of

Table 3
Magnetic resonance image protocol

Standard protocol	• T1-weighted sagittal • Proton density and T2 pulse sequences in both the axial[a] and sagittal planes
Additional sequences	• STIR • T1-weighted images before and after contrast media injection

Abbreviation: STIR, short tau inversion recovery.
[a] Axial sections should be obtained for at least the L5-S1, L4-5, and L3-4 levels; additional axial sections can be obtained through adjacent or more cephalad levels as indicated.

Table 4
Pfirrmann classification

Grade I	• Homogeneous disk with bright signal intensity • Normal disk height
Grade II	• Inhomogeneous disk with hyper-intense white signal • Nucleus and annulus are clearly differentiated, and a gray horizontal band could be present • Normal disk height
Grade III	• Inhomogeneous disk with an intermittent gray signal intensity • Unclear distinction between nucleus and annulus • Normal or slightly decreased disk height
Grade IV	• Inhomogeneous disk with a hypo-intense dark gray signal intensity • No more distinction between the nucleus and annulus • Disk height is slightly or moderately decreased
Grade V	• Inhomogeneous disk with a hypo-intense black signal intensity • Disk space is collapsed with no more difference between the nucleus and annulus

Data from Pfirrmann CW, Metzdorf A, Zanetti M et-al. Magnetic resonance classification of lumbar intervertebral disc degeneration. Spine. 2001;26 : 1873-8.

annulus fibrosus and posterior longitudinal ligament, or not contained, with a tear of outer fibers of annulus fibrosus and posterior longitudinal ligament.[22]

Although these measurements are useful as guidelines, there is a lack of correlation between symptoms and spinal canal narrowing on MR imaging or CTI, whereas the degree of impingement on the nerve root seems to be more reliable.[23,24]

IMAGE-GUIDED PERCUTANEOUS TREATMENTS

Selection of patients is mandatory to achieve successful treatment.[25]

Patients must be interviewed before their procedures in order to select and plan the treatment.[17]

Focused clinical history and physical examination need to be correlated with the imaging findings[17]; the procedure details and expected results must be described in detail to the patient in order to obtain the requested procedure approval or have a different one proposed, with a written informed consent signed at the end of the interview.[17]

Image-Guided Steroid Injection

Although the efficacy of steroid injection is controversial, no comprehensive guidelines are available, and corticosteroid infiltration is widely used in the treatment of spinal pain to reduce the local inflammation and subsequently the pain.[26]

The goal of image-guided steroid injection is to target and deliver the drug at the level of the area involved in inflammation, sparing the surrounding structures; hence, image-guided injections are preferred to blind procedures to avoid needle displacement: non–fluoroscopically guided caudal epidural injections have a rate of inaccurate placement ranging from 25% to 53% and lumbar interlaminar epidural injections have a rate of inaccurate placement ranging from 17% to 30%.[12,26–28]

Image guidance can be performed with fluoroscopy or CT guidance, and MR guidance and ultrasonography guidance have been described in the literature[29,30]; moreover, the recent introduction of fusion imaging is gaining an important role in image-guided techniques, perfectly matching an inexpensive technique, such as US, with MR and/or CT images.

Image guidance improves the efficacy of spinal injection while reducing the risk of complications.[26]

Recently, particulate corticosteroids have been associated with neurologic damage during transforaminal cervical and lumbar injections, probably related to direct intra-arterial administration resulting in embolic occlusion followed by ischemia or infarction of neural tissue; for this reason, nonparticulate formulations of steroids are preferred, especially in cervical transforaminal injection.[31–33]

Selection of patients is mandatory to achieve good outcomes with spinal injection.[25]

Periradicular steroid injection is indicated in patients with medical therapy–resistant radicular symptoms (positive Lasègue sign and slump test; decreased tendon reflex, sensation, and motor response; and specific dermatomal pain distribution) caused by disc decompression shown with CTI/MR imaging at the corresponding level[25] (Fig. 3).

Patients with neurogenic claudication or radiculopathy are suitable for interlaminar epidural steroid providing short-term (2 weeks to 6 months) symptom relief; however, there is conflicting evidence concerning long-term efficacy, and some investigators advocate the multiple-injection regimen of radiographically guided transforaminal epidural steroid injection or caudal injections to produce medium-term relief in patients with radiculopathy or NIC.[12]

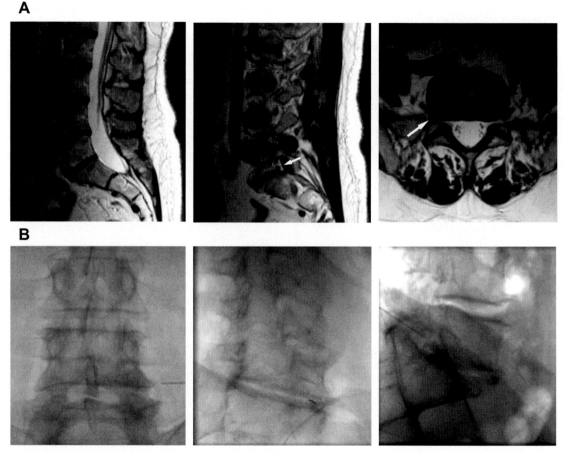

Fig. 3. Periradicular infiltration. (*A*) Sagittal and axial T2-weighted images show a right foraminal stenosis and L5-S1 disc herniation (*arrows*). (*B*) Fluoroscopic anteroposterior (AP), oblique, and laterolateral (LL) views show the correct placement of the needle at the level of L4-L5 right foraminal space.

For lumbar-level injections, patients are placed supine: the epidural lateral space is the target for central stenosis, whereas the foramen is the landmark for lateral stenosis.[26,33]

Epidural infiltration is performed via an interlaminar approach using a 20-gauge or 22-gauge needle; after passing the ligamentum flavum, the epidurogram with 1 mL of iodine contrast is suggested to confirm the needle tip position within the epidural space.[12,26,33] When the needle is correctly placed, 1.5 mL of long-acting steroid solution mixed with 1 mL of lidocaine 1% can be injected.

In cases of severe spinal canal stenosis, hydrocortisone is preferred because long-acting synthetic steroids may transiently worsen the symptoms because of their hyperosmotic effect[26] (**Fig. 4**).

Foraminal infiltration is performed via an oblique posterolateral approach, slipping along the lateral border of l-z joints, targeting the lower part of the foramen in order to avoid the nerve root and the arterial vessel[26,33]; 0.5 mL of iodine contrast can be injected in order to check the position of the 22-gauge needle, and subsequently 1.5 mL of long-acting steroid solution mixed with 1 mL of lidocaine 1% is injected slowly (see **Fig. 3**).

Image-Guided Percutaneous Techniques for Disc Decompression

The percutaneous minimally invasive treatments of radicular and discogenic pain caused by disc herniation are based on the rationale that intradiscal pressure letup is related to the reduction of irritation of the nerve root and the pain receptors in the annulus and peridiscal area[11]; this goal can be achieved by reducing the volume of the nucleus pulposus using chemical, thermal, or mechanical sources.[10]

Indications for percutaneous disc ablative procedures are represented by failure of medical (including steroid infiltrations) and physical treatment prolonged for at least 6 weeks in contained discal herniation (Pfirrmann grade 1–3); provocative discography should be performed before

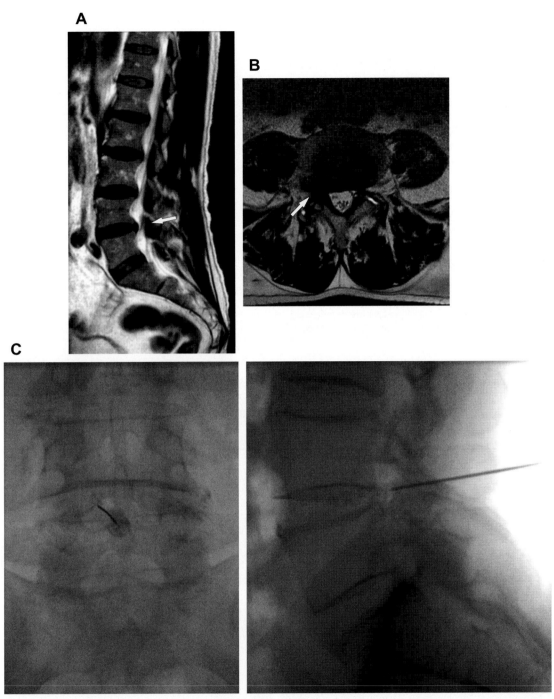

Fig. 4. Epidural infiltration. (*A*) Sagittal and (*B*) axial T2-weighted images show an L4-L5 disc herniation (*arrows*). (*C*) Fluoroscopic AP and LL views shows the correct placement of the needle at the level of L4-L5 epidural space.

any percutaneous intervertebral disc ablative technique in order to evoke the typical patient pain and plan the procedure.[10]

Contraindications are[10]:

- Absolute contraindications:
  - Sequestered (free) disc fragment
  - Segmental instability (spondylolisthesis)
  - Stenosis of neural foramen or spinal canal
  - Asymptomatic intervertebral disc bulging discovered as incidental finding in CTI or MR imaging
  - Untreated, ongoing, active infection and/or discitis

- Pregnancy (radiation exposure of the fetus must be avoided)
- Relative contraindications:
  - Hemorrhagic diathesis (should be corrected before the operation)
  - Anticoagulant therapy (should be interrupted before the operation)
  - Severe degenerative disc disease with more than two-thirds of disc height decrease
  - Prior surgical treatment at the same level
  - Primary or metastatic malignancy

Imaging-guided percutaneous decompression techniques can be divided based on the method used to reduce the volume of nucleus pulposus and subsequently the inflammation and the related pain.

- Percutaneous mechanic disc decompression
  - Percutaneous disc decompression (PDD) is able to remove a small portion of nucleus pulposus using a single-use device based on the physical principle of Archimedes'

pump; PDD series showed good clinical outcomes in selected populations, with success rates up to 75% in radicular and discogenic pain (**Figs. 5** and **6**).[10,34]

- Percutaneous laser disc decompression
  - Percutaneous laser disc decompression (PLDD) is the vaporization of a small portion of nucleus pulposus performed with a laser fiber introduced into the nucleus pulposus, resulting in reduced disc volume and pressure (**Fig. 7**).[10,35,36]

    PLDD has a high reported success rate (78%), with improvement of function at the end of the procedure, but it has also been shown to be effective in many cases, with immediate and sustained pain relief reported (up to 71% at 53 months of follow-up).[37]
  - Percutaneous laser disc coagulation therapy (PDCT) uses targeted so-called plasma light (range of 550–1800 nm) condensed at the tip of the fiber with a dome shape; the temperature ranges from 160°C (center of

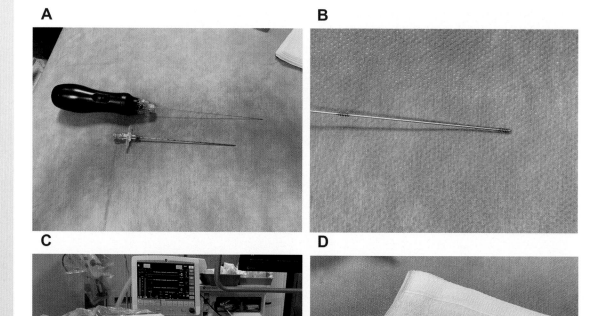

Fig. 5. Mechanical decompression disc removal system. (*A*) Mechanical decompression system kit with 17-G needle for percutaneous disc introduction. (*B*) Mechanical decompression probe tip with "infinite" screw design. (*C*) Mechanical decompression during percutaneous discectomy. (*D*) The disc material after percutaneous discectomy.

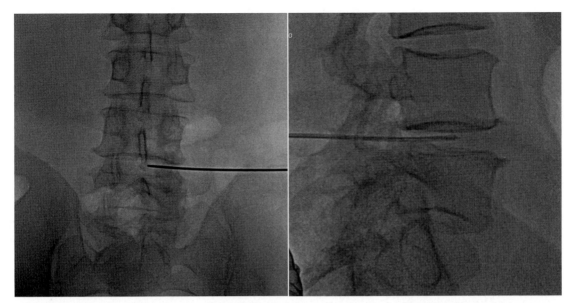

Fig. 6. Fluoroscopic AP and LL images show mechanical decompression probe tip during treatment.

the fiber) to 164°C (3 mm around the fiber) for coagulation, evaporation, and disc decompression, and less than 40°C at more than 3 mm around the fiber, sparing the nerve roots, with a higher safety profile than PLDD (**Fig. 8**).[38,39]

○ Euthermic discolysis with the holmium: yttrium-aluminum-garnet (Ho:YAG) laser extracts pieces but also the fluid portion of the nucleus pulposus, sparing the peripheral portion (average temperature, <45°C) and without affecting the vitality of the residual fibroblasts, thus avoiding disc collapse; subsequently, a compensatory hyperplasia can develop following the removal of the hyperbaric stress.[10]

Ho:YAG laser series reported pain relief and improvement of quality of life with a success rate of 80% and high safety profile because it delivers less energy in comparison with conventional PLDD, which adopts a nonselective laser for the vaporization; euthermic discolysis with the Ho:YAG laser seems particularly recommended in young patients and with a single-level disease.[40]

• PDD with radiofrequency (RF)

○ Disc nucleoplasty (NP) (coablation) is a RF ablation with focused high energy able to destroy intramolecular bonds within the nucleus; it is a non–heat-driven process, so thermal damage and tissue necrosis is avoided[41] (**Fig. 9**).

NP series reported a success rate of 80% with a complication rate of 1.8% in large

A   B

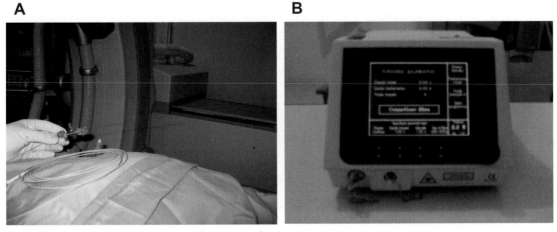

Fig. 7. PLDD system. (*A*) PLDD probe. (*B*) PLDD machine.

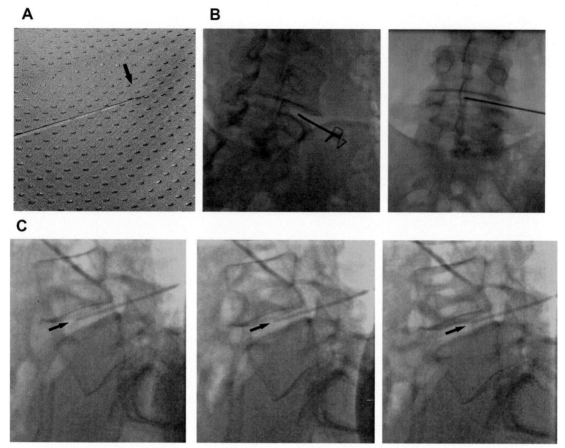

Fig. 8. PDCT percutaneous treatment. (A) PDCT system equipped with 0.4-cm plasma optical fiber (arrow). (B) Fluoroscopic oblique (left) and posteroanterior (PA) (right) views show correct needle cannula placement. (C) Fluoroscopic lateral view shows the 3-points treatment technique for lumbar herniation; a total of 1500 J (500 3 J) has been administered first in the center of disc, and subsequently 6 mm behind the center of the disc, and then close to the annulus. Note the tip of the fiber is radiotransparent and comes out 5 mm from the working cannula (arrow).

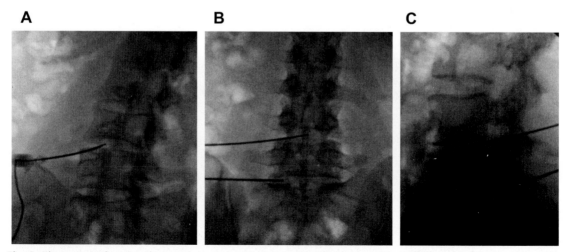

Fig. 9. Placement of nucleoplasty system probe. Fluoroscopic oblique view (A), AP (B), and LL (C) views show the correct placement of nucleoplasty probe under fluoroscopic guidance at the level of L4-L5 and L5-S1.

studies, with about an 1.8% adverse event reported.[42]

○ Continuous RF (CRF) or pulsed RF (PRF) generates an electrical current (able to obtain necrosis of target tissue) through a generator with 2 electrodes: an active electrode placed in the center of the disc and a dispersive electrode positioned on the patient's skin; the sequence and number of pulse used depend on operator.[10,43]

  ■ CRF is represented by the constant output of pulses delivered through an electrode placed on the pathologic tissue.

  ■ PRF consists of short RF pulses applied in the target area with an interval of pauses able to reach a temperature of less than 42°C (temperature of tissue necrosis) (**Fig. 10**).

PRF seems to be more effective than CRF in discogenic LBP but its efficacy decreases during follow-up (from 22.9% at 6 months to 13.1% at 12 months); other studies reported a good efficacy of PRF in chronic sciatic pain.[44]

○ Quantum molecular resonance disc decompression (QMR) is a new RF that combines different frequencies: alternating current with high-frequency waves dispensed through a bipolar electrode (fundamental wave at 4 MHz followed by waves at 8, 12, and 16 MHz). The aim of the frequencies is to destroy the molecular bonds of the nucleus pulposus, sparing the adjacent tissue.[11]

• Chemodiscolisys

○ Chemodiscolisys with ethanol gel is chemonucleolysis using radiopaque gelified ethanol containing ethyl alcohol and cellulose derivative products associated with a contrast agent (tungsten); the injection of ethanol gel within the nucleus pulposus causes molecular scission of proteoglycans and glycosaminoglycans leading to degradation of these components and a loss of

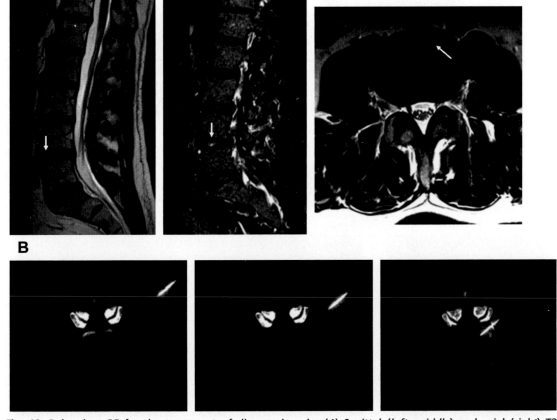

Fig. 10. Pulse dose RF for the treatment of discogenic pain. (*A*) Sagittal (*left, middle*) and axial (*right*) T2-weighted and short tau inversion recovery images show an L4-L5 disc prolapse with anterior annular tear at the level of the anterior portion (*arrows*). (*B*) Insertion of RF needle probe under CT guidance; axial CT images show the correct position of RF probe within the disc (*central portion*) for the treatment of discogenic pain.

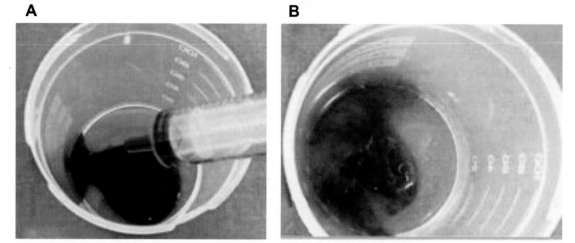

Fig. 11. Radiopaque gelified ethanol reaction with water. (*A*) A radiopaque gelified ethanol liquid solution without water. (*B*) After injection of some water the radiopaque gelified ethanol became solid with a consistency similar to soft silicon.

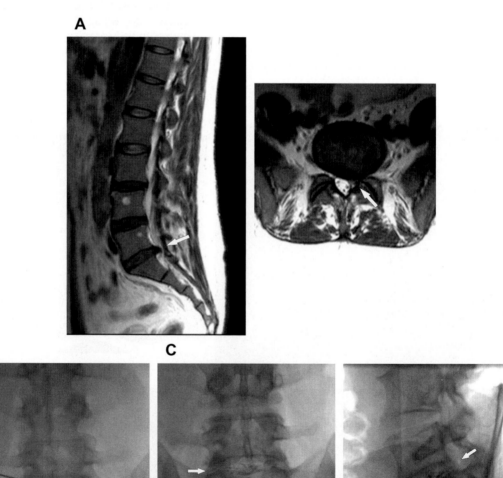

Fig. 12. Radiopaque gelified ethanol procedure at the level of lumbar spine. (*A*) Sagittal (*left*) and axial (*right*) T2-weighted images show a left subarticular disc herniation at the level of L4-L5 (*arrows*). (*B*) AP view shows correct position of the Chiba needle inside the disc under fluoroscopy. (*C*) Subsequent injection of radiopaque gelified ethanol with optimum distribution within the disc (*arrows*).

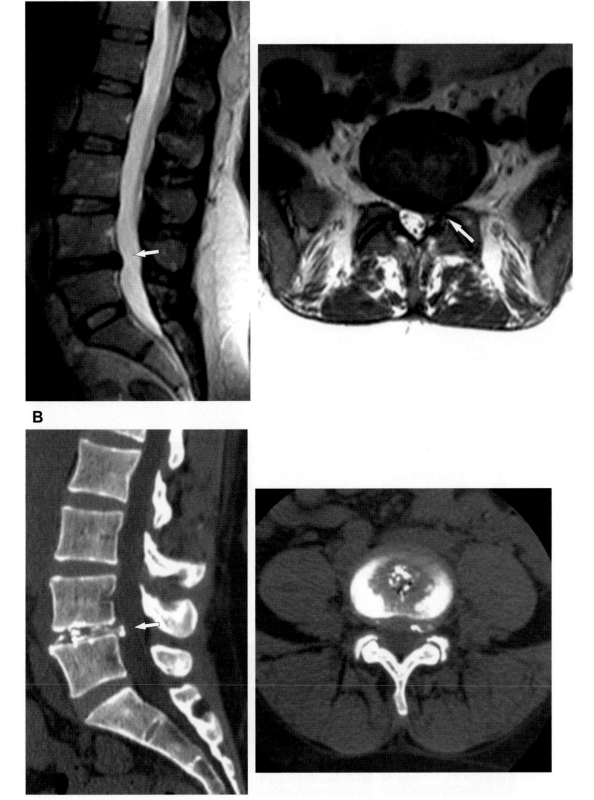

Fig. 13. Radiopaque gelified ethanol procedure at the level of lumbar spine. (*A*) Sagittal (*left*) and axial (*right*) T2-weighted images show a left subarticular and intraforaminal disc herniation at the level of L4-L5 (*arrows*). (*B*) Sagittal reformatted CT image (*left*) of radiopaque gelified ethanol procedure shows the correct distribution of radiopaque ethanol gel within the affected disc (*arrow*); the axial CT image (*right*) clearly shows the correct distribution of radiopaque gelified ethanol because of the presence of radiopaque tungsten within the ethanol gel solution.

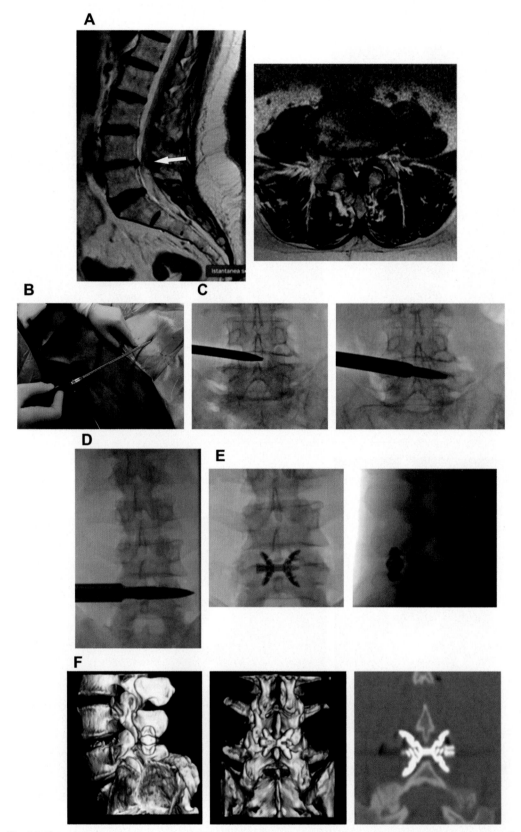

Fig. 14. Percutaneous IPD placement. (*A*) Sagittal (*left*) and axial (*right*) T2-weighted images show central canal and foraminal stenosis at level L4-L5 with compression of cauda equina and nerve roots associated with important disc bulging and facet joint degeneration (*arrow*). (*B*) Fascial dilatator placement under local anesthesia. (*C*)

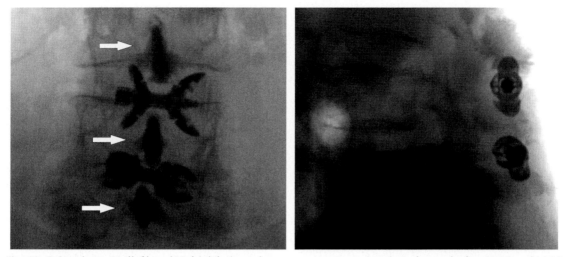

Fig. 15. Spinoplasty. PA (*left*) and LL (*right*) views show percutaneous spinoplasty (*arrows*) after L3-L4 and L4-L5 double-IPD placement.

their water-retaining capacity, resulting in dehydration and chemical decompression of the disc[10] (**Figs. 11–13**).

○ Chemodiscolisys with oxygen-ozone is a chemodiscolysis using oxygen-ozone that is able to reduce inflammation because of the oxidizing effect on pain-producing mediators; moreover, the injection of ozone can also inhibit synthesis and secretion of algogen molecules, causing rapid pain relief. The ozone has direct action on the mucopolysaccharides of the nucleus pulposus with rupture of water molecules and shrinkage of the disc exerting compression on the nerve roots; moreover, it improves microcirculation because of resolution of venous stasis and lack of oxygenated blood supply following mechanical compression of the herniated disc and disc protrusion on the vessel components.

• Intradiscal electrothermal therapy (IDET)

○ The procedure is performed placing a thermal catheter in the posterior annulus by an introducer needle connected to a generator, which is electrically heated to 90°C for 17 minutes, leading to thermocoagulation of nerve fibers and nociceptors[45]; it is an effective procedure only in selected cases of discogenic pain, with a high success rate up to 81% and a 2% adverse event rate.[46]

A 17-gauge Crawford needle is used for NP, PDD, QMR, and IDET; an 18-gauge or 21-gauge Chiba needle for PLDD; an 18-gauge Chiba for chemodiscolisys with ethanol gel and YAG Laser; and a 21-gauge Chiba needle is necessary for chemodiscolisys with oxygen-ozone.[47,48]

The intradiscal advancement of the needle is monitored fluoroscopically by oblique, anteroposterior, and lateral projections, because the tip has to reach the nucleus pulposus central portion; when crossing the annulus it is possible to feel a mild/hard-elastic resistance, and the patient may experience a pain sensation, because it represents the only innervated zone.[10]

Image-Guided Procedures for Lumbar Stenosis

Interspinous process devices (IPDs) are able to decrease facet join overload through a shock-absorber mechanism, shifting the forces to the posterior column and reducing the discal pressure; moreover, segmental enlargement of the spinal canal with unload of facet joint and posterior annulus resulting in restoration of normal foraminal height are described, in cadaveric studies, after IPD placement.[49]

IPDs provide stability, especially in extension, maintaining the spine motion in all directions.

The main indication for IPD is NIC caused by degenerative LSS with a failure of medical and physical therapy for at least 6 weeks.[50]

Fluoroscopic PA views show the correct placement of fascial dilatator. (*D*) Fluoroscopic PA view shows the placement of interspinous space dilatator needed to choose the correct size of IPD. (*E*) Fluoroscopic PA (*left*) and LL (*right*) views show the correct placement of percutaneous interspinous spacer. (*F*) 3D volume rendering and 2D multiplanar reconstruction CT reconstructions show the correct placement of percutaneous interspinous spacer.

Contraindications to IPD are[50]:

- Efficacy of medical and physical treatment
- Coagulation disorders
- Local/systemic infection
- High grade of spondylolisthesis
- Fractures
- Prior surgical treatments at the same level

The IPD procedure is performed under local anesthesia and mild/deep sedation with continuous monitoring of oxygen saturation, blood pressure, and electrocardiogram. IPD placement is accomplished under fluoroscopic guidance through a 1-cm skin incision with a unilateral approach as a standalone decompressive procedure preserving the thoracolumbar fascia and thus supraspinous legament (**Fig. 14**); the procedure is performed in a day care surgery regimen and the patient is able to return to daily activities.

IPDs have been shown to be more effective than conservative treatment of DLSS.[50–52]

Treatment failure seemed to be significantly lower in the implant group.[52]

However, complications, such as dislocation, erosion of the spinous process, and fracture of the spinous process, seemed to be more frequent for the IPD group compared with conservative treatment[52]; nevertheless, the spinoplasty procedure has been described for the treatment/prevention of fracture or remodeling of spinous processes (**Fig. 15**).[53,54]

Although IPD series describe several benefits in the short term, further prospective randomize studies are needed to evaluate efficacy in the long term.

REFERENCES

1. Abdi S, Datta S, Trescot AM, et al. Epidural steroids in the management of chronic spinal pain: a systematic review. Pain Physician 2007;10: 185–212.
2. Ravindra VM, Senglaub SS, Rattani A, et al. Degenerative lumbar spine disease: estimating global incidence and worldwide volume. Global Spine J 2018; 8:784–94.
3. US Burden of Disease Collaborators. The state of US health, 1999-2010: burden of diseases, injuries, and risk factors. JAMA 2013;310:591–608.
4. Hoy D, March L, Woolf A, et al. The global burden of neck pain: estimates from the global burden of disease 2010 study. Ann Rheum Dis 2014;73: 1309–15.
5. Hoy D, March L, Brooks P, et al. The global burden of low back pain: estimates from the Global Burden of Disease 2010 study. Ann Rheum Dis 2014;73: 968–74.
6. Gaskin DJ, Richard P. The economic costs of pain in the United States. J Pain 2012;13:715–24.
7. Backstrom KM, Whitman JM, Flynn TW. Lumbar spinal stenosis-diagnosis and management of the aging spine. Man Ther 2011;16:308–17.
8. Arbit E, Pannullo S. Lumbar stenosis. A clinical review. Clin Orthop Relat Res 2001;384:137–43.
9. Kaye AD, Manchikanti L, Abdi S, et al. Efficacy of epidural injections in managing chronic spinal pain: a best evidence synthesis. Pain Physician 2015;18:E939–1004.
10. Kelekis AD, Filippiadis DK, Martin JB, et al. Standards of practice: quality assurance guidelines for percutaneous treatments of intervertebral discs. Cardiovasc Intervent Radiol 2010;33:909–13.
11. Kelekis AD, Somon T, Yilmaz H, et al. Interventional spine procedures. Eur J Radiol 2005;55:362–83.
12. Available at: https://www.spine.org/ResearchClinical Care/QualityImprovement/ClinicalGuidelines. Accessed March 3, 2019.
13. Cavanaugh JM, Ozaktay AC, Yamashita HT, et al. Lumbar facet pain: biomechanics, neuroanatomy and neurophysiology. J Biomech 1996;29:1117–29.
14. Lee SY, Kim TH, Oh JK, et al. Lumbar stenosis: a recent update by review of literature. Asian Spine J 2015;9:818–28.
15. Lee CK, Rauschning W, Glenn W. Lateral lumbar spinal canal stenosis: classification, pathologic anatomy and surgical decompression. Spine (Phila Pa 1976) 1988;13:313–20.
16. Rydevik B, Brown MD, Lundborg G. Pathoanatomy and pathophysiology of nerve root compression. Spine (Phila Pa 1976) 1984;9:7–15.
17. Palmer WE. Spinal injections for pain management. Radiology 2016;281:669–88.
18. Bischoff RJ, Rodriguez RP, Gupta K, et al. A comparison of computed tomography-myelography, magnetic resonance imaging, and myelography in the diagnosis of herniated nucleus pulposus and spinal stenosis. J Spinal Disord 1993;6:289–95.
19. Ullrich CG, Binet EF, Sanecki MG, et al. Quantitative assessment of the lumbar spinal canal by computed tomography. Radiology 1980;134:137–43.
20. Pfirrmann CW, Metzdorf A, Zanetti M, et al. Magnetic resonance classification of lumbar intervertebral disc degeneration. Spine 2001;26:1873–8.
21. Griffith JF, Wang YX, Antonio GE, et al. Modified Pfirrmann grading system for lumbar intervertebral disc degeneration. Spine 2007;32:E708–12.
22. Fardon DF, Williams AL, Dohring EJ, et al. Lumbar disc nomenclature: version 2.0: recommendations of the combined task forces of the North American Spine Society, the American Society of Spine Radiology and the American Society of Neuroradiology. Spine J 2014;14:2525–45.
23. Zeifang F, Schiltenwolf M, Abel R, et al. Gait analysis does not correlate with clinical and MR

imaging parameters in patients with symptomatic lumbar spinal stenosis. BMC Musculoskelet Disord 2008;9:89.

24. Sirvanci M, Bhatia M, Ganiyusufoglu KA, et al. Degenerative lumbar spinal stenosis: correlation with Oswestry Disability Index and MR imaging. Eur Spine J 2008;17:679–85.

25. Buy X, Gangi A. Percutaneous treatment of intervertebral disc herniation. Semin Intervent Radiol 2010; 27:148–59.

26. Marcia S, Zini C, Hirsch JA, et al. Steroids spinal injections. Semin Intervent Radiol 2018;35:290–8.

27. Renfrew DL, Moore TE, Kathol MH, et al. Correct placement of epidural steroid injections: fluoroscopic guidance and contrast administration. AJNR Am J Neuroradiol 1991;12:1003–7.

28. Deli M, Fritz J, Mateiescu S, et al. Saline as the sole contrast agent for successful MRI-guided epidural injections. Cardiovasc Intervent Radiol 2013;36:748–55.

29. Provenzano DA, Narouze S. Sonographically guided lumbar spine procedures. J Ultrasound Med 2013; 32:1109–16.

30. Scanlon GC, Moeller-Bertram T, Romanowsky SM, et al. Cervical transforaminal epidural steroid injections: more dangerous than we think? Spine (Phila Pa 1976) 2007;32:1249–56.

31. Okubadejo GO, Talcott MR, Schmidt RE, et al. Perils of intravascular methylprednisolone injection into the vertebral artery. an animal study. J Bone Joint Surg Am 2008;90:1932–8.

32. Rathmell JP, Benzon HT, Dreyfuss P, et al. Safeguards to prevent neurologic complications after epidural steroid injections: consensus opinions from a multidisciplinary working group and national organizations. Anesthesiology 2015;122:974–84.

33. Shim E, Lee JW, Lee E, et al. Fluoroscopically guided epidural injections of the cervical and lumbar spine. Radiographics 2017;37:537–61.

34. Onik GM. Percutaneous diskectomy in the treatment of herniated lumbar disks. Neuroimaging Clin N Am 2000;10:597–607.

35. Singh V, Manchikanti L, Benyamin RM, et al. Percutaneous lumbar laser disc decompression: a systematic review of current evidence. Pain Physician 2009;12:573–88.

36. Singh V, Derby R. Percutaneous lumbar disc decompression. Pain Physician 2006;9:139–46.

37. Gangi A, Dietemann JL, Ide C, et al. Percutaneous laser disc decompression under CT and fluoroscopic guidance: Indications, technique and clinical experience. Radiographics 1996;16:89–96.

38. Kim SH, Kim SC, Cho KH. Clinical outcomes of percutaneous plasma disc coagulation therapy for lumbar herniated disc disease. J Korean Neurosurg 2012;51:8–13.

39. Yucetas SC, Gezgin I, Yildirim CH, et al. Evaluation of long-term clinical results of percutaneous plasma

disk coagulation treatment in lumbar and cervical disk herniation. Neurosurg Q 2016;26:219–24.

40. Agarwal S, Bhagwat AS. Ho: Yag laser-assisted lumbar disc decompression: a minimally invasive procedure under local anesthesia. Neurol India 2003; 51:35–8.

41. Kapural L, Hayek S, Malak O, et al. Intradiscal thermal annuloplasty versus intradiscal radiofrequency ablation for the treatment of discogenic pain: a prospective matched control trial. Pain Med 2005;6: 425–31.

42. Ren DJ, Liu XM, Du SY, et al. Percutaneous nucleoplasty using coblation technique for the treatment of chronic nonspecific low back pain: 5-years followup. Chin Med J 2015;128:1893–7.

43. Manchikanti L1, Abdi S, Atluri S, et al. An update of comprehensive evidence-based guidelines for interventional techniques in chronic spinal pain. Part II: guidance and recommendations. Pain Physician 2013;16:S49–283.

44. Van Boxem K, de Meij N, Patijn J, et al. Predictive factors for successful outcome of pulsed radiofrequency treatment in patients with intractable lumbosacral radicular pain. Pain Med 2016;17:1233–40.

45. Singh K, Ledet E, Carl A. Intradiscal therapy: a review of current treatment modalities. Spine 2005; 30:S20–6.

46. Derby R, Eek B, Chen Y, et al. Intradiscal electrothermal annuloplasty (IDET): a novel approach for treating chronic discogenic back pain. Neuromodulation 2000;3:82–8.

47. Bellini M, Romano DG, Leonini S, et al. Percutaneous injection of radiopaque gelified ethanol for the treatment of lumbar and cervical intervertebral disk herniations: experience and clinical outcome in 80 patients. AJNR Am J Neuroradiol 2015;36: 600–5.

48. Muto M, Andreula C, Leonardi M. Treatment of herniated lumbar disc by intradiscal and intraforaminal oxygen-ozone (O2-O3) injection. J Neuroradiol 2004;31:183–9.

49. Richards JC, Majumdar S, Lindsey DP, et al. The treatment mechanism of an interspinous process implant for lumbar neurogenic intermittent claudication. Spine (Phila Pa 1976) 2005;30:744–9.

50. Anderson PA, Tribus CB, Kitchel SH. Treatment of neurogenic claudication by interspinous decompression: application of the X STOP device in patients with lumbar degenerative spondylolisthesis. J Neurosurg Spine 2006;4:463–71.

51. Hsu KY, Zucherman JF, Hartjen CA, et al. Quality of life of lumbar stenosis-treated patients in whom the X STOP interspinous device was implanted. J Neurosurg Spine 2006;5:500–7.

52. Zucherman JF, Hsu KY, Hartjen CA, et al. A multicenter, prospective, randomized trial evaluating the X STOP interspinous process

decompression system for the treatment of neurogenic intermittent claudication: two-year follow-up results. Spine (Phila Pa 1976) 2005;30: 1351–8.

53. Bonaldi G, Bertolini G, Marrocu A, et al. Posterior vertebral arch cement augmentation (spinoplasty) to prevent fracture of spinous processes after interspinous spacer implant. AJNR Am J Neuroradiol 2012;33:522–8.

54. Manfré L. Posterior arch augmentation (spinoplasty) before and after single and double interspinous spacer introduction at the same level: preventing and treating the failure? Interv Neuroradiol 2014; 20:626–31.

Spontaneous Intracranial Hypotension
Pathogenesis, Diagnosis, and Treatment

Peter G. Kranz, MD*, Linda Gray, MD, Michael D. Malinzak, MD, PhD, Timothy J. Amrhein, MD

KEYWORDS

- Spontaneous intracranial hypotension • CSF leak • Myelography • CSF-venous fistula
- Epidural blood patch

KEY POINTS

- Spontaneous intracranial hypotension (SIH) is a treatable cause of headache; imaging plays a critical role in both diagnosis and treatment.
- Spinal cerebrospinal fluid (CSF) leaks are the cause of SIH. Three main mechanisms for leak have been recognized: meningeal diverticula, ventral dural tears, and CSF-venous fistulas.
- Brain MR imaging with contrast should be the first diagnostic test performed when SIH is suspected.
- Spine imaging can be conceptually divided into initial imaging techniques and problem-solving techniques, and is important for guiding treatment.

INTRODUCTION

Spontaneous intracranial hypotension (SIH) is an important and treatable secondary cause of headache. Imaging is central to the care of the patients with SIH: brain and spine imaging are critical for diagnosis, and treatment often involves image-guided procedures. This article discusses the clinical presentation and pathogenesis of SIH, reviews findings associated with SIH on various imaging modalities, and describes treatment options.

CLINICAL PRESENTATION

The most common presentation of SIH is orthostatic headache. Classically, there is a strong relation between headache severity and upright position, similar to the more familiar headache after lumbar puncture. In practice, the positional component is variable in intensity. Many patients complain of headaches that predominantly occur during the second half of the day.[1] The orthostatic nature of the headache may decrease with time, and up to one-quarter of patients present with nonorthostatic headaches.[2] Some patients may have no headache at all.[3]

Onset of symptoms is usually abrupt, with headache present every day thereafter. Activities involving sharp increases in intraabdominal pressure, such as vigorous coughing or sneezing, or vigorous twisting or stretching activities, may coincide with symptom onset.

Auditory symptoms may accompany headache, including tinnitus or muffled hearing.[4] Occasionally patients with brain sagging due to SIH may

Disclosure Statement: The authors have nothing to disclose.
Department of Radiology, Division of Neuroradiology, Duke University Medical Center, DUMC Box 3808, Durham, NC 27710, USA
* Corresponding author.
E-mail address: peter.kranz@duke.edu
; @PeterGKranz (P.G.K.); @TimAmrheinMD (T.J.A.)

Neuroimag Clin N Am 29 (2019) 581–594
https://doi.org/10.1016/j.nic.2019.07.006

present with dementia, a process termed fronto-temporal sagging brain syndrome.[5] Obtundation and coma requiring emergent intervention is a rare complication.[6,7]

Other entities may cause headache that is worse when upright, such as postural orthostatic tachycardia syndrome, cervicogenic headaches, and craniocervical instability.[8] Abrupt-onset daily headaches can be seen with new daily persistent headache. The combination of orthostatic headache and abrupt onset, however, should increase particular suspicion for SIH.

DIAGNOSTIC CRITERIA

The most widely recognized diagnostic criteria for SIH are provided by the *International Classification of Headache Disorders*, 3rd edition (ICHD-3).[9] These criteria are listed in **Box 1**. Objective evidence of SIH includes abnormal brain imaging, demonstration of cerebrospinal fluid (CSF) leakage on spinal imaging, or CSF pressure of less than 6 cm H_2O. Thus, brain and spine imaging play a critical role in the diagnosis of SIH.

Although the ICHD-3 provides a high level of specificity for the diagnosis of SIH, the criteria may miss some patients with SIH. Further refinements to diagnostic criteria can be expected as a greater understanding of SIH pathophysiology develops.

CEREBROSPINAL FLUID PRESSURE

Low CSF pressure was originally considered to be the defining feature of SIH, with many patients in early reports exhibiting CSF opening pressures of 6 cm H_2O or less.[10,11] However, more recent evidence reveals that most patients with SIH have CSF opening pressures that are not low. CSF pressure in the normal range (7–20 cm H_2O) is found in many or most patients, and on occasion, CSF pressures may be greater than 20 cm H_2O despite an active CSF leak.[12] Low CSF pressure should, therefore, be thought of as a relatively specific but insensitive indicator of SIH. Furthermore, these investigations suggest that low CSF pressure is not in fact the defining pathophysiology of SIH but that it may instead be low CSF volume.[3]

PATHOGENESIS OF SPONTANEOUS SPINAL CEREBROSPINAL FLUID LEAKS

SIH is caused by leakage of CSF from the spine. Although CSF leaks can also arise from the skull base, these types of leaks do not typically cause orthostatic headache, are more commonly associated with high (rather than low) CSF pressure, and

do not cause brain imaging manifestations of SIH.[13]

Spinal CSF leaks are currently recognized to occur through 3 main mechanisms: meningeal diverticula, ventral dural tears, and CSF-venous fistulas (CVFs) (**Fig. 1**). In a large series of subjects with SIH, diverticula were the most common (42%), followed by ventral dural tears (27%), and CVF (3%); the remaining 28% were of indeterminate cause.[14] Since publication of that series, CVFs have become increasingly recognized, and it is likely that their prevalence will be found to be

---

Box 1
International Classification of Headache Disorders, 3rd edition, criteria for headache attributed to low cerebrospinal fluid pressure

Diagnostic criteria

A. Any headache[a] fulfilling criterion C

B. Either or both of the following
   i. Low cerebrospinal fluid (CSF) pressure (<60 mm)
   ii. Evidence of CSF leakage on imaging[b]

C. Headache has developed in temporal relation to the low CSF pressure or CSF leakage, or led to its discovery[c]

D. Not better accounted for by another ICHD-3 diagnosis.

Notes

a. 7.2 Headache attributed to low cerebrospinal fluid (CSF) pressure is usually but not invariably orthostatic. Headache that significantly worsens soon after sitting upright or standing, and/or improves after lying horizontally, is likely to be caused by low CSF pressure; however, this cannot be relied on as a diagnostic criterion.

b. Brain imaging showing brain sagging or pachymeningeal enhancement, or spine imaging (MR imaging, CT or digital subtraction myelography) showing extradural CSF are diagnostic.

c. Evidence of causation may depend on onset in temporal relation to the presumed cause, together with exclusion of other diagnoses.

From Headache Classification Committee of the International Headache Society (IHS) The International Classification of Headache Disorders, 3rd edition. Cephalalgia 2018;38:1-211.

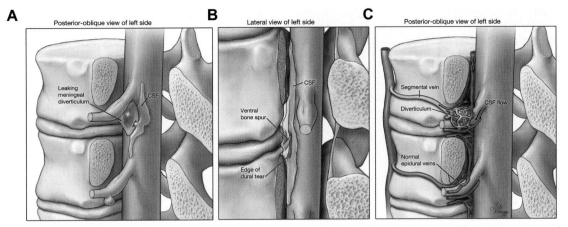

Fig. 1. Causes of SIH. The most common causes of spontaneous spinal CSF leaks include: (*A*) fragile meningeal diverticula, usually associated with nerve root sleeves; (*B*) ventral dural tears, often caused by calcified disk protrusions or osteophytes; and (*C*) CVFs.

higher as techniques develop to identify them more reliably.

Meningeal Diverticula

Meningeal diverticula were among the first-recognized causes of spontaneous spinal CSF leaks. On surgical exploration, they have been found to represent areas of dural dehiscence that permit protrusion of the leptomeninges though the dural defect, creating a fragile outpouching prone to rupture.[15] They are found most commonly in the thoracic or upper lumbar spine, either along a nerve root sleeve or at the nerve root axilla where it joins the thecal sac (**Fig. 2**). Some diverticula involve large meningeal tears that allow rapid egress of CSF, whereas others produce slow weeping of CSF with the Valsalva

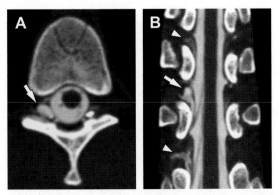

Fig. 2. CSF leak due to meningeal diverticulum. Axial (*A*) and coronal (*B*) CT myelogram images show a diverticulum (*arrow*) of the lateral thecal sac located at the axilla of the nerve root sleeve. Leaked CSF is visible in the epidural space (*arrowheads*).

maneuver.[16] Connective tissue disorders, such as Marfan syndrome or Ehlers-Danlos syndrome, may predispose patients to the formation of these defects.[17]

On imaging, leaking diverticula can mimic perineural cysts found in normal patients; however, the presence of a broad base along the thecal sac or location at the axilla of the nerve root in the context of SIH should suggest a pathologic diverticulum. Other imaging features, such as the number, size, or complexity of any given perineural cystic structure have not been shown to distinguish normal perineural cysts from leaking diverticula.[18] The presence of perineural cysts alone in the absence of leaked epidural fluid is not sufficient to establish a diagnosis of SIH because such cysts are found commonly in normal patients.[18] Sacral Tarlov cysts, a commonly encountered incidental finding defined histologically by the presence of nerve fibers in the cyst wall, are not usually associated with spontaneous CSF leakage.[19]

Ventral Dural Tears

Ventral dural tears are most commonly caused by calcified disk protrusions or sharp endplate osteophytes that incise the dura, producing a longitudinally oriented tear (**Fig. 3**). They account for approximately one-quarter of cases of SIH and are most commonly found in the in the thoracic or lower cervical spine, where calcified disks are most common.[14] Leaks due to ventral tears are often rapid, resulting in extensive epidural CSF collections. The spur may protrude into the tear, preventing healing, and necessitating a surgical resection of the spur for dural closure.[20]

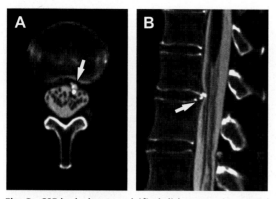

Fig. 3. CSF leak due to calcified disk protrusion. Axial (*A*) and sagittal (*B*) CT myelogram images show a calcified disk protrusion (*arrow*) penetrating into the thecal sac.

Cerebrospinal Fluid–Venous Fistula

CVF is a more recently recognized cause of SIH, first described in 2014.[21] In this entity, there is a direct connection between the spinal subarachnoid space and a draining paraspinal vein that allows rapid loss of CSF into the venous circulation (**Fig. 4**).

CSF is normally reabsorbed at the level of spinal nerve roots, with transport of CSF across the wall of arachnoid villi regulated by vacuoles.[22] In contrast, CSF volume loss due to CVFs is unregulated, resulting in CSF volume depletion and intracranial hypotension. Flow across the fistula is unidirectional because CSF pressure is physiologically maintained at a greater pressure than venous pressure.[23]

Similar to other leak types, the thoracic spine is the most common location for CVFs, with lumbar and cervical locations uncommonly encountered.[24] The fistula is often located along the

nerve root sleeve and is associated with a perineural diverticulum in approximately 80% of cases (**Fig. 5**).[24] Drainage is commonly seen into a segmental spinal vein, which runs along the lateral midportion of the vertebral body; however, drainage may also be seen into intercostal or muscular branches. Venous filling within the spinal canal in the internal vertebral epidural venous plexus may mimic a subtle epidural leak of CSF.[24]

IMAGING IN SPONTANEOUS INTRACRANIAL HYPOTENSION
Brain Imaging

Brain MR imaging with contrast is the most sensitive single imaging test for diagnosing SIH and should be the first study performed. Imaging findings of SIH on brain MR imaging (**Box 2**) are all fundamentally linked to the same underlying problem of low CSF volume.

The Monro-Kellie doctrine states that, within the fixed volume of the rigid cranial vault, the total volume of brain, blood, and CSF must remain constant.[25] If the volume of 1 of these components decreases, there must be a compensatory increase in volume of 1 of the others. Because the brain is relatively incompressible, when CSF volume decreases, blood volume must increase. This results in enlargement of the vascular spaces with the dura, leading to increased dural thickness and enhancement, dilation of the dural venous sinuses, and dilation of vessels within the pituitary gland. As volume depletion continues beyond the compensatory ability of the vascular structures, fluid may be pulled out of the intravascular space and into the subdural space, leading to subdural effusions.

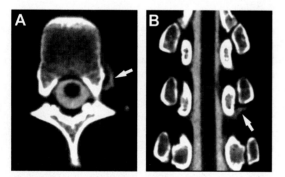

Fig. 4. CVF. Axial (*A*) and coronal (*B*) CT myelogram images show increased attenuation of a vein (*arrows*) draining from the neural foramen into a segmental paravertebral vein. This hyperdense paraspinal vein sign indicates the presence of a CVF.

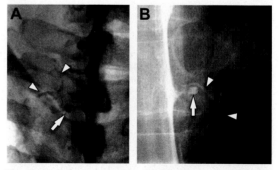

Fig. 5. CVF seen on dynamic myelography. Dynamic myelograms from 2 different patients show CVFs (*arrowheads*) arising from an upper thoracic (*A*) and a lower thoracic (*B*) nerve root sleeve. In both patients, the CVF is associated with a diverticulum of the distal nerve root (*arrow*).

> **Box 2**
> **Brain imaging findings of spontaneous intracranial hypotension**
>
> - Dural (pachymeningeal) enhancement
> - Brain sagging
> - Venous distension sign
> - Subdural collections
> - Pituitary engorgement

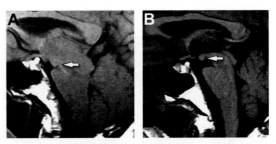

Fig. 7. Brain sagging due to SIH. (*A*) Sagittal precontrast T1-weighted MR image before treatment of SIH shows caudal displacement of the brainstem and third ventricular floor. The mammillary bodies (*arrow*) have descended below the level of the dorsum sella, the suprasellar cistern is effaced, and the optic chiasm is draped over the sella. (*B*) Posttreatment sagittal precontrast T1-weighted MR image shows resolution of brain sagging, with elevation of the third ventricular floor and mammillary bodies (*arrow*).

Dural enhancement

Dural enhancement in SIH has 2 cardinal features: it is smooth and it is diffuse (**Fig. 6**). Other conditions that cause dural enhancement, such as metastatic disease, granulomatous disease, or prior subdural hematoma, are either nodular or irregular (ie, not smooth) or localized to 1 region (ie, not diffuse).[26] The dural enhancement associated with SIH should not be mistaken for infectious meningitis, which usually involves the leptomeninges but not the dura. Diffuse, smooth dural enhancement in the context of orthostatic headache almost always indicates SIH.

Brain sagging

Brain sagging is marked by a downward displacement of the brainstem and basal structures of the brain (**Fig. 7**). The third ventricular floor normally slopes upward as one moves posteriorly from the optic chasm toward the maxillary bodies; however, in SIH, the slope may become flattened or downward sloping.[27] The mammillary bodies descend toward the pons, resulting in a vertical reduction of the mamillopontine distance. In some cases, the mammillary bodies may descend below the plane of the dorsum sella. Flattening of the ventral pons and effacement of the prepontine cistern may also be present.

Cerebellar tonsillar ectopia may be present as a result of brain sagging (**Fig. 8**). However, care must

be taken not to mistake this for Chiari I malformation. Chiari I is a deformity caused by an abnormally small posterior fossa but is not associated with other signs of brain sagging.[26,28,29] The term acquired Chiari should be avoided because true Chiari I malformations cannot be acquired in adulthood, and confusion surrounding this term may lead to inappropriate suboccipital decompression, a treatment that will not help patients with headaches due to SIH.

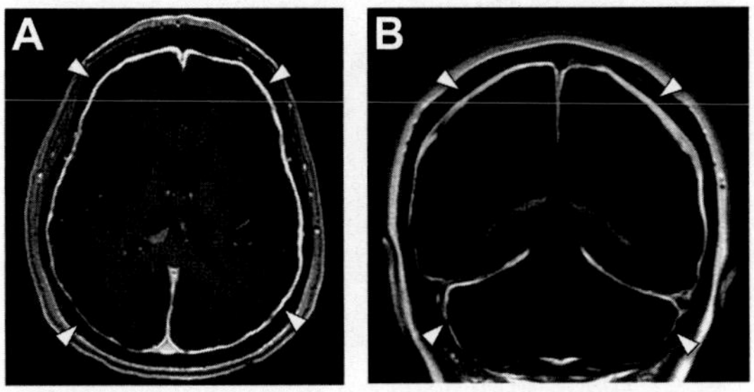

Venous distension sign

Described by Farb and colleagues[30] in 2007, the venous distension sign refers to a rounded contour

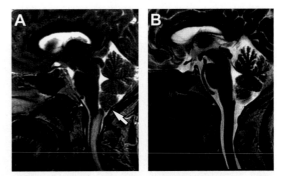

Fig. 8. Cerebellar tonsillar ectopia associated with brain sagging in SIH. (*A*) Sagittal T2-weighted MR image before treatment shows cerebellar tonsillar ectopia (*arrow*) and presyrinx edema in the cervical spinal cord. Note the descent of the mammillary bodies, another indicator of brain sagging. (*B*) Sagittal T2-weighted MR image after epidural blood patch (EBP) shows elevation of the cerebellar tonsils, resolution of the spinal cord edema, and elevation of the mammillary bodies.

Fig. 6. Dural enhancement in SIH. Axial (*A*) and coronal (*B*) postcontrast T1-weighted MR images show diffuse, smooth dural enhancement (*arrowheads*). This pattern of enhancement is characteristic of SIH.

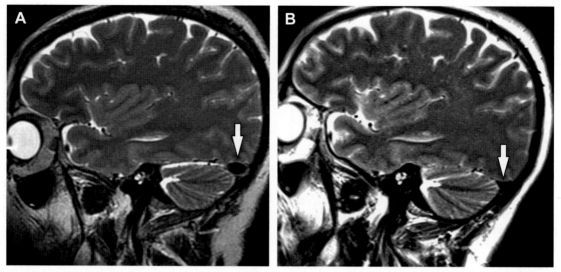

Fig. 9. Venous distension sign. (*A*) Sagittal T2-weighted MR image before treatment. A rounded contour of the transverse venous sinus (*arrow*), with convex margins, termed the venous distension sign. (*B*) Sagittal T2-weighted MR image after EBP. Normalization of the contour of the sinus (*arrow*), which now show straight or mildly concave margins.

of the midportion of the dominant transverse sinus (**Fig. 9**). Normally, the sinus has straight or concave margins, producing a triangular or arrowhead-type appearance on sagittal images. However, in SIH, intracranial CSF volume depletion may lead a compensatory increase in blood volume, producing a convex, outwardly bulging margin of the sinus.

Subdural collections
Subdural collections are the least common brain imaging feature of SIH (**Fig. 10**).[31] However, because they are readily identified on noncontrast

head computed tomography (CT), they should prompt consideration of the diagnosis when subdural collections are encountered in young patients without a history of trauma.

Subdural collections in SIH are usually bilateral (~90%).[31] They may be simple in appearance or hemorrhagic. If drainage of the subdural collections is performed before treatment of the spinal CSF leak, they will recur in most cases.[31,32]

Pituitary engorgement
The pituitary gland may become enlarged and appear hyperenhancing on postcontrast MR

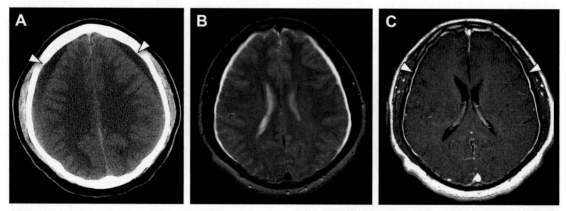

Fig. 10. Subdural collections due to SIH. (*A*) Axial noncontrast CT image from a patient presenting with orthostatic headache shows bilateral subdural hemorrhages (*arrowheads*) containing a mixture of low-density fluid and dependently layering blood products. (*B*) Axial T2-weighted MR image redemonstrates the subdural collections. (*C*) Axial postcontrast T1-weighted MR image shows diffuse, smooth dural enhancement (*arrowheads*). The cause of SIH was found to be a CVF (not shown).

imaging due to dilation of the vasculature within the gland (**Fig. 11**).[3] In some cases, this appearance has been mistaken for a pituitary tumor.

Prevalence of cranial imaging findings

The mnemonic SEEPS has been suggested to help clinicians remember the cranial findings of SIH: subdural fluid collections, enhancement of the pachymeninges, engorgement of the venous structures, pituitary hyperemia, and sagging of the brain.[33] Of these features, the authors have found dural enhancement, brain sagging, and the venous distention sign to be the most sensitive and specific signs.

One investigation found that dural enhancement was present in 83% of cases of SIH, venous distention sign in 75%, and brain sagging in 61%.[34] Dural enhancement in SIH tends to decrease with time.[35]

Of note, approximately 10% of patients with SIH have normal brain imaging. Therefore, the absence of brain MR imaging findings of SIH should not be used to exclude the condition if it is suspected clinically.[26,34]

Spine Imaging in Spontaneous Intracranial Hypotension

Approach: initial imaging versus problem-solving

Spine imaging plays an important role in the workup of SIH because demonstration of a leak both confirms the diagnosis and helps guide treatment.

The appearance of a spinal CSF leak on imaging highly depends on the rate of CSF leakage from the dural defect, which varies from patient to patient and depends, in part, on the cause of the leak (ie, meningeal diverticulum, ventral dural

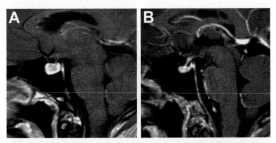

Fig. 11. Pituitary engorgement in SIH. (*A*) Sagittal postcontrast T1-weighted image in a patient with SIH before treatment shows expansion and homogenous enhancement of the pituitary gland, a consequence of increased intracranial blood volume compensating for CSF volume loss. (*B*) Sagittal postcontrast T1-weighted image after treatment shows normalization of pituitary gland volume.

tear, or CVF).[36] Leaks due to larger dural defects cause rapid egress of CSF into the epidural space, resulting in a large collection that may extend longitudinally over many vertebral segments. These leaks are referred to as high-flow or fast leaks. Smaller dural defects result in an epidural collection that does not span more than 1 vertebral body, referred to as low-flow or slow leaks. CVFs often present without any epidural fluid collections and are only detectable by identifying intrathecal contrast extending into a draining vein.

Many techniques for spinal imaging have been described in SIH; however, it is useful to think of these in 2 groups: initial imaging techniques and problem-solving techniques. The initial imaging study needs to have high sensitivity for epidural fluid collections and should be as widely available outside of specialty centers as possible; CT myelography (CTM) and MR imaging are best suited for this purpose. If a high-flow leak is found to be present on initial imaging, a subsequent imaging study tailored to the suspected site of leak (ie, problem-solving study) may be needed to definitively localize the origin of the leak. Dynamic techniques such as dynamic myelography, digital subtraction myelography (DSM), and dynamic CTM are useful in these instances.

Computed tomography myelography

CTM is often regarded as the gold standard for the detection of spinal CSF leaks.[37] It can identify high-flow CSF leaks, many low-flow CSF leaks, and CVFs.[36,38] Advantages of CTM include high spatial resolution, excellent contrast resolution between CSF (including leaked CSF) and surrounding tissues, exceptional depiction of calcified disks and osteophytes, wide availability, and good familiarity with the technique among radiologists. Disadvantages include the need to perform a dural puncture and the use of ionizing radiation.

Refinements to standard CTM technique help optimize this modality for the detection of CSF leaks. First, it is important to achieve adequate contrast concentration within the CSF in order to improve detection of subtle leaks. The authors use 10 mL of myelographic contrast medium that contains 300 mg/mL iodine (iopamidol; Isovue-M 300, Bracco Diagnostics, Princeton, NJ, USA). Second, it is critical to scan as quickly as possible after injection of contrast in order to maintain high concentration of contrast in the spinal canal and to minimize spread of contrast away from the site of leak in the event of a high-flow leak (**Fig. 12**). This can be facilitated by performing the lumbar puncture and contrast

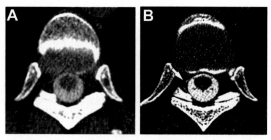

Fig. 12. Importance of myelographic technique in detecting subtle CSF leaks. (*A*) Axial CT myelogram image from a patient with SIH does not show evidence of a CSF leak. Slice thickness in this image is 2.5 mm, and the scan was performed approximately 20 minutes after intrathecal injection of contrast. (*B*) Axial CT myelogram image from the same spinal level in the same patient but scanned immediately after contrast injection with a slice thickness of 0.625 mm shows a subtle CSF leak in the right epidural space (*arrow*).

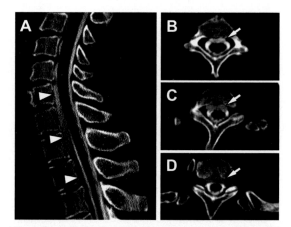

Fig. 13. Utility of rapid scanning in high-flow CSF leaks. (*A*) Sagittal CT myelogram image of the cervicothoracic junction from a patient with a high-flow cervical CSF leak shows a longitudinally-extensive ventral epidural fluid collection (*arrowheads*). (*B–D*) Corresponding axial CT myelogram images from progressively lower vertebral levels shows a decreasing concentration of myelographic contrast (*arrows*) in the epidural collection as one moves more inferiorly, farther from the source of the leak. This ventral collection will progressively fill in with contrast if scanning is more delayed, making localization of the leak origin more difficult.

injection on the CT table using CT-fluoroscopy.[39] Third, thin-section imaging and minimization of motion via attention to good breath-holding technique is important for detecting subtle leaks and CVFs. The authors routinely use submillimeter axial slices with 1 mm coronal reformatted images.

High-flow leaks are easily identified on CTM; however, when very rapid, it may be difficult to localize the exact site of origin. Early scanning may limit the spread of contrast from the leak site, creating a gradient of contrast that becomes progressively less densely opacified the farther one moves from the origin (**Fig. 13**).

MR imaging

MR imaging is also widely used as an initial spinal imaging test in SIH. The use of heavily T2-weighted sequences and fat suppression may improve detection of leaked epidural fluid.[40]

The main advantages of spinal MR imaging include wide availability, noninvasive nature, and lack of ionizing radiation. Disadvantages include decreased sensitivity for low-flow leaks, inability to detect CVFs, decreased contrast resolution compared with CTM, inability to detect subtle osseous pathologic features, and technical artifacts.

On MR imaging, a leak is identified as fluid signal within the spinal canal outside of the thecal sac separated from the subarachnoid space by a thin dark line representing the dura (**Fig. 14**). Leaked CSF may spread over several vertebral levels and may exit the spinal canal via spread through 1 or more neural foramina. The presence of fluid in multiple neural foramina should not be

mistakenly interpreted as multiple CSF leaks. In reality, multiple sites of leakage from the thecal sac are extremely rarely, if indeed ever, present. Localization of the exact leak site is often impossible on MR imaging when the epidural collection is extensive.

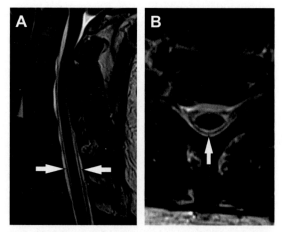

Fig. 14. MR imaging findings of spinal CSF leak. Sagittal (*A*) and axial (*B*) T2-weighted MR images from a patient with SIH and a high-flow CSF leak shows extensive epidural fluid separated from the subarachnoid space by the thin black line of the dura (*arrows*).

Dynamic imaging studies

In order to deal with the challenge of localizing the origin of high-flow CSF leaks, several imaging techniques have been developed that use intrathecal iodinated contrast and high-temporal resolution imaging to capture the moment when the contrast first begins to leak into the epidural space. Fluoroscopy-based techniques have been described that use real-time observation, either with or without digital subtraction, termed dynamic myelography and DSM, respectively.[24,41] Both techniques use a tilting fluoroscopy table to assist flow of contrast material to the site of leak (**Fig. 15**). Digital subtraction suppresses background tissues and increases conspicuity of subtle leaks; its use requires the patient to be completely still and undergo a long breath hold, and may require general anesthesia.

Dynamic CT-based techniques have also been described.[42,43] In these techniques, the patient's entire spine is scanned while contrast is injected and the patient's hips are elevated on a foam wedge in order to capture the leak site. Multiple sequential scans are carried out as contrast migrates cranially until the leak site is visualized. Radiation exposure is the main concern with CT-based dynamic techniques.

Both fluoroscopy-based and CT-based dynamic techniques are optimally performed with some suspicion for what surface (ie, ventral, right lateral, left lateral) of the thecal sac the leak is originating from, so that the patient can be positioned such that contrast layers dependently over that surface (**Fig. 16**). Consequently, these dynamic studies are not typically useful as initial imaging tests.

Optimal studies to detect cerebrospinal fluid–venous fistulas

CVFs were first reported in 2014[21] and are thus a relatively newly described cause of SIH. Most investigations have reported their identification on planar or cross-sectional imaging using intrathecal iodinated contrast media, using techniques such as CTM, DSM, and dynamic myelography.[38,44] Most CVFs occur without concurrent associated epidural CSF leaks,[24] and thus they are especially difficult to identify on conventional and heavily T2-weighted MR imaging, which is better suited to identifying epidural fluid.

DSM has been shown to detect CVFs in approximately one-fifth of SIH patients with initially negative spinal imaging.[44] On DSM, the CVF is seen as a vessel filling with myelographic contrast, usually originating from a nerve root sleeve.

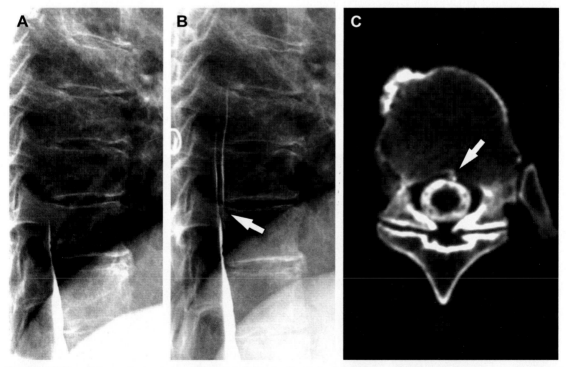

Fig. 15. Utility of dynamic myelography in localizing leak origin. (*A, B*) Sequentially obtained lateral images of the thoracic spine with the patient positioned prone during dynamic myelogram on a tilting fluoroscopy table shows a split in the column of contrast (*arrow*) into intrathecal and epidural components, marking the level of a ventral dural tear. (*C*) Axial CT myelogram image of the level of leak shows a calcified disk protrusion (*arrow*), the cause of the tear.

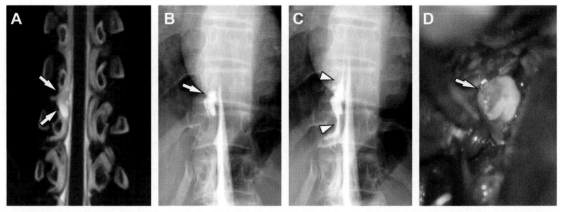

Fig. 16. Utility of dynamic myelography in leak localization. Coronal image (*A*) from a CT myelogram in a patient with SIH shows extensive leaked epidural contrast and a diverticulum arising inferior to a lower thoracic nerve root sleeve (*arrows*). Sequentially obtained images of the thoracic spine (*B, C*) with the patient positioned in right lateral decubitus during dynamic myelogram on a tilting fluoroscopy table shows filling of the diverticulum (*arrow*) followed by rapid leakage of contrast into the epidural space (*arrowheads*). (*D*) Intraoperative photograph of the lateral aspect of the thecal sac shows the diverticulum to be a thin, fragile herniation of the leptomeningeal layer (*arrow*) through a lateral dural defect.

An analogous finding seen on CTM is increased attenuation of a paraspinal vein, termed the hyperdense paraspinal vein sign (**Fig. 17**).[38] Paraspinal vein attenuation values of greater than 70 HU have been shown to be reliable indicators of CVFs on CTM.[24] The findings can be subtle and easily overlooked if not actively sought. One study found that, among SIH subjects whose CTMs were previously interpreted as negative, CVFs were identifiable in retrospect in 7% of cases.[45]

At present, no studies have demonstrated the ability of conventional or heavily T2-weighted MR imaging to detect CVFs.

MR imaging with intrathecal gadolinium

Intrathecal injection of gadolinium-based contrast agents (GBCAs) has also been explored for CSF leak detection. One study evaluating the utility of T1-weighted MR myelography (MRM) after intrathecal injection of GBCA (an off-label use) found a higher rate of CSF leak detection on MRM compared with CTM.[46] Although generally well-tolerated in appropriate doses, overdose of intrathecal GBCAs has been associated with neurologic injury, and few long-term safety data are available.[47,48] Although it may be helpful in select cases, the authors have not found much additional diagnostic yield from MRM compared

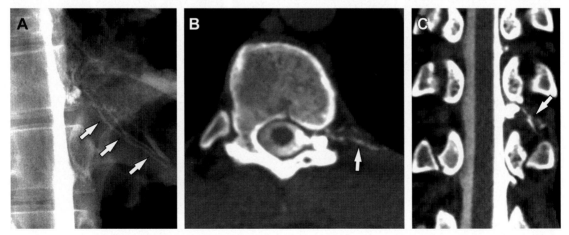

Fig. 17. CVF. (*A*) Anteroposterior radiograph of the thoracic spine with the patient positioned in left lateral decubitus during dynamic myelogram shows extensive filling of venous branches (*arrows*) with myelographic contrast lateral to the spine. Axial (*B*) and coronal (*C*) CT myelogram images from the corresponding spinal level shows hyperattenuating veins (*arrows*), known as the hyperdense paraspinal vein sign.

with good-quality CTM and rarely use this technique any longer.

Nuclear medicine cisternography

Radionuclide cisternography has been used for several decades to evaluate for skull base and spinal CSF leaks. After injection of radiotracer into the lumbar thecal sac, planar imaging is performed at 1, 2, 4, and 24 hours. Areas of radiotracer activity outside of the thecal sac constitute direct evidence of CSF leak. Indirect signs of CSF leak include early uptake of tracer activity within the kidneys and bladder by 4 hours, and absence of activity over the cerebral convexities by 24 hours.[49] Nuclear medicine cisternography is less commonly used currently due to its relatively poor spatial resolution, advances in cross-sectional techniques, and limited sensitivity and specificity.

TREATMENT OF SPONTANEOUS INTRACRANIAL HYPOTENSION

Treatment options for SIH consist of conservative therapy, epidural blood patch (EBP), and surgery. There is a paucity of evidence in the literature regarding treatment outcomes, with most studies consisting of single-arm, retrospective case series of 1 treatment modality that do not use standardized outcome measures or uniform follow-up intervals. Recommendations for treatment are, therefore, mostly based on expert opinion and small uncontrolled case series.

Conservative Therapy

Conservative therapy in SIH consists of bed rest, oral hydration, and oral caffeine administration. No headache medications have yet been reported to be widely effective in treating SIH. It is often stated in the literature that most cases of SIH have a benign course and resolve with bed rest, although few studies systematically address this assumption. One study of 13 subjects, including 8 treated exclusively with conservative measures (complete bed rest, hydration, and analgesia), found that 61% still had mild to moderate headache at 6 months, and half of subjects still had headache symptoms at 2 years.[50] Some patients clearly improve with conservative therapy alone; however, the actual efficacy and optimal duration of bed rest has not been proven. One must also consider the potential social and economic costs of prolonged bed rest.

Epidural Blood Patch

EBP is the most commonly performed intervention for spinal CSF leaks. Its mechanism of action is thought to be direct tamponade of the leak or by decreasing the compliance of the thecal sac, which shifts the CSF pressure gradient cranially.

It can be performed as a targeted patch if the site of leak is known (**Fig. 18**) or as a nontargeted (also referred to as blind) patch. Nontargeted patches are most commonly performed in the lumbar spine or at the thoracolumbar junction.

EBP is usually performed with autologous blood. Fibrin sealant, a biological product developed to facilitate dural repair during surgery, has been injected (an off-label use) in addition to or in place of blood.[51]

Estimates of the efficacy of EBP vary significantly between investigations, with response rates to initial EBP ranging from 36% to 90%.[52–58] One study found complete headache relief was more likely in subjects treated with EBP compared with conservative therapy (77% vs 40%, respectively, P<.05).[56]

Several investigators have suggested that targeted EBP may be more successful than nontargeted patching. One study of 25 subjects found a trend toward greater headache improvement with targeted patching.[57] Another larger study of 56 subjects found significantly higher rates of improvement in patients treated with targeted EBP compared with nontargeted patching (87% vs 52%, respectively, P<.05).[54]

Surgery

Surgery is generally reserved for patients with well-localized CSF leaks who fail EBP. Leaks associated with nerve root sleeve diverticula are typically easier to access than ventral leaks and may be treated via primary dural repair, clipping of the leaking root sleeve, or epidural packing.[15,59] Ventral leaks are less accessible and harder to expose surgically, especially when approached extradurally. Posterior transdural approaches that open the thecal sac posteriorly can allow for direct visualization of the ventral dural tears and permit resection of any associated osteophyte.[20] Such approaches are technically challenging and may require careful displacement of the spinal cord but permit primary repair of the dura (**Fig. 19**).

Cerebrospinal Fluid–Venous Fistula Treatment

Surgery seems to be the most successful treatment of CVFs, with high cure rates reported in early case series.[44] Epidural patching for CVFs is less effective than for epidural leaks. One series found only 3 of 22 CVFs were successfully treated with epidural patching alone.[24]

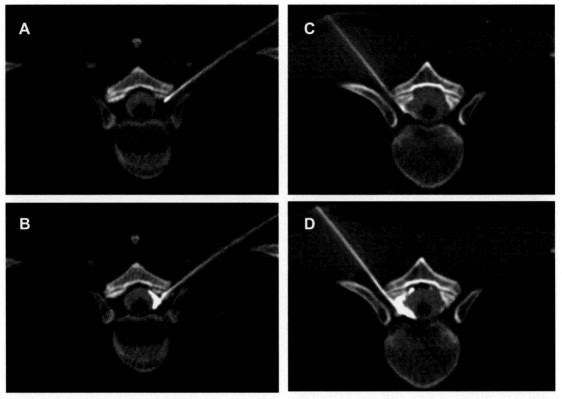

Fig. 18. Targeted EBPs using CT guidance. Axial CT-fluoroscopy images in 2 different patients before (*A, C*) and following (*B, D*) EBP placement using a transforaminal approach. In both patients, CSF leaks were associated with thoracic nerve root sleeves at the patched level. Contrast is mixed with blood in order to help assess epidural spread of the patch, as well as extent of mass effect on the thecal sac.

Rebound Intracranial Hypertension

After blood patching or surgical repair, some patients will experience an increase in CSF pressures to supraphysiologic levels.[60] This

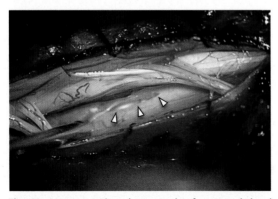

Fig. 19. Intraoperative photograph of a ventral dural tear (*arrowheads*) resulting in a high-flow CSF leak. A posterior transdural approach was used and the spinal cord gently rotated in order to allow direct visualization and repair of the defect. (Photograph courtesy of Dr. Vinay Deshmukh.)

phenomenon, termed rebound intracranial hypertension (RIH), is characterized by a new headache phenotype consisting of headache worse when lying down or nonorthostatic headache, often accompanied by nausea and blurry vision.[61] Typically RIH begins within the first 36 hours after blood patching.[61,62]

Recognition of this complication is important because treatment of RIH involves lowering CSF pressure, the opposite intent of treatment of SIH. Management typically includes head elevation and oral acetazolamide. Severe cases may require therapeutic lumbar puncture.[61]

SUMMARY

Knowledge of clinical symptoms of SIH and the role imaging plays in diagnosis and treatment is central to recognition and management of patients with spinal CSF leaks. Selection of appropriate imaging requires an understanding of the different causes of leaks and imaging findings associated with those causes, which in turn facilitates appropriate treatment.

REFERENCES

1. Leep Hunderfund AN, Mokri B. Second-half-of-the-day headache as a manifestation of spontaneous CSF leak. J Neurol 2012;259:306–10.

2. Mea E, Chiapparini L, Savoiardo M, et al. Headache attributed to spontaneous intracranial hypotension. Neurol Sci 2008;29(Suppl 1):S164–5.

3. Mokri B. Spontaneous cerebrospinal fluid leaks: from intracranial hypotension to cerebrospinal fluid hypovolemia–evolution of a concept. Mayo Clin Proc 1999;74:1113–23.

4. Arai M, Takada T, Nozue M. Orthostatic tinnitus: an otological presentation of spontaneous intracranial hypotension. Auris Nasus Larynx 2003;30:85–7.

5. Wicklund MR, Mokri B, Drubach DA, et al. Frontotemporal brain sagging syndrome: an SIH-like presentation mimicking FTD. Neurology 2011;76:1377–82.

6. Sayao AL, Heran MK, Chapman K, et al. Intracranial hypotension causing reversible frontotemporal dementia and coma. Can J Neurol Sci 2009;36:252–6.

7. Schievink WI, Moser FG, Pikul BK. Reversal of coma with an injection of glue. Lancet 2007;369:1402.

8. Mokri B, Low PA. Orthostatic headaches without CSF leak in postural tachycardia syndrome. Neurology 2003;61:980–2.

9. Headache Classification Committee of the International Headache Society (IHS) The International Classification of Headache Disorders, 3rd edition. Cephalalgia 2018;38:1–211.

10. Mokri B, Hunter SF, Atkinson JL, et al. Orthostatic headaches caused by CSF leak but with normal CSF pressures. Neurology 1998;51:786–90.

11. Chung SJ, Kim JS, Lee MC. Syndrome of cerebral spinal fluid hypovolemia: clinical and imaging features and outcome. Neurology 2000;55:1321–7.

12. Kranz PG, Tanpitukpongse TP, Choudhury KR, et al. How common is normal cerebrospinal fluid pressure in spontaneous intracranial hypotension? Cephalalgia 2016;36:1209–17.

13. Schievink WI, Schwartz MS, Maya MM, et al. Lack of causal association between spontaneous intracranial hypotension and cranial cerebrospinal fluid leaks. J Neurosurg 2012;116:749–54.

14. Schievink WI, Maya MM, Jean-Pierre S, et al. A classification system of spontaneous spinal CSF leaks. Neurology 2016;87:673–9.

15. Cohen-Gadol AA, Mokri B, Piepgras DG, et al. Surgical anatomy of dural defects in spontaneous spinal cerebrospinal fluid leaks. Neurosurgery 2006;58. ONS-238–45. [discussion: ONS-245].

16. Mokri B. Expert commentary: role of surgery for the management of CSF leaks. Cephalalgia 2008;28: 1357–60.

17. Mokri B, Maher CO, Sencakova D. Spontaneous CSF leaks: underlying disorder of connective tissue. Neurology 2002;58:814–6.

18. Kranz PG, Stinnett SS, Huang KT, et al. Spinal meningeal diverticula in spontaneous intracranial hypotension: analysis of prevalence and myelographic appearance. AJNR Am J Neuroradiol 2013;34:1284–9.

19. Nabors MW, Pait TG, Byrd EB, et al. Updated assessment and current classification of spinal meningeal cysts. J Neurosurg 1988;68:366–77.

20. Beck J, Raabe A, Schievink WI, et al. Posterior approach and spinal cord release for 360° repair of dural defects in spontaneous intracranial hypotension. Neurosurgery 2018;84(6):E345–51.

21. Schievink WI, Moser FG, Maya MM. CSF-venous fistula in spontaneous intracranial hypotension. Neurology 2014;83:472–3.

22. Edsbagge M, Tisell M, Jacobsson L, et al. Spinal CSF absorption in healthy individuals. Am J Physiol Regul Integr Comp Physiol 2004;287:R1450–5.

23. Andersson N, Malm J, Eklund A. Dependency of cerebrospinal fluid outflow resistance on intracranial pressure. J Neurosurg 2008;109:918–22.

24. Kranz PG, Amrhein TJ, Gray L. CSF venous fistulas in spontaneous intracranial hypotension: imaging characteristics on dynamic and CT myelography. AJR Am J Roentgenol 2017;209(6):1360–6.

25. Mokri B. The Monro-Kellie hypothesis: applications in CSF volume depletion. Neurology 2001;56: 1746–8.

26. Kranz PG, Gray L, Amrhein TJ. Spontaneous intracranial hypotension: 10 myths and misperceptions. Headache 2018;58:948–59.

27. Shah LM, McLean LA, Heilbrun ME, et al. Intracranial hypotension: improved MRI detection with diagnostic intracranial angles. AJR Am J Roentgenol 2013;200:400–7.

28. Raybaud C, Jallo GI. Chiari 1 deformity in children: etiopathogenesis and radiologic diagnosis. Handb Clin Neurol 2018;155:25–48.

29. Milhorat TH, Nishikawa M, Kula RW, et al. Mechanisms of cerebellar tonsil herniation in patients with Chiari malformations as guide to clinical management. Acta Neurochir (Wien) 2010;152:1117–27.

30. Farb RI, Forghani R, Lee SK, et al. The venous distension sign: a diagnostic sign of intracranial hypotension at MR imaging of the brain. AJNR Am J Neuroradiol 2007;28:1489–93.

31. Takahashi K, Mima T, Akiba Y. Chronic subdural hematoma associated with spontaneous intracranial hypotension: therapeutic strategies and outcomes of 55 cases. Neurol Med Chir (Tokyo) 2016;56:69–76.

32. Wan Y, Xie J, Xie D, et al. Clinical characteristics of 15 cases of chronic subdural hematomas due to spontaneous intracranial hypotension with spinal cerebrospinal fluid leak. Acta Neurol Belg 2016;116:509–12.

33. Schievink WI. Spontaneous spinal cerebrospinal fluid leaks and intracranial hypotension. JAMA 2006;295:2286–96.

34. Kranz PG, Tanpitukpongse TP, Choudhury KR, et al. Imaging signs in spontaneous intracranial hypotension: prevalence and relationship to CSF pressure. AJNR Am J Neuroradiol 2016;37:1374–8.

35. Kranz PG, Amrhein TJ, Choudhury KR, et al. Time-dependent changes in dural enhancement associated with spontaneous intracranial hypotension. AJR Am J Roentgenol 2016;207:1283–7.

36. Kranz PG, Luetmer PH, Diehn FE, et al. Myelographic techniques for the detection of spinal CSF leaks in spontaneous intracranial hypotension. AJR Am J Roentgenol 2016;206:8–19.

37. Wendl CM, Schambach F, Zimmer C, et al. CT myelography for the planning and guidance of targeted epidural blood patches in patients with persistent spinal CSF leakage. AJNR Am J Neuroradiol 2012; 33:541–4.

38. Kranz PG, Amrhein TJ, Schievink WI, et al. The "hyperdense paraspinal vein" sign: a marker of CSF-venous fistula. AJNR Am J Neuroradiol 2016;37: 1379–81.

39. Kranz PG, Gray L, Taylor JN. CT-guided epidural blood patching of directly observed or potential leak sites for the targeted treatment of spontaneous intracranial hypotension. AJNR Am J Neuroradiol 2011;32:832–8.

40. Tsai PH, Fuh JL, Lirng JF, et al. Heavily T2-weighted MR myelography in patients with spontaneous intracranial hypotension: a case-control study. Cephalalgia 2007;27:929–34.

41. Hoxworth JM, Patel AC, Bosch EP, et al. Localization of a rapid CSF leak with digital subtraction myelography. AJNR Am J Neuroradiol 2009;30: 516–9.

42. Luetmer PH, Schwartz KM, Eckel LJ, et al. When should I do dynamic CT myelography? Predicting fast spinal CSF leaks in patients with spontaneous intracranial hypotension. AJNR Am J Neuroradiol 2012;33:690–4.

43. Thielen KR, Sillery JC, Morris JM, et al. Ultrafast dynamic computed tomography myelography for the precise identification of high-flow cerebrospinal fluid leaks caused by spiculated spinal osteophytes. J Neurosurg Spine 2015;22:324–31.

44. Schievink WI, Moser FG, Maya MM, et al. Digital subtraction myelography for the identification of spontaneous spinal CSF-venous fistulas. J Neurosurg Spine 2016;24:960–4.

45. Clark MS, Diehn FE, Verdoorn JT, et al. Prevalence of hyperdense paraspinal vein sign in patients with spontaneous intracranial hypotension without dural CSF leak on standard CT myelography. Diagn Interv Radiol 2018;24:54–9.

46. Chazen JL, Talbott JF, Lantos JE, et al. MR myelography for identification of spinal CSF leak in spontaneous intracranial hypotension. AJNR Am J Neuroradiol 2014;35:2007–12.

47. Arlt S, Cepek L, Rustenbeck HH, et al. Gadolinium encephalopathy due to accidental intrathecal administration of gadopentetate dimeglumine. J Neurol 2007;254:810–2.

48. Park KW, Im SB, Kim BT, et al. Neurotoxic manifestations of an overdose intrathecal injection of gadopentetate dimeglumine. J Korean Med Sci 2010; 25:505–8.

49. Mokri B. Radioisotope cisternography in spontaneous CSF leaks: interpretations and misinterpretations. Headache 2014;54:1358–68.

50. Kong D-S, Park K, Nam DH, et al. Clinical features and long-term results of spontaneous intracranial hypotension. Neurosurgery 2005;57:91–6.

51. Gladstone JP, Nelson K, Patel N, et al. Spontaneous CSF leak treated with percutaneous CT-guided fibrin glue. Neurology 2005;64:1818–9.

52. He FF, Li L, Liu MJ, et al. Targeted epidural blood patch treatment for refractory spontaneous intracranial hypotension in China. J Neurol Surg B Skull Base 2018;79:217–23.

53. Wu JW, Hseu SS, Fuh JL, et al. Factors predicting response to the first epidural blood patch in spontaneous intracranial hypotension. Brain 2017;140: 344–52.

54. Cho KI, Moon HS, Jeon HJ, et al. Spontaneous intracranial hypotension: efficacy of radiologic targeting vs blind blood patch. Neurology 2011;76: 1139–44.

55. Ferrante E, Arpino I, Citterio A, et al. Epidural blood patch in Trendelenburg position pre-medicated with acetazolamide to treat spontaneous intracranial hypotension. Eur J Neurol 2010;17:715–9.

56. Chung SJ, Lee JH, Im JH, et al. Short- and long-term outcomes of spontaneous CSF hypovolemia. Eur Neurol 2005;54:63–7.

57. Sencakova D, Mokri B, McClelland RL. The efficacy of epidural blood patch in spontaneous CSF leaks. Neurology 2001;57:1921–3.

58. Berroir S, Loisel B, Ducros A, et al. Early epidural blood patch in spontaneous intracranial hypotension. Neurology 2004;63:1950–1.

59. Schievink WI, Reimer R, Folger WN. Surgical treatment of spontaneous intracranial hypotension associated with a spinal arachnoid diverticulum. Case report. J Neurosurg 1994;80:736–9.

60. Mokri B. Intracranial hypertension after treatment of spontaneous cerebrospinal fluid leaks. Mayo Clin Proc 2002;77:1241–6.

61. Kranz PG, Amrhein TJ, Gray L. Rebound intracranial hypertension: a complication of epidural blood patching for intracranial hypotension. AJNR Am J Neuroradiol 2014;35:1237–40.

62. Philipps J, Busse O. From low to high: late-onset intracranial hypertension after treatment of spontaneous intracranial hypotension. J Neurol 2007;254: 956–7.

Introduction to Diagnostic and Therapeutic Spinal Angiography

Philippe Gailloud, MD

KEYWORDS

- Spinal angiography • Endovascular treatment • Embolization • Liquid embolic agent
- Spinal vascular malformation

KEY POINTS

- Diagnostic spinal angiography is the gold standard modality for the imaging of the spinal vasculature.
- Diagnostic spinal angiography is a safe technique with extremely low risks of neurologic complication.
- Adequate catheterization and radioprotection techniques are essential to keeping the contrast and radiation doses low.
- Endovascular therapy is now a valid alternative to surgery for the treatment of spinal vascular malformations.

INTRODUCTION

This article reviews the basic principles of diagnostic and therapeutic spinal angiography (SA) as practiced by the author; one should keep in mind that factors such as the choice of a diagnostic catheter shape or an embolic agent are in part guided by personal preferences and experience.

DIAGNOSTIC SPINAL ANGIOGRAPHY
Indications

SA is the gold standard imaging modality for the investigation of the spinal vasculature. Besides the diagnostic portion of therapeutic procedures, its main indications include the characterization of spinal vascular malformations (SVMs) and tumors, and the evaluation of the spinal cord supply before complex aortic or vertebral procedures. The role of SA in the diagnosis and management of spinal ischemia is currently underappreciated.

Preparation

Diagnostic SA is an outpatient procedure most often performed under local anesthesia and conscious sedation; pediatric patients and those unable to lay flat on the angiography table require general anesthesia. Basic coagulation and kidney function testing are routinely obtained. Intravenous heparin is administered to patients without acute hemorrhage. Intravenous glucagon reduces the artifacts caused by peristaltic motion in nondiabetic patients.[1]

Technique

Adequate SA technique reduces the contrast load, the radiation dose, and the risk of complication. SA is performed via a transfemoral arterial access (4F in children, 5F in adults); the need for a radial or brachial approach is exceptional (**Fig. 1**). The catheterization method depends on the selected catheter shape, on locoregional anatomic factors (eg,

Disclosure Statement: Consultant for Cerenovus, Research grant from Siemens Medical.
Division of Interventional Neuroradiology, The Johns Hopkins Hospital, 1800 East Orleans Street, Baltimore, MD 21287, USA
E-mail address: phg@jhmi.edu

Neuroimag Clin N Am 29 (2019) 595–614
https://doi.org/10.1016/j.nic.2019.07.008
1052-5149/19/© 2019 Elsevier Inc. All rights reserved.

neuroimaging.theclinics.com

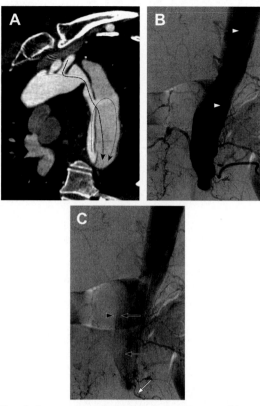

Fig. 1. Preoperative evaluation of a 58-year-old man with aortic dissection and conus medullaris ischemia. (*A*) Computed tomography angiography, oblique reconstruction along the aortic arch plane, documenting the true and false lumens of the aortic aneurysm, as well as 2 small interconnections. The catheter paths to the false lumen from a transfemoral (*dotted line*) or left brachial (*dashed line*) access are indicated. The transfemoral path was attempted, but the pressure generated by the catheter was felt to be too significant for the fragile false lumen wall. (*B*) Abdominal aortogram, early arterial phase, posteroanterior projection; a 5F pigtail catheter (*arrowheads*) was advanced through a left brachial access into the bottom of the false aneurysm sac. (*C*) Same injection, late arterial phase, documenting the artery of Adamkiewicz (*arrows*), originating from the left L2 ISA, and supplying the anterior spinal artery (*arrowhead*). (© 2019 Philippe Gailloud.)

severe aortic atheroma), and on the indication. Complete SA investigates all the vessels that can supply an SVM, including all the intersegmental arteries (ISA) of aortic origin (in general T3–L4), the subclavian artery and its branches, the carotid arteries, and the pelvic vasculature (ie, the median and lateral sacral arteries). Limited SA addresses specific questions, for example, the follow-up of a treated anomaly or the precise morphology of an SVM detected by noninvasive techniques

(keeping in mind, however, the possibility of multiple anomalies).

The selection of a diagnostic catheter shape is guided by individual anatomic characteristics and by the operator's experience; most angiograms require the use of multiple catheters (**Fig. 2**). ISAs must be investigated by selective catheterization; nonselective injections (ie, thoracic and lumbar aortograms) may help to identify patent ISAs in patients with severe aortic disease but cannot exclude an SVM.[2] Selective ISA catheterization is often easier to perform (in particular for inexperienced operators) one side at a time, in a caudocranial sequence, taking advantage of the longitudinal alignment of the intersegmental ostia. Catheters with reverse curves (eg, Simmons or Mikaelsson), notably stiff ones, require caution because they can damage aortic side branches (**Fig. 3**).

Accurate identification of the branches investigated during SA—best achieved with the help of a radio-opaque ruler alongside the vertebral column—is essential; it decreases the procedure duration and the radiation exposure, and helps to prevent the omission of important vessels as well as unwarranted multiple injections of the same branch.

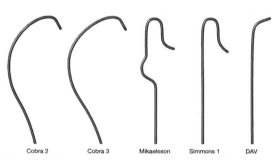

Cobra 2   Cobra 3   Mikaelsson   Simmons 1   DAV

Fig. 2. Catheter shapes commonly used during diagnostic SA. Our catheter of choice for the aortic portion of SA and for the exploration of the contralateral common and internal iliac arteries is the Cobra 2 (*1*). The Cobra 3 (*2*) is useful for patients with a wider upper thoracic aorta. Simmons 1 (*3*) and Mikaelsson (*4*) catheters are used for the homolateral iliac arteries, for the median sacral artery, and for lumbar ISAs with a steep angle of origin, notably L3 and L4. The exploration of the cervical circulation (subclavian branches and carotid arteries) benefits from a short, simple curve such as a DAV (*5*). Other shapes may be necessary, depending on individual patients' characteristics (eg, atheromatous plaque, anatomic variants). Five-French catheters are used in adults, 4F systems in children; a 3F Mayo catheter is an excellent option for SA in small children. Many other catheters may be useful in specific situations (eg, pigtail, renal double curve, Rösch inferior mesenteric, Sos). (© 2019 Johns Hopkins University.)

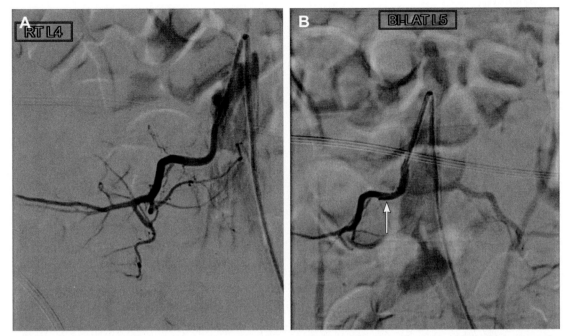

Fig. 3. SA in a 48-year-old man with progressive myelopathy referred for second opinion. (*A*) Digital subtraction angiography (DSA), right L4 ISA injection, posteroanterior projection; the branch; selected with a Mikaelsson catheter, is unremarkable. (*B*) DSA, right L4 ISA injection, posteroanterior projection; the same vessel was catheterized again and a new angiogram performed (incorrectly labeled as L5), revealing an arterial dissection (*arrow*). Based on the location of the dissection flap, it is likely that the tip of the catheter was inadvertently advanced into the curved segment of the ISA, where it caused the arterial wall injury. This case illustrates the hazard associated with the manipulation of reverse curve catheters and the need for careful documentation of the branches investigated during SA. (© 2019 Philippe Gailloud.)

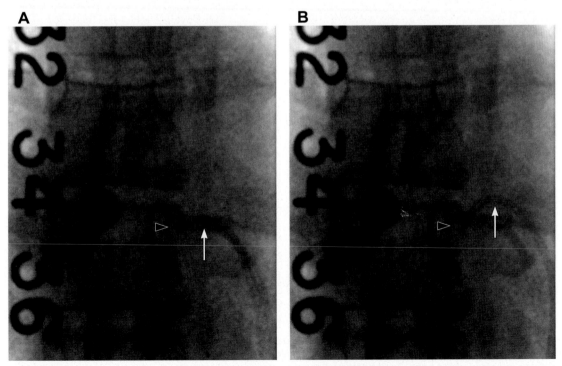

Fig. 4. Diagnostic SA in a 34-year-old woman. Once a catheter has engaged an ISA (*A, arrowhead*), its tip shows a slight upward deflection (*B, white arrow*) that obviates the need to inject contrast to locate an ostium or confirm the catheter position before an angiographic acquisition. (© 2019 Philippe Gailloud.)

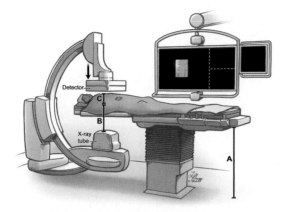

Fig. 5. Control of geometric factors during SA. Optimization of the geometric factors consists in increasing the table height (A) and the patient–source distance (B), and decreasing the patient–detector distance (C). Note that the image offered by a wide display setting is equivalent to the image provided by a conventional multiscreen display with a higher magnification level; in our suite, this difference is of 2 zoom factors, with a dose reduction of up to 60%.[7] (© 2016 Lydia Gregg.)

SA requires optimal contrast management, particularly in children (maximum doses of 2 and 4 mL/kg for diagnostic and therapeutic procedures, respectively). As Kendall noted, "the use of non-ionic contrast media has virtually removed the morbidity of spinal angiography."[3] We use diluted contrast, with concentrations ranging between 50% and 75%, depending on age and body habitus.

Instead of puffing contrast to locate branches or check the catheter position, Djindjian and associates[4] recommended to rely on the slight deflection of the catheter tip observed when it engages an ostium (**Fig. 4**). It is also important, when exchanging syringes, to let the contrast still within the catheter dead space drip out until blood appears at the hub, a maneuver that decreases both the contrast load and the risk of dissection from subendothelial injections.

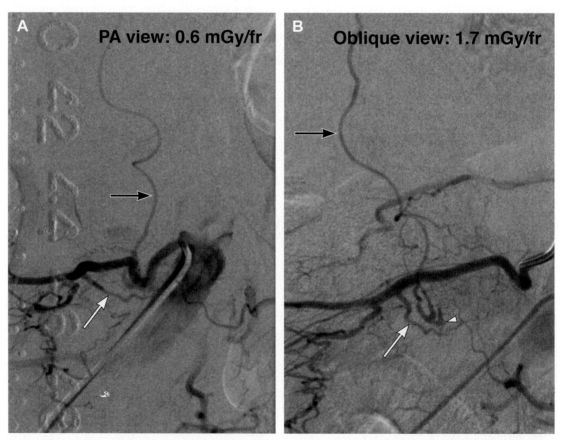

PA view: 0.6 mGy/fr

Oblique view: 1.7 mGy/fr

Fig. 6. Right L3 SA in a 69-year-old woman. The dose increase associated with oblique projections depends on the thickness of the tissues crossed by the x-ray beam. In this example, the posteroanterior projection (*A*) showed retrograde opacification of the right L3 radiculomedullary vein (*black arrow*), consistent with a spinal epidural arteriovenous fistula supplied by a retrocorporeal artery (*white arrow*), but the shunt itself was not well-appreciated. The lesion was better analyzed by an oblique view (*B*), which identified the connection (*arrowhead*) between a short posteromedian osseous branch and an isolated pouch of the anterior epidural plexus. The dose increase caused by the obliquity, all other parameters being unchanged, was of 280% (0.6–1.7 to µGy/frame). (© 2019 Philippe Gailloud.)

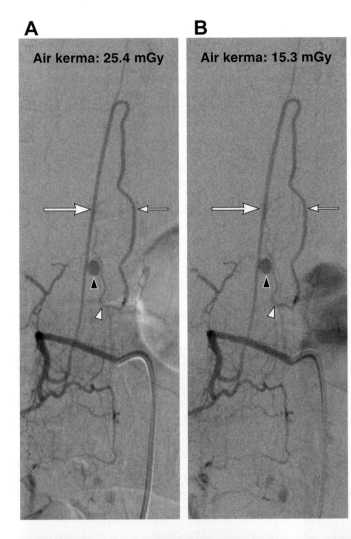

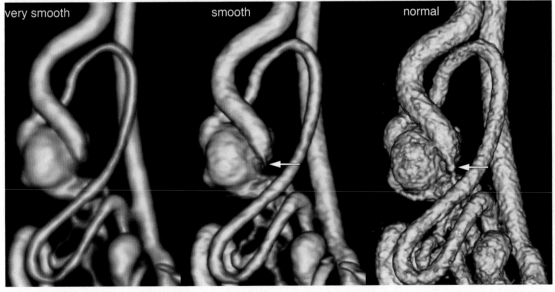

Fig. 7. Left T12 angiography in a 36-year-old man with multiple spinal hemangioblastomas. A right L1 injection was performed with (*A*) and without (*B*) antiscatter grids, all other parameters being kept identical (eg, acquisition duration, magnification, copper filtration, etc). A dose reduction of approximately 40% was achieved in that patient without loss of diagnostic information. Of note, we perform gridless SA without air gap, that is, without increasing the patient–detector distance. Both injections document the artery of Adamkiewicz (*large arrow*), the anterior spinal artery (*small arrow*), and a dorsal hemangioblastoma (*black arrowhead*) supplied by the posterior spinal circulation via the periconal arterial anastomotic circle (*white arrowhead*). Additional hemangioblastomas are seen within the cauda equina, in the lower part of the field of view. (© 2019 Philippe Gailloud.)

Fig. 8. Three-dimensional angiography of left T12 in 7-year-old girl with a high-flow perimedullary arteriovenous fistula. The rotational angiogram was reconstructed with 3 different algorithms: the normal algorithm provides less appealing but more accurate information than the smooth and very smooth reconstructions. In particular, the continuation of the anterior spinal artery distal to the site of the arteriovenous shunt (*arrow*), clearly delineated by the normal algorithm, is only suggested or undetectable with the smooth and very smooth reconstructions, respectively. (© 2019 Philippe Gailloud.)

Radioprotection

Dose-reducing methods are critical during angiography, particularly in children.[5] Radioprotection techniques are adapted to the patient's habitus and the clinical indication. Angiographic images must be diagnostic rather than esthetically pleasing, a difference measured in radiation exposure.

Low-dose protocols

Operators can nowadays create personal protocols that may be selected using table-side controls within the angiography suite, even during a procedure. The dose generated per acquired frame is easily customized: besides 3.0 µGy/frame (factory default), our protocols include 0.8, 1.2, 1.8, and 2.4 µGy/frame. Low-dose protocols are

selected based on age, habitus, and the concomitant use of other dose-reducing methods. We most often perform SA with 1.8 or 2.4 µGy/frame in adults and 1.2 or 1.8 µGy/frame in children.

Pulsed fluoroscopy keeps radiation exposure low. We find 2 pulses/s sufficient for diagnostic SA and 3 pulses/s for therapeutic procedures. Liquid embolic agents are injected under "blank roadmap" fluoroscopy at 7.5 pulses/s.

Variable frame rates protocols and high frame rate protocols

The information recorded during an SA acquisition decreases with time, the venous phase being most often limited to the observation, sometimes considerably delayed, of a few venous structures. VFR protocols can thus reduce radiation exposure without impacting the quality of the study. Our

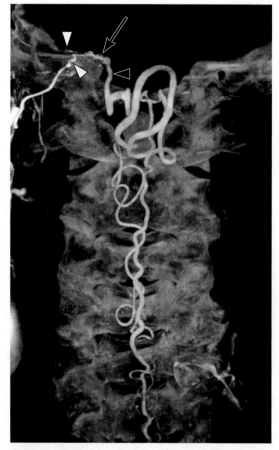

Fig. 9. Preoperative FPCA in a 62-year-old man with progressive myelopathy. The dataset was acquired during a 20-second injection of the left external carotid artery; this coronal reconstruction shows a low-flow arteriovenous fistula of the foramen magnum (*arrow*) supplied by multiple external carotid branches (*white arrowheads*) and draining into a single vein (*black arrowhead*) connected to the anterior and posterior spinal venous systems. (© 2019 Philippe Gailloud.)

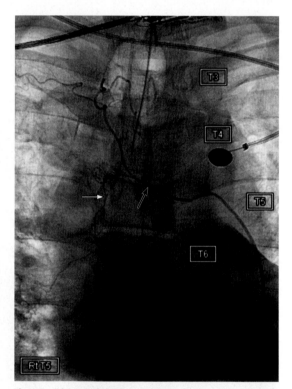

Fig. 10. Diagnostic SA in a 76-year-old man with progressive myelopathy. The vertebral levels are appropriately indicated but the injected right T3 intercostobronchial trunk (*black arrow*) is labeled as right T5. Incorrect identification of ISAs by their origin rather than their destination is a frequently encountered anatomic error. It can lead to the omission of important vessels (in this instance, the actual right T5 ISA) and misguide a subsequent surgical approach. The presence of a bronchial branch (*white arrow*) may have represented an additional misleading factor, which emphasizes the importance of a detailed knowledge of the vascular anatomy relevant to SA. (© 2019 Philippe Gailloud.)

spinal VFR protocol includes 2 frames/s for 3 seconds, 1 frame/s for 2 seconds, and 0.5 frame/s thereafter. The dose reduction achieved by a 10-s VFR acquisition (10 images) compared with standard protocols using 2, 3, or 4 frames/s (20, 30, or 40 images) is of 50%, 67%, and 75%, respectively.

Fast frame rate protocols (4 or 6 frames/s) are necessary to analyze the dynamic characteristics of fast-flow SVMs; they result, however, in substantial radiation exposure and must be used parsimoniously.

Collimation
Although collimation slightly increases the air kerma, it considerably decreases the dose area product, limiting radiation exposure to the patient's neighboring organs and to the angiography team. Collimation also improves the image quality by reducing the impact of scattered x-rays.

Geometric and electronic magnification
Both geometric and electronic magnification increase the radiation dose. Being mostly a single plane procedure, SA offers ideal control on geometric magnification (**Fig. 5**). Oblique and lateral acquisitions increase radiation exposure[6]; although a few oblique or lateral views may be necessary to clarify a specific anatomic relationship, the routine use of lateral acquisitions must be avoided during SA (**Fig. 6**).

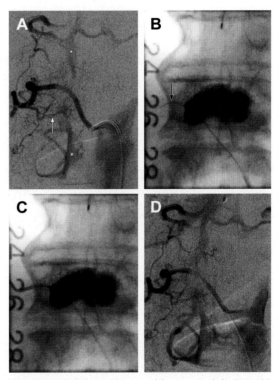

Fig. 12. SEAVF in a 70-year-old man. A right T11 ISA angiogram performed during the presurgical embolization of a renal cell metastatic disease revealed an SEAVF at the site of a prior percutaneous vertebroplasty, supplied by branches of the retrocorporeal artery (*arrow*) and draining into the epidural plexus (*asterisks*) (*A*). The vessel configuration was favorable to the use of a multipurpose catheter shape. An 0.035 guide wire (*arrow*) was gently advanced into the ISA (*B*), and a 4F multipurpose catheter threaded over the wire (*C*). A new angiogram confirmed that the multipurpose catheter conformed well to the vessel shape, providing a stable platform for subsequent embolization (*D*). (© 2019 Philippe Gailloud.)

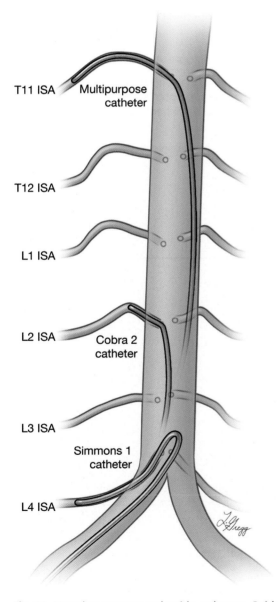

Fig. 11. Vascular anatomy and guide catheters. Guide catheters adapted to the morphology of the targeted ISA improve the stability of the embolization platform. (© 2019 Johns Hopkins University.)

Electronic magnification is an important determinant of radiation exposure. With our equipment, for example, increasing magnification by switching the input field size from 42 cm (zoom 1) to 22 cm (zoom 3) doubles the dose.[7] High magnification is at times necessary, for example, during precise microwire and microcatheter manipulations, but its impact on radiation exposure must be kept in mind, in particular when combined with oblique views.

The best approach to optimize magnification and radiation dose combines low magnification with tight collimation. Recently introduced large monitors with various configuration options represents a powerful radioprotection tool by decreasing the need for magnification (see **Fig. 5**).[7]

Gridless spinal angiography

We perform SA without antiscatter grids in a large fraction of our adult population, based on patients' habitus, and in most children (**Fig. 7**). Grids can be reinserted for a specific portion of the study; for example, grids may be required at the abdominal level but not at the thoracic level. Grids removal offers on average a dose reduction of about 30% without loss of information (Philippe Gailloud, unpublished data, 2017).

Additional factors

Various other factors affect image quality and radiation exposure. For example, copper filtration lowers the dose but excessive filtration reduces the image quality. Using a micro focal spot size improves sharpness with a negligible dose increase but decreases the x-ray tube life expectancy.[8]

Three-Dimensional Angiography Techniques

Three-dimensional angiography techniques provide important morphologic information but result in substantial radiation exposure and must be

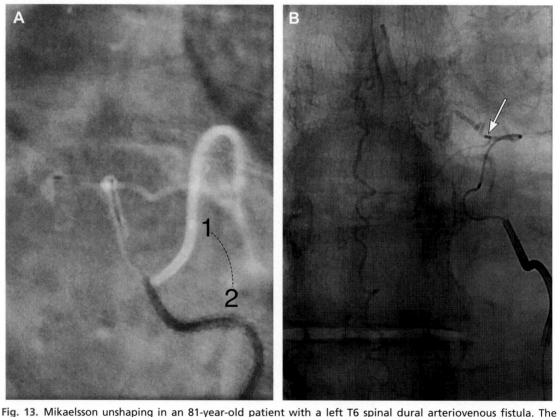

Fig. 13. Mikaelsson unshaping in an 81-year-old patient with a left T6 spinal dural arteriovenous fistula. The roadmap image (*A*) shows the original configuration of the 5F Mikaelsson catheter. Because it did not offer enough stability to advance the 1.7F microcatheter distally, the Mikaelsson catheter was unshaped by gently pulled it down until its tip aligned with and advanced into the proximal portion of the ISA (position 1 to position 2). This maneuver is also possible without a microcatheter guiding the progression of the reverse catheter tip, but then carries risk of damaging the ISA. Subsequent superselective angiography of the feeding branch of the arteriovenous fistula (*B*) confirms the adequate position of the microcatheter tip (*arrow*) and shows the unshaped but stable Mikaelsson catheter. (© 2019 Philippe Gailloud.)

used thoughtfully. Three-dimensional spinal digital subtraction angiography uses standard cranial protocols, with a power injector rate of 1 mL/s for selective ISA rotational acquisitions; we prefer hand injections in children. The x-ray delay is tailored to the lesion's hemodynamic characteristics: a 2-second delay is adequate for fast shunts, but the visualization of the drainage pathways of slower anomalies can require delays of up to 10 seconds. Three-dimensional spinal digital subtraction angiography datasets can be reconstructed in native or subtracted modes; depending on the indication, 3-dimensional digital angiography can achieve a 50% dose reduction by eliminating the mask acquisition. Three-dimensional angiography can be deceptive, notably when reconstructions privilege visual appeal over accuracy (**Fig. 8**).

Flat panel catheter angiotomography (FPCA)[9,10] has transformed the investigation of the spinal venous system. FPCA provides high-resolution multiplanar reconstructions unaffected by respiratory or intestinal motion artifacts.[11,12] It consists of a 20-second rotational angiogram showing arteries and veins simultaneously. Selective ISA studies require the injection of a mixture of 25% contrast and 75% saline at a rate of 1 mL/s; a long x-ray delay (ie, 10 seconds) may be necessary to ensure adequate venous opacification. FPCA is most often performed, in our practice, to evaluate SVMs without shunts or characterize low-flow lesions before surgery (**Fig. 9**).[13] The radiation exposure is higher with FPCA than 3-dimensional spinal digital subtraction angiography, limiting its role in children.

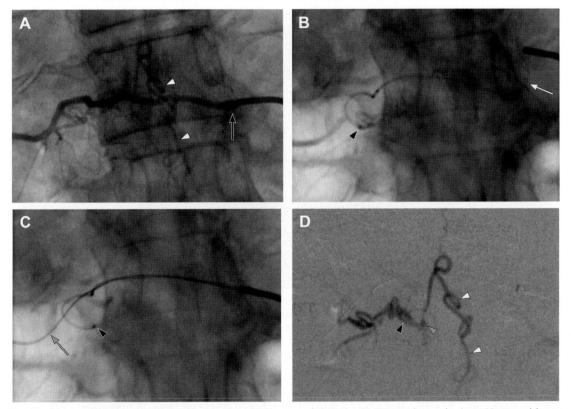

Fig. 14. The buddy wire technique for spinal embolization. (*A*) Right T9 ISA angiography in a 68-year-old man with a right T9 spinal dural arteriovenous fistula; the catheter is unstable because of an ostial stenosis. Note the poststenotic dilation (*black arrow*) and the dilated perimedullary veins draining the fistula (*white arrowheads*). (*B*) A 1.7F microcatheter has been advanced into the spinal branch of the ISA, but its tip (*black arrowhead*) is not distal enough for efficient embolization; the guide catheter has been dislodged from its ostial position (*white arrow*), preventing further microcatheter manipulations. (*C*) After repositioning the guide catheter, a second wire was threaded alongside the microcatheter into the posterior intercostal artery (*gray arrow*). Thanks to that extra support, the microcatheter tip could be advanced further (*black arrowhead*). (*D*) Superselective angiography confirms the adequate position of the microcatheter, and documents the arteriovenous shunt (*gray arrowhead*), the feeding radiculomeningeal branch (*black arrowhead*), and the draining perimedullary veins (*white arrowheads*). (© 2019 Philippe Gailloud.)

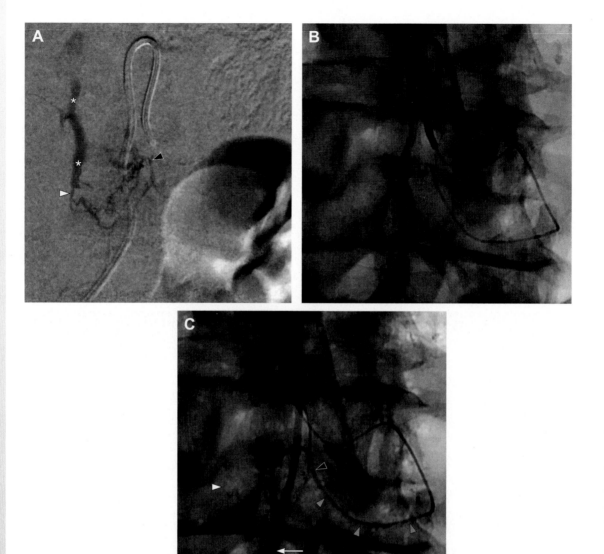

Fig. 15. Microcatheter retention. (*A*) A superselective injection (posteroanterior projection), performed with a 1.7F microcatheter tip (*black arrowhead*) in the distal end of the left retrocorporeal artery of L4, documents a right L4 SEAVF (*) via retrograde opacification of a right retrocorporeal network converging to a discrete feeder (*white arrowhead*). (*B*). Same injection, subtracted view, documenting the path of the microcatheter. (*C*) Postembolization spot film. NBCA reached the distal feeding pedicle (*white arrowhead*) but failed to fill the epidural pouch; increased resistance was encountered during retraction of the microcatheter, which broke proximally; the white arrow indicates the broken proximal end of the microcatheter free flowing within the aortic lumen. Several elements may have contributed to the catheter retention: (i) the small size of the catheterized branches and the development of vasospasm, which was believed to be the dominant factor in this case; (ii) NBCA reflux along the microcatheter (highlighted by *gray arrowheads*), which is in our experience not sufficient to account for a retained microcatheter with slow setting NBCA; and (iii) the suboptimal NBCA concentration (3 parts ethiodol, 1 part glue) instead of a more diluted mixture (at least 4 parts ethiodol in our current practice for this type of injection). Vessel tortuosity and multiple proximal microcatheter loops, other possible risk factors, played no role here. This technical complication, the only instance of microcatheter retention in our NBCA experience (cranial and spinal) of over 20 years, had no clinical repercussion. (© 2019 Philippe Gailloud.)

Pediatric Spinal Angiography

A few peculiarities of pediatric SA deserve to be mentioned:

i. Children have conspicuous anastomotic pathways, both within the spinal canal and around the vertebral column, which protect them against ischemia during spinal or aortic surgery but represent dangerous anastomoses during embolization.

ii. SA documents more radiculomedullary arteries in children than in adults; the retrograde opacification of one or more of these radiculomedullary arteries during the injection of a single ISA is common and may falsely suggests a steal phenomenon.

iii. The anterior spinal artery has a similar diameter in newborns and adults[14]; it is markedly sinuous at the level of the conus medullaris in very young patients.[15]

iv. The circulation time is faster and the venous system more conspicuous in children. The brisk filling of prominent venous structures can render the diagnosis of subtle anomalies difficult; in this context, it is worth remembering that the vertebral body blush normally precedes the opacification of the epidural venous system.

v. Vertebral angiography in children can document a normal cervical cord blush.[16]

Intraoperative Spinal Angiography

Intraoperative SA allows to assess the efficacy of a surgical procedure before skin closure; it is safe and fast in experienced hands.[17] Because intraoperative spinal SA is performed in the prone position, it requires the placement of a long femoral arterial sheath with an extra-arterial segment taped to the side of the thigh for access during the surgical intervention; popliteal access is an alternative.[18]

Complications

Diagnostic SA is nowadays a safe procedure[19]; in particular, neurologic complications are extremely rare, in large parts thanks to the introduction of nonionic contrast agents in the 1980s.[3] Our ongoing prospective SA safety database of more than 280 diagnostic spinal angiograms (diagnostic studies performed since June 2013 including a minimum of 4 vertebral levels with the injection of

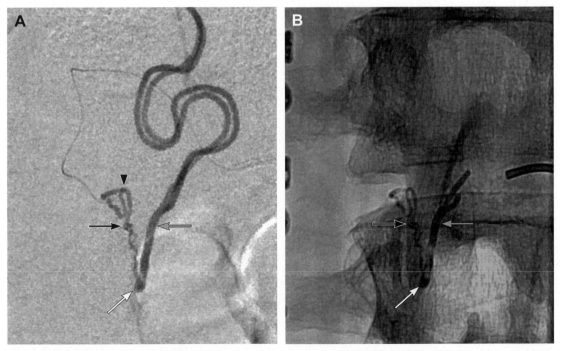

Fig. 16. NBCA embolization of a right L1 spinal dural arteriovenous fistula (SDAVF) in a 60-year-old man with the microcatheter tip in a wedged position. (*A*) A 1.7F microcatheter tip (*black arrowhead*) is wedged into the radiculomeningeal artery supplying the SDAVF (*black arrow*); superselective angiography documents the shunt (*white arrow*) and its draining radiculomedullary vein (*gray arrow*). (*B*). Postembolization spot film showing the NBCA cast extending from the feeding artery (*black arrow*) to the proximal segment of the draining vein (*gray arrow*). (© 2019 Philippe Gailloud.)

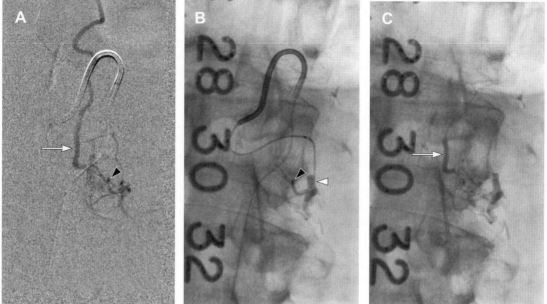

Fig. 17. NBCA embolization of a left L1 spinal dural arteriovenous fistula (SDAVF) in a 57-year-old man with NBCA with the microcatheter tip in a nonwedged position. (*A*) A 1.7F microcatheter tip seems to be in an adequate position within the radiculomedullary artery supplying the SDAVF (*black arrowhead*); a complex network of minute branches is seen converging toward a single shunt and draining vein (*white arrow*). (*B*) Spot film taken during the NBCA injection, showing limited progression of the liquid embolic agent that fails to reach the venous side of the shunt and substantial reflux along the microcatheter (*white arrowhead*). In this situation, the injection is paused and resumed after a short delay of about 30 to 45 seconds. (*C*). Postembolization spot film after further injection through the same microcatheter after a short pause. The NBCA cast now extends into the proximal segment of the draining vein (*white arrow*). (© 2019 Philippe Gailloud.)

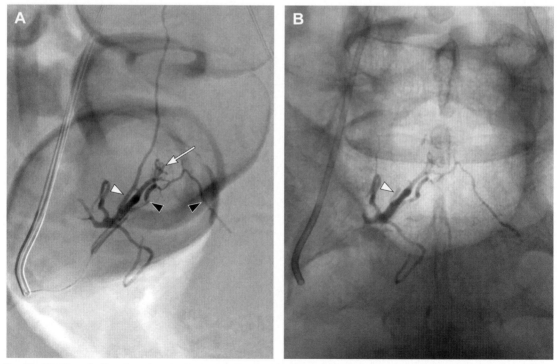

Fig. 18. NBCA embolization of an S1 SEAVF in a 64-year-old man with the 5% dextrose push technique. (*A*). Right S1 angiography documenting an arteriovenous fistula near the S1 basivertebral foramen (*arrow*), supplied by bilateral retrocorporeal branches (*black arrowheads*), and draining into an isolated epidural pouch connected to a right S1 radiculomedullary vein (*white arrowhead*). The lesion was embolized with NBCA during simultaneous injection of 5% dextrose through the guide catheter (push technique). (*B*). Postembolization spot film showing the NBCA cast within the bilateral feeding arteries, the epidural pouch and the proximal segment of the draining radiculomedullary vein (*white arrowhead*). (© 2019 Philippe Gailloud.)

at least 1 significant radiculomedullary artery) has no instance of neurologic complication (Philippe Gailloud, unpublished data, 2019).

Diagnostic Errors

Diagnostic errors were defined by Graber as "those diagnoses that are missed, wrong, or delayed, as detected by some subsequent definitive test or finding."[20] Being the gold standard modality for the spinal vasculature, SA should be expected to be highly sensitive; it is in reality a frequent source of diagnostic errors. Genuine false-negative results are rare; the problem lies essentially with inadequate studies and erroneous interpretations. A study analyzing negative SA in patients later treated for an SVM showed that more than one-half of the missed lesions (55%) were documented but not recognized by the operator.[21] In another 30% of cases, the vessel supplying the SVM was not investigated, either because the procedure was intentionally limited (eg, no

pelvic injections) or the branch was misidentified and not injected (**Fig. 10**). The last 15% were caused by operator-dependent technical mistakes, including poor or nonselective injections. The quality of a negative angiogram must thus be carefully assessed before it is used to rule out an SVM. The threshold to seek second opinions or repeat angiography when an initial study was incomplete should be low.

THERAPEUTIC SPINAL ANGIOGRAPHY
Indications

Spinal endovascular techniques have broadened the scope of SA from diagnostic tool to efficient therapeutic option, either as a standalone modality or in combination with surgery. Current indications for therapeutic SA principally involve the management of SVMs with arteriovenous shunts and the preoperative embolization of hypervascular tumors of the spine (eg, metastases) and spinal cord (eg, hemangioblastomas). Burgeoning or

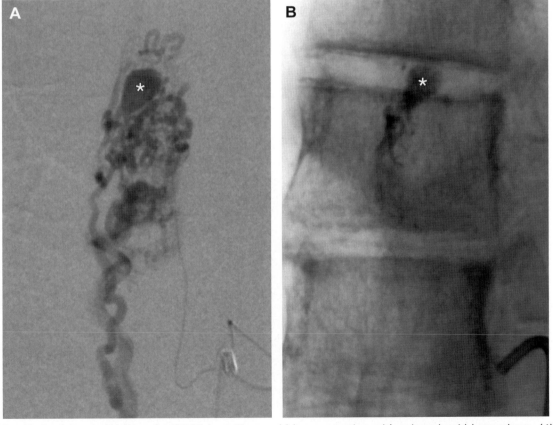

Fig. 19. Partial embolization of a SAVM in a 13-year-old boy presenting with subarachnoid hemorrhage. (*A*) Superselective injection of the posterior spinal arterial network through a 1.2F microcatheter advanced through a left posterior radiculomedullary artery documenting the SAVM nidus as well as a feeding artery aneurysm (*asterisk*) held responsible for the hemorrhage. (*B*) Postembolization spot film showing the NBCA cast, including the targeted aneurysm (*asterisk*). (© 2019 Philippe Gailloud.)

future applications include the endovascular treatment of spinal cord ischemia (eg, intra-arterial thrombolysis) or the endovascular delivery of therapeutic agents (intra-arterial chemotherapy or stem cell therapy).

Vascular Access

Vascular access for therapeutic SA is gained, like for diagnostic studies, via a femoral route, using 4F to 6F systems depending on the patient's age and the indication. Radial access may, in exceptional circumstances, be necessary.[22] A venous approach can be used in some instances, notably to treat a high-flow spinal epidural arteriovenous fistula (SEAVF).

The morphology of the targeted vessel influences the guide catheter selection: a Cobra shape may work well for a midthoracic access but be unstable at the lumbar level, where a reverse curve (Simmons or Mikaelsson) is often preferred. A 4F multipurpose catheter is a great option for right-

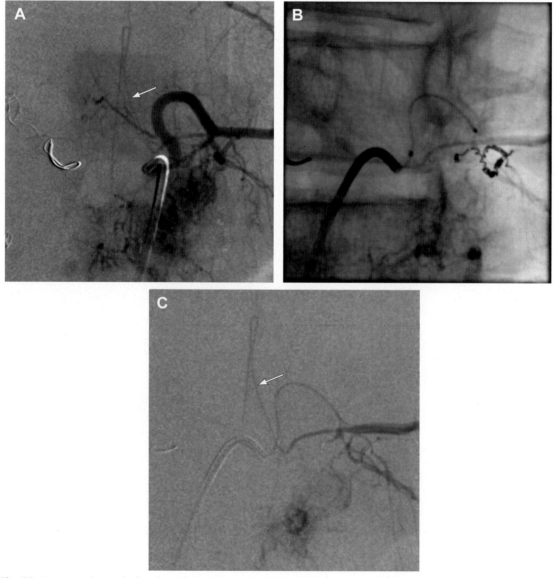

Fig. 20. Preoperative embolization of metastases in a 72-year-old woman. (*A*) Digital subtraction angiography (DSA), left T10 injection, posteroanterior projection, documenting a tumoral blush and the artery of Adamkiewicz (*white arrow*). (*B*) DSA, left T10 injection postembolization, nonsubtracted view; the presence of an important radiculomedullary artery changed the embolization plan from NBCA to detachable microcoils. (*C*) DSA, same injection, subtracted view; residual blush is noted but the artery of Adamkiewicz is patent. (© 2019 Philippe Gailloud.)

sided thoracic ISAs (**Fig. 11**). Advancing the guiding catheter into the targeted ISA over a microcatheter or over a regular 0.035 guidewire improves stability (**Fig. 12**).[23] A reverse curve catheter in an unsteady position can be carefully unshaped to align with the proximal segment of the ISA and gain in stability (**Fig. 13**). The use of a buddy wire can also offer additional support (**Fig. 14**).

The selection of a microcatheter depends on the targeted lesion (eg, low-flow vs high-flow shunt) and the choice of embolic material (liquid agent, microcoils); microcatheter sizes range in our practice between 1.2F and 1.9F. Besides compatibility with the microcatheter, the selection of a microwire mostly depends on operators' preferences.

Embolic Agents

The targeted pathology and the operator's experience affect the choice of embolic material, which includes liquid agents such as N-butyl 2-cyanoacrylate (NBCA) and ethylene-vinyl alcohol copolymer, both used off-label at the spinal level, and detachable microcoils. We do not use calibrated particles. Our liquid agent of choice is NBCA, which offers lower recanalization rates,[24,25] better distal progression,[26,27] reduced radiation exposure (shorter embolization), as well as a lower risk of microcatheter retention[28] (**Fig. 15**).

The embolization of spinal dural arteriovenous fistulas and low-flow SEAVFs requires a liquid embolic agent, because the treatment is only successful when it addresses the proximal segment of the draining vein (**Figs. 16** and **17**). The 5% dextrose push technique helps to deliver NBCA distally when the microcatheter is not in a wedged position[29]; it is also useful when treating SEAVFs with venous pouches interposed between the shunt and the draining radiculomedullary vein (**Fig. 18**). The adjunct use of microcoils can protect nontarget territories during proximal embolization when superselective catheterization of the radiculomeningeal feeder has failed. The injection of liquid agents through a dual lumen microballoon, reported with ethylene-vinyl alcohol copolymer,[30] is also possible with NBCA despite the theoretic incompatibility between that agent and the microballoon material (Heck, personal communication). SDAVFs and SEAVFs supplied by an ISA that provides a radiculomedullary artery are best treated surgically.

Spinal arteriovenous malformations (SAVMs) and high-flow perimedullary arteriovenous fistulas are also embolized with liquid agents, alone or in combination with microcoils. The treatment of SAVMs is challenging; partial embolization seems

to decrease the risk of hemorrhage,[31,32] whereas extensive embolization ($\geq$90%) has higher complication rates without improved outcomes.[32] The specific targeting of a feeding artery or nidal aneurysm may decrease the risk of (re)hemorrhage (**Fig. 19**). A new generation of particles, delivered one by one, has also shown efficacy for SAVMs.[33] Spinal provocative testing using amytal (50 mg) and lidocaine (40 mg) can evaluate the functional

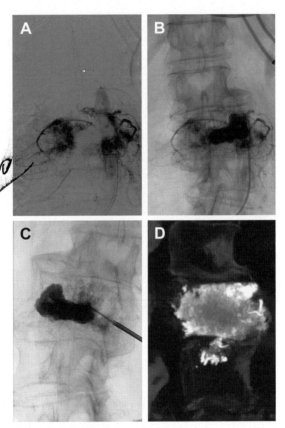

Fig. 21. Preoperative embolization of a vertebral hemangioma in a 68-year-old woman. (*A*) Digital subtraction angiography (DSA), bilateral L1 ISA trunk injection, posteroanterior projection, showing an extensive tumoral blush partially obscured by intravertebral bone cement placed during a prior percutaneous vertebroplasty. A prominent left posterior radiculomedullary artery is noted (*arrow*). (*B*) DSA, same injection, unsubtracted view. (*C*) Spot film obtained during NBCA injection; a 13-Gauge vertebroplasty needle was placed into the posterior aspect of the vertebral body via a right pedicular approach. Two 20-cm-long spinal needles were successively advanced coaxially into various parts of the vertebra for NBCA injection. (*D*). Flat panel tomography, sagittal reconstruction, showing the distribution of the NBCA within the L3 vertebral body, with extension to the upper aspect of the L4 vertebra. The patient experienced complete pain relief and the surgery was postponed. (© 2019 Philippe Gailloud.)

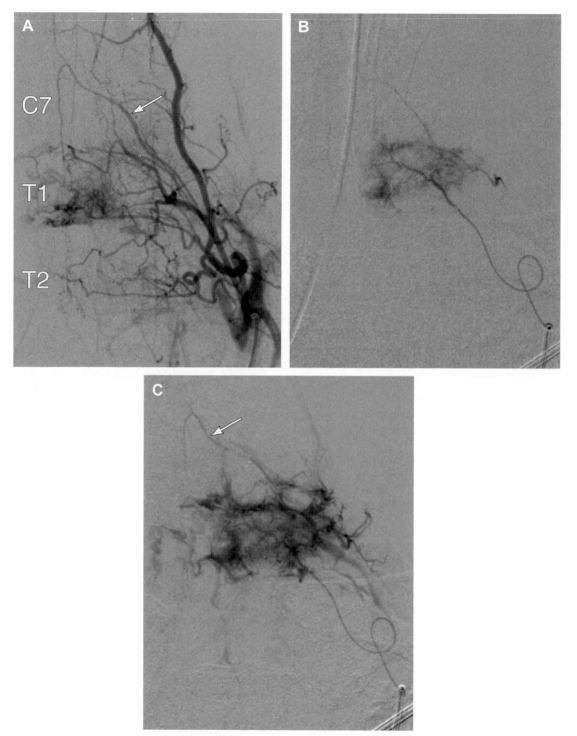

Fig. 22. Preoperative embolization of a T1 metastasis. (*A*) Left costocervical trunk injection, posteroanterior projection, documenting a tumoral blush at T1 and a prominent radiculomedullary artery at C7 with anterior and posterior contributions (inferior artery of the cervical enlargement, *arrow*). (*B*) Left T1 superselective injection showing the tumoral blush. The 1.7F microcatheter is in a wedged position. (*C*) Later phase of the same injection better delineating the blush and opacifying the radiculomedullary branch through the tumoral bed. The potential for intratumoral dangerous anastomoses must be kept in mind when considering embolization with a liquid embolic agent, notably in the cervicothoracic junction and when the microcatheter is wedged. (© 2019 Philippe Gailloud.)

importance of a feeding pedicle before emboliza-tion[34,35]; prone to false-positive and false-negative results, provocative testing has advo-cates and detractors.[36] The treatment of SAVMs is in our practice staged.

High-flow SEAVFs are most often treated with detachable coils, either by a transarterial or trans-venous approach. Preoperative embolization of hypervascular tumors is performed with a combi-nation of NBCA and detachable coils. It is critical to establish a map of the spinal cord supply before embolizing a spine tumor and to plan the proced-ure accordingly (**Fig. 20**).[37] In selected situations, embolization with a liquid embolic agent by direct puncture offers a valuable alternative to a transar-terial approach (**Fig. 21**).[38]

Dangerous Anastomoses

The concept of dangerous anastomoses is crit-ical at the spinal level; the superposition of numerous vessels in the posteroanterior projec-tion renders their detection challenging, particu-larly at the cervicothoracic junction. Dangerous anastomoses may use normal anatomic path-ways or occur through abnormal vessel, the tu-moral bed for example (**Fig. 22**). A hand injection with a 1-mL syringe may reveal dangerous branches not appreciated during an injection performed with a 3-mL syringe; howev-er, because the pressure generated with a 1-mL syringe can be sufficient to rupture a small branch when the microcatheter tip is in a wedged position, it is in general safer to use a 3-mL syringe first (**Fig. 23**).

Complications

Spinal cord ischemia
Spinal cord ischemia is a dreaded complication of therapeutic SA. Its avoidance relies for a large part on a thorough analysis of the spinal vascular

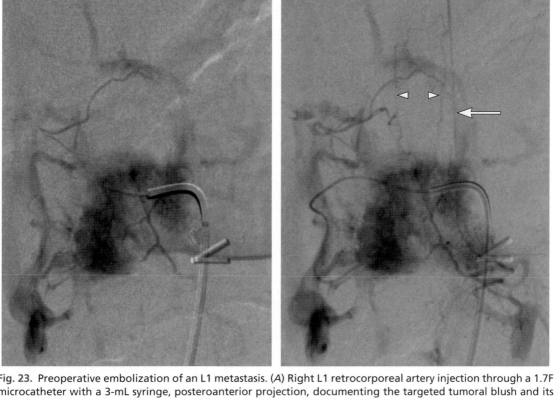

Fig. 23. Preoperative embolization of an L1 metastasis. (*A*) Right L1 retrocorporeal artery injection through a 1.7F microcatheter with a 3-mL syringe, posteroanterior projection, documenting the targeted tumoral blush and its venous drainage. (*B*) A second in injection performed with a 1-mL syringe shows passage of contrast into a left posterior radiculomedullary artery (*arrow*) via the retrocorporeal network, with opacification of the left and right posterior spinal arteries (*arrowheads*). (© 2019 Philippe Gailloud.)

supply before embolization. The risk associated with the treatment of low-flow fistulas is low; ischemia principally occurs when a radiculomedullary branch arising from the radicular artery supplying the lesion is hidden or overlooked.[39] SAVMs are associated with higher complication risks because of their intraparenchymal location and exclusive spinal arterial supply. Ischemia may result from a direct injury to the cord supply (ie, nontarget embolization or excessive reflux) or from indirect thromboembolic cerebral complications, notably when targeting branches of the vertebral artery.

Vessel rupture and perforation

Vessel perforation may occur during wire manipulation in the typically small and tortuous branches supplying SDAVFs and SEAVFs; it may be caused by a sudden change in the parent artery conformation triggered by the catheterization itself. Extradural perforations may oblige to consider a surgical alternative when access to the lesion has been lost but they often do not prevent successful completion of the embolization (**Fig. 24**). Intradural ruptures are, in contrast, severe complications with potentially catastrophic consequences.

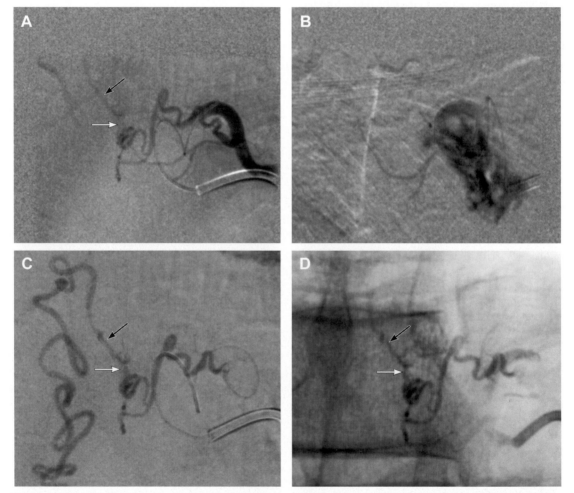

Fig. 24. NBCA embolization of a left T7 spinal dural arteriovenous fistula (SDAVF) in a 60-year-old man. (*A*) Digital subtraction angiography (DSA), left T7 injection, posteroanterior projection, showing a left T7 SDAVF (*arrow*) and its venous drainage (*black arrow*). (*B*) DSA, superselective left T7 injection via a 1.7F microcatheter, posteroanterior projection; the microcatheter tip is extraluminal and the injection results in extradural/paravertebral contrast extravasation. The microcatheter was slightly withdrawn and a new angiogram obtained; because no further extravasation was observed, heparin was not reversed and the procedure resumed. (*C*) DSA, superselective injection of the left T7 radiculomeningeal artery supplying the SDAVF (same legends). (*D*) Postembolization spot film documenting the NBCA cast, including the shunt (*white arrow*) and the proximal segment of the draining radiculomedullary vein (*black arrow*). In this case, NBCA was allowed to reflux on purpose to secure the site of a prior extravasation. (© 2019 Philippe Gailloud.)

Spinal venous thrombosis

Spinal venous thrombosis can complicate the successful treatment of a vascular malformation, notably a low-flow fistula with dilated perimedullary veins and limited outflow pathways.[40] Thrombosis may occur early, within 48 hours of the procedure, or be delayed by several months; prophylactic anticoagulation is therefore critical.[41] Our protocol includes heparinization during and after embolization (at least 24 hours, generally 48 hours), and various combination of long-term antiplatelet and/or anticoagulation therapy.

REFERENCES

1. Maglinte DD, Chernish SM. The optimal dose of glucagon: what is enough. Radiology 1992;183(2): 326–7.

2. Gailloud P. Diagnostic inefficiency of nonselective spinal angiography (flush aortography) in the evaluation of the normal and pathological spinal vasculature. Curr Probl Diagn Radiol 2016;45(3):180–4.

3. Kendall B. Spinal angiography with iohexol. Neuroradiology 1986;28(1):72–3.

4. Djindjian R, Hurth M, Houdart E. Angiography of the spinal cord. Baltimore (MD): University Park Press; 1970.

5. Pearl MS, Torok C, Wang J, et al. Practical techniques for reducing radiation exposure during cerebral angiography procedures. J Neurointerv Surg 2015;7(2):141–5.

6. Mahesh M. Fluoroscopy: patient radiation exposure issues. Radiographics 2001;21(4):1033–45.

7. Gailloud P. A large display is a powerful tool to reduce radiation exposure during single-plane fluoroscopically guided procedures. AJR Am J Roentgenol 2015;204(4):W483–5.

8. Gorham S, Brennan PC. Impact of focal spot size on radiologic image quality: a visual grading analysis. Radiography 2010;16(4):304–13.

9. Zellerhoff M, Scholz B, Ruehrnschopf E-P, et al. Low contrast 3D reconstruction from C-arm data Paper presented at: SPIE. Medical Imaging 2005: Physics of Medical Imaging 2005.

10. Akpek S, Brunner T, Benndorf G, et al. Three-dimensional imaging and cone beam volume CT in C-arm angiography with flat panel detector. Diagn Interv Radiol 2005;11(1):10–3.

11. Chen J, Ethiati T, Gailloud P. Flat panel catheter angiotomography of the spinal venous system: an enhanced venous phase for spinal digital subtraction angiography. AJNR Am J Neuroradiol 2012; 33(10):1875–81.

12. Pearl MS, Chen JX, Gregg L, et al. Angiographic detection and characterization of "cryptic venous anomalies" associated with spinal cord cavernous malformations using flat-panel catheter angiotomography. Neurosurgery 2012;71(1 Suppl Operative):125–32.

13. Gregg L, Gailloud P. Transmedullary venous anastomoses: anatomy and angiographic visualization using flat panel catheter angiotomography. AJNR Am J Neuroradiol 2015;36(7):1381–8.

14. Suh T, Alexander L. Vascular system of the human spinal cord. Arch Neurol Psychiatry 1939;41: 659–77.

15. Harwood-Nash DH, Fitz CR. Neuroradiology in Infants and children. Saint Louis (MO): The C.V. Mosby Company; 1976.

16. Harwood-Nash DC. The cerebrogram and the spinal cordogram. Am J Roentgenol Radium Ther Nucl Med 1972;114(4):773–80.

17. Orru E, Sorte DE, Wolinsky JP, et al. Intraoperative spinal digital subtraction angiography: indications, technique, safety, and clinical impact. J Neurointerv Surg 2017;9(6):601–7.

18. Villelli NW, Lewis DM, Leipzig TJ, et al. Intraoperative angiography via the popliteal artery: a useful technique for patients in the prone position. J Neurosurg Spine 2018;29(3):322–6.

19. Chen J, Gailloud P. Safety of spinal angiography: complication rate analysis in 302 diagnostic angiograms. Neurology 2011;77(13):1235–40.

20. Graber M. Diagnostic errors in medicine: a case of neglect. Jt Comm J Qual Patient Saf 2005;31(2): 106–13.

21. Barreras P, Heck D, Greenberg B, et al. Analysis of 30 spinal angiograms falsely reported as normal in 18 patients with subsequently documented spinal vascular malformations. AJNR Am J Neuroradiol 2017;38(9):1814–9.

22. Orru E, Tsang COA, Klostranec JM, et al. Transradial approach in the treatment of a sacral dural arteriovenous fistula: a technical note. J Neurointerv Surg 2019;11:e4.

23. Fanning NF, Pedroza A, Willinsky RA, et al. Segmental artery exchange technique for stable 4F guiding-catheter positioning in embolization of spinal vascular malformations. AJNR Am J Neuroradiol 2007;28(5):875–6.

24. Gokhale S, Khan SA, McDonagh DL, et al. Comparison of surgical and endovascular approach in management of spinal dural arteriovenous fistulas: a single center experience of 27 patients. Surg Neurol Int 2014;5:7.

25. Adamczyk P, Amar AP, Mack WJ, et al. Recurrence of "cured" dural arteriovenous fistulas after Onyx embolization. Neurosurg Focus 2012;32(5): E12.

26. Blackburn SL, Kadkhodayan Y, Ray WZ, et al. Onyx is associated with poor venous penetration in the treatment of spinal dural arteriovenous fistulas. J Neurointerv Surg 2014;6(7):536–40.

27. Roccatagliata L, Kominami S, Krajina A, et al. Spinal cord arteriovenous shunts of the ventral (anterior) sulcus: anatomical, clinical, and therapeutic considerations. Neuroradiology 2017;59(3):289–96.

28. Qureshi AI, Mian N, Siddiqi H, et al. Occurrence and management strategies for catheter entrapment with onyx liquid embolization. J Vasc Interv Neurol 2015; 8(3):37–41.

29. Gailloud P. The 5% dextrose push technique for use with NBCA Glue. In: Gonzalez LF, Albuquerque FC, McDougall C, editors. Neurointerventional techniques. Tricks of the trade. New York: Thieme; 2014. p. 158–61.

30. Nakae R, Nagaishi M, Hyodo A, et al. Embolization of a spinal dural arteriovenous fistula with ethylene-vinyl alcohol copolymer (Onyx) using a dual-lumen microballoon catheter and buddy wire technique. Surg Neurol Int 2017;8:166.

31. Gross BA, Du R. Spinal glomus (type II) arteriovenous malformations: a pooled analysis of hemorrhage risk and results of intervention. Neurosurgery 2013;72(1):25–32 [discussion: 32].

32. Saliou G, Tej A, Theaudin M, et al. Risk factors of hematomyelia recurrence and clinical outcome in children with intradural spinal cord arteriovenous malformations. AJNR Am J Neuroradiol 2014;35(7):1440–6.

33. Collin A, Labeyrie MA, Lenck S, et al. Long term follow-up of endovascular management of spinal cord arteriovenous malformations with emphasis on particle embolization. J Neurointerv Surg 2018; 10(12):1183–6.

34. Niimi Y, Berenstein A, Setton A, et al. Symptoms, vascular anatomy and endovascular treatment of spinal cord arteriovenous malformations. Interv Neuroradiol 2000;6(Suppl 1):199–202.

35. Niimi Y, Sala F, Deletis V, et al. Provocative testing for embolization of spinal cord AVMs. Interv Neuroradiol 2000;6(Suppl 1):191–4.

36. Rodesch G, Hurth M, Alvarez H, et al. Embolization of spinal cord arteriovenous shunts: morphological and clinical follow-up and results–review of 69 consecutive cases. Neurosurgery 2003;53(1):40–9 [discussion: 49–50].

37. Westbroek EM, Ahmed AK, Pennington Z, et al. Hypervascular metastatic spine tumor angiographic relationships with the artery of Adamkiewicz and other radiculomedullary arteries. World Neurosurg 2019. [Epub ahead of print].

38. Garzon-Muvdi T, Iyer R, Goodwin CR, et al. Percutaneous embolization and spondylectomy of an aggressive L2 hemangioma. Spine J 2016;16(3): e167–8.

39. Mascalchi M, Cosottini M, Ferrito G, et al. Posterior spinal artery infarct. AJNR Am J Neuroradiol 1998; 19(2):361–3.

40. Niimi Y, Berenstein A, Setton A, et al. Embolization of spinal dural arteriovenous fistulae: results and follow-up. Neurosurgery 1997;40(4):675–82 [discussion: 682–3].

41. Knopman J, Zink W, Patsalides A, et al. Secondary clinical deterioration after successful embolization of a spinal dural arteriovenous fistula: a plea for prophylactic anticoagulation. Interv Neuroradiol 2010; 16(2):199–203.

Spinal Vascular Anatomy

Philippe Gailloud, MD

KEYWORDS

• Angiography • Vascular anatomy • Spinal arteries • Spinal veins • Spinal cord vascularization

KEY POINTS

- The vascularization of the spinal cord depends on the intersegmental artery and its derivates.
- Thoracic and lumbar ISA keep a primitive configuration between T3 and L4 (those are ISAs, not nerves).
- Intersegmental artery derivates include the vertebral artery (C1-C6), the supreme intercostal artery (C7–T1), and the sacral arteries (S1-S4).
- The spinal cord is supplied by a small number of constant radiculomedullary arteries, including the superior and inferior arteries of the cervical enlargement, the artery of von Haller, and the artery of Adamkiewicz.

THE SPINAL ARTERIAL SYSTEM

The Intersegmental Artery and Its Branches

Developmental anatomy

The primitive intersegmental arteries (ISAs) first emerge from the unfused primitive dorsal aortas at the 6-somite stage 1; 14 to 16 pairs of ISAs of aortic origin persist in adults (T2/T3 to L3/L4). The first 6 cervical ISAs combine with the proatlantal artery (ProA) to form the subclavian artery, the vertebral artery (VA), and the vertebrobasilar junction (**Fig. 1**). At the lumbosacral level, the aorta becomes the median sacral artery (MSA),[1] whereas the first 4 sacral ISAs form the lateral sacral arteries. Despite these variations, a typical intersegmental pattern that includes an aortic stem and 3 branches (spinal, lateral, and dorsal) remains identifiable at any level.

Primitive intersegmental loops run from one dorsal aorta to the ipsilateral posterior cardinal vein; their proximal and distal limbs differentiate into ISAs and veins. Rami sprouting from the arterial limb connect to homologous branches from adjoining ISAs to form a capillary plexus along the neural tube. The dorsal branches of the primitive aortas and their capillary plexuses form the primary elements of the ISA: the aortic stem and its spinal branch. The dorsal and lateral branches are secondary vessels appearing later (**Fig. 2**).[2]

The intersegmental ostia are well-aligned longitudinally but frequently asymmetric transversally. Lumbar and low thoracic ostia are close to the midline, mid and upper thoracic ostia deviate leftward, a trend that increases with age. The proximity of the low lumbar intersegmental ostia explains their tendency to form bilateral trunks.[3]

Paraspinal arterial anastomoses and unilateral intersegmental trunks

ISAs form a complex paraspinal arterial network. This network is an important source of collateral supply and takes part in the formation of unilateral intersegmental trunks, that is, stems branching off 2 or more ipsilateral ISAs, most commonly in the lower lumbar and upper thoracic regions. A complete unilateral trunk includes spinal, lateral, and dorsal branches for each involved ISA. An incomplete trunk often lacks its spinal and dorsal branches, which originate from the aorta as a separate vessel identified as an isolated dorsospinal artery.[4–7]

Disclosure Statement: The author is a consultant for Cerenovus and received a research grant from Siemens Medical.

Division of Interventional Neuroradiology, The Johns Hopkins Hospital, 1800 East Orleans Street, Baltimore, MD 21287, USA

E-mail address: phg@jhmi.edu

neuroimaging.theclinics.com

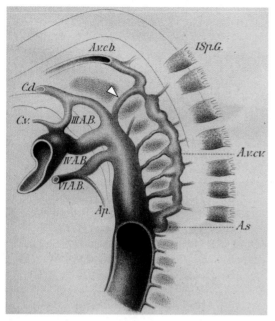

Fig. 1. Development of the VA in rabbits. The ProA (*arrowhead* added to original figure) and the subclavian artery (A.S) are interconnected by a succession of anastomoses linking the first 5 cervical ISAs (A.v.cv.). The ProA accompany the first cervical nerve,[11,82,83] whereas the subclavian artery is derived from the sixth cervical ISA.[84] Other depicted structures include the first cervical ganglion (I.Sp.G.), the internal carotid artery (C.d.), the external carotid artery (C.v.), the third, fourth and sixth aortic arches (III A.B., IV A.B., VI A.B.), the basilar artery (A.v.c.B.), and the pulmonary artery (A.p.). (*From* Hochstetter F. Uber die Entwicklung der A. Vertebralis beim Kaninchen, nebst Bemerkungen über die Entstehung des Ansa Vieussenii. *Morphol Jahrb.* 1890;16:572-586.)

Locoregional modifications of the intersegmental pattern

The vertebral artery The ProA provides anterior and posterior radiculomedullary arteries (RMAs) that respectively become the distal VA and the vertebral root of the posterior spinal artery (PSA).[8–10] The distal VA divides into ascending and descending rami. The left and right ascending rami fuse over the midline to form the proximal basilar artery; the left and right descending rami converge medially to form the anterior spinal artery (ASA) (**Fig. 3**). The cervical VA consists of a succession of longitudinal anastomoses connecting the subclavian artery to the distal VA (**Fig. 4**).[11]

The site of origin of the VA depends on the primitive ISA forming its proximal segment; it is most often the sixth cervical ISA (ie, the subclavian artery), but any cervical or upper thoracic ISA can be involved. Persistent cervical ISAs are identified by their relation with the transverse canal: a

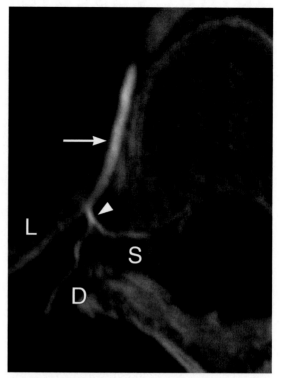

Fig. 2. The ISA. A typical ISA is made of an aortic stem (*arrow*) and 3 branches. The dorsal branch is essentially muscular; the name of the lateral branch varies by region (intercostal, subcostal, lumbar). A small trunk for the dorsal and spinal branches, the dorsospinal trunk (*arrowhead*), is formed when the lateral branch takes off proximally. D, dorsal; L, lateral; S, spinal. (© 2019 Philippe Gailloud.)

persistent seventh cervical ISA always passes through the C7 transverse foramen but may originate from the supreme intercostal artery or from the aorta, distal to the left subclavian artery (**Fig. 5**). Persistent second cervical ISAs are extremely rare.[12,13] Persistent third, fourth, and particularly fifth cervical ISAs are more common, either in isolation or as part of a proximal VA duplication.

Thoracic VAs are divided into ascending and descending types.[14] In general, descending thoracic VAs form a trunk with a cervical VA.[15] Ascending thoracic VAs originate from a thoracic ISA and continue cranially as a cervical VA[16] (see **Fig. 5**). Injury to a thoracic VA supplying the posterior fossa can be catastrophic; an enlarged costotransverse space (T1, T2) may be the only warning sign on preoperative imaging.[14]

The supreme intercostal artery The supreme intercostal artery arises from the subclavian artery as an individual vessel or as a trunk with the deep cervical artery. It most often provides the seventh

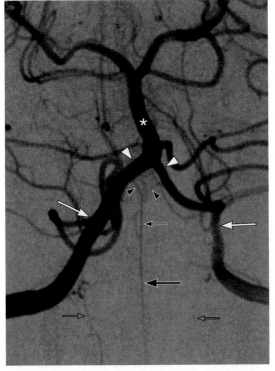

Fig. 3. The distal VA and the basilar artery. The distal VA (*large white arrows*) is formed by the anterior radiculomedullary branch of the ProA; it divides into ascending (*white arrowheads*) and descending (*black arrowheads*) rami. The basilar artery (*asterisk*) and the ASA (*large black arrow*) are formed by the fusion of these ascending and descending rami, respectively. The descending rami of the posterior radiculomedullary branch of the ProA form the posterior vertebrospinal trunks (*gray arrows*). The small black arrow indicates a focal ASA duplication. (© 2019 Philippe Gailloud.)

cervical and first thoracic ISAs[17] but can also branch off, in order of decreasing frequency, the second, third, and fourth thoracic ISAs.

The lumbosacral region The aorta continues below the iliac bifurcation as the MSA.[1] The MSA courses over the anterior aspect of the sacrum and occasionally provides a prominent renal or rectal branch.[18] There are 5 pairs of lumbar ISAs; the fifth pair arises from the MSA, as does the fourth pair when the iliac bifurcation is above L4 (**Fig. 6**). The diminutive L5 ISA is supplemented by the iliolumbar artery. The 4 sacral ISAs most commonly form 2 trunks, the superior S1 and inferior (S2, S3, S4) lateral sacral arteries.[19]

The Spinal Division of the Intersegmental Artery

In its complete form, the spinal division of the ISA provides the retrocorporeal, radicular, and

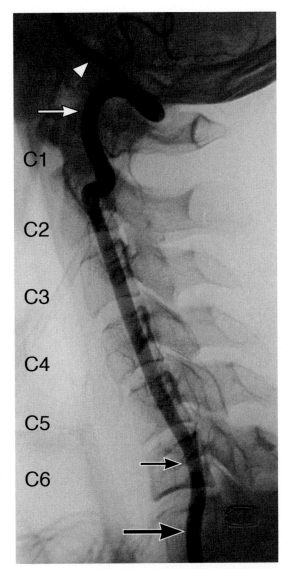

Fig. 4. The VA. The normal adult VA is a composite vessel consisting of 3 portions of different embryonic origin: a proximal segment made of a persistent sixth cervical ISA (*large arrow*), an intermediate segment formed by a chain of anastomoses established between the first 5 cervical ISAs, and a distal segment derived from the ProA. Seamless transitions connect the proximal and intermediate segments below the transverse foramen of C6 (*small black arrow*), and the intermediate and distal segments above the transverse foramen of C1 (*small white arrow*). The anterior radiculomedullary branch of the ProA is particularly prominent; it becomes the distal VA (*arrowhead*). (© 2019 Philippe Gailloud.)

prelaminar arteries. The retrocorporeal artery has ascending and descending branches that pass beneath the posterior longitudinal ligament to connect with opposite and adjacent arteries, and form a diamond-shaped anastomotic network.[20,21] This

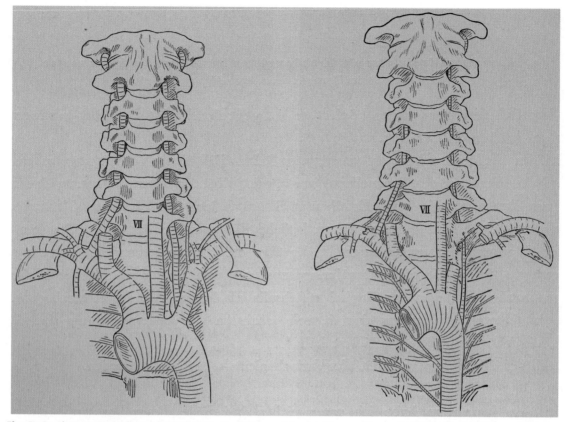

Fig. 5. Persistent cervical and thoracic ISA. (*Left*) A persistent left seventh cervical ISA takes off from the aorta distal to the subclavian artery; it is identified by its passage through the seventh transverse foramen. (*Right*) A persistent first thoracic ISA also takes off from the aorta distal to the subclavian artery; it is identified by its passage through the first costotransverse space. This variant is also known as a thoracic VA (ascending type). (*From* Adachi B. *Das Arteriensystem der Japaner.* Kyoto and Tokyo: Kaiserlich-japanische Universität zu Kyoto, in kommission bei "Maruzen Co."; 1928.)

network represents an important source of collateral supply; it is prominent in children but regresses with age (**Fig. 7**). The prelaminar arteries form a similar network over the anterior aspect of the posterior arch.

The Vertebral Body Vascularization

Anterolateral osseous branches
The anterolateral osseous arteries arise from the ISA stem and penetrate the periphery of the vertebral body. They are more numerous on the right because of the leftward deviation of the aorta.[22] Ascending and descending anterolateral branches connect with similar vessels from adjacent levels to form a periosteal network over the anterior and lateral aspects of the vertebral column.

Posteromedial osseous branches
One or 2 large posteromedial osseous arteries arise from the ascending branch of the retrocorporeal artery; they penetrate the vertebral body

through the basivertebral foramen or, less often, through an accessory canal (see **Fig. 7**).[20,23]

The vascularization of the posterior arch
The posterior arch is supplied by the prelaminar artery and by the dorsal branch of the ISA, which sends small rami to the lamina, the posterior vertebral joint, and the spinous process. The dorsal branch also takes part in the formation of a complex arterial network within the paraspinal musculature.[24]

The prelaminar network provides a central artery that penetrates the base the spinous process, and bilateral laminar arteries that pierce the lamina and bifurcate into ascending and descending branches for the apophyseal joints. The posterior elements, less robustly supplied than the vertebral body, are more prone to ischemia during surgical procedures.[24]

The vascularization of C2
The vascularization of the odontoid process comes from the anterior and posterior ascending

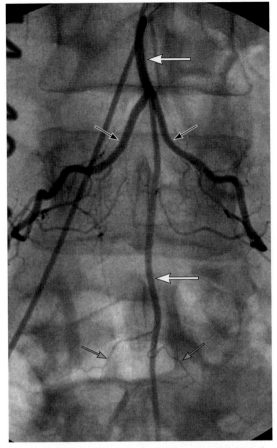

Fig. 6. Selective MSA angiography. The MSA is the continuation of the abdominal aorta: in this case, a prominent MSA (*white arrows*) provides the L4 (*black arrows*) and L5 (*gray arrows*) ISAs. Note the diminutive nature of the L5 ISAs, which share their territories with the iliolumbar arteries and L4 ISAs.[23] (© 2019 Philippe Gailloud.)

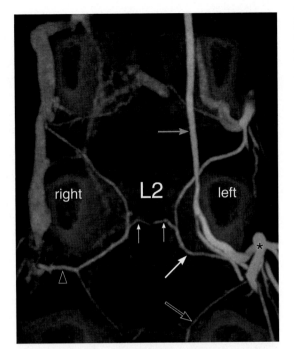

Fig. 7. The retrocorporeal network. Three-dimensional angiography of the left L2 ISA in an 8-year-old boy. The left L2 ISA (*asterisk*) supplies a prominent retrocorporeal network via ascending (*large white arrow*) and descending (*black arrow*) retrocorporeal branches. The retrocorporeal artery of right L2 is well-appreciated (*black arrowhead*). The posteromedian osseous arteries (*small white arrows*) come from the ascending branches and enter the basivertebral foramen. A prominent posterior RMA (*gray arrow*) supplies a spinal vascular malformation sitting above the field of view. (© 2019 Philippe Gailloud.)

branches of the VA[25,26] (**Fig. 8**). The main contributor is the posterior ascending artery (or anterior meningeal artery of the VA[27,28]), a cranial extension of the retrocorporeal artery of C2.[29] The left and right posterior ascending arteries connect above the odontoid process to form the apical arcade.[25] The anterior ascending artery is a tributary of the ISA stem of C2. Branches of the ascending pharyngeal artery also participate, notably those passing through the hypoglossal canal.[30]

The hemivertebral blush

Selective ISA angiography routinely documents a vertebral body blush. Initially central, this blush becomes hemivertebral in adults as the dominant osseous supply shifts from posteromedial to anterolateral osseous branches. A linear contrast uptake follows the upper and lower vertebral endplates in children; it gradually diminishes before disappearing with the closure of the growth plates at age 20 years (**Fig. 9**). The hemivertebral blush fades in later life as fat replaces the bone marrow.

The Radiculomedullary Arteries

All the primitive RMAs take part in the formation of the longitudinal spinal arteries, but only a few remain functionally important in adults[8,31,32]: 8 anteriorly and 16 posteriorly, on average.[8] This regression is an adaptation of the vascular supply to the metabolic demand of the spinal gray matter.[33] Although the marked dominance of the arteries of the cervical and lumbosacral enlargements is well-established, it is important to remember that any ISA can participate in the spinal cord supply.[34]

The relative ascent of the conus medullaris within the spinal canal explains the near vertical course of the lumbosacral RMAs. Thoracic anterior RMAs overwhelmingly originate from the left side, a prevalence apparently linked to geometric

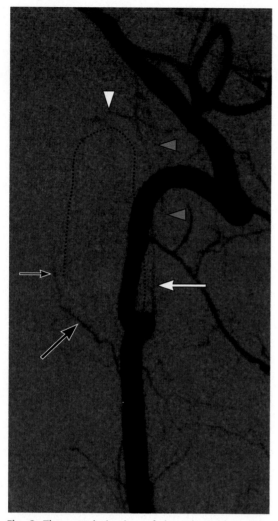

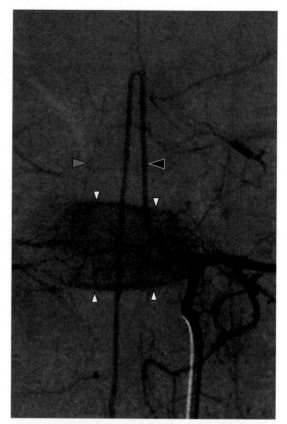

Fig. 9. Vertebral blush in a 5-year-old child. The central blush observed during selective angiography of a left T9 ISA spread to both sides of the midline (indicated by the position of the ASA). Note the linear contrast uptake marking the active vertebral growth plates (*white arrowheads*). The ISA provides a robust anterior RMA (artery of Adamkiewicz, *black arrowhead*); a contralateral posterior RMA (*gray arrowhead*) is opacified via collaterals. (© 2019 Philippe Gailloud.)

Fig. 8. The vascularization of the odontoid process. The anterior ascending branch (*small black arrow*) comes from the remnant of the C2 aortic stem (*large black arrow*). The posterior ascending branch (*white arrow*) is derived from the C2 retrocorporeal artery; with its contralateral counterpart, it forms the apical arcade (*white arrowhead*) above the odontoid process (*dotted line*). The posterior ascending branch is ventral to the ASA (*gray arrowheads*) on lateral projections. (© 2019 Philippe Gailloud.)

Anterior and posterior vertebrospinal trunks

The distal segment of the VA provides anterior and posterior radicular arteries that each end in ascending and descending rami. The anterior descending rami (anterior vertebrospinal trunks) converge medially to form the ASA; their territory does normally not exceed 1 or 2 cord segments. The posterior descending rami (posterior vertebrospinal trunks) remain unfused and continue caudally as the posteromedial spinal arteries (PmedSAs) and posterolateral spinal arteries (PlatSAs) in front and behind the posterior spinal nerve rootlets, respectively.

The superior and inferior arteries of the cervical enlargement

At least 2 RMAs supply the cord between C3 and T2. The superior artery of the cervical enlargement originates from 1 of the VAs between C3

factors (ie, selection of the shortest path). Posterior RMAs are evenly distributed in all regions, possibly because of the lack of fusion of the PSAs. Significant anterior and posterior RMAs can originate from a single radicular artery (ie, artery of Lazorthes). Variations in which an RMA territory extends beyond its normal boundaries are common; an anterior vertebrospinal trunk can supply the entire cervical cord. **Fig. 10** illustrates the locoregional variations in the designation of anterior RMAs.

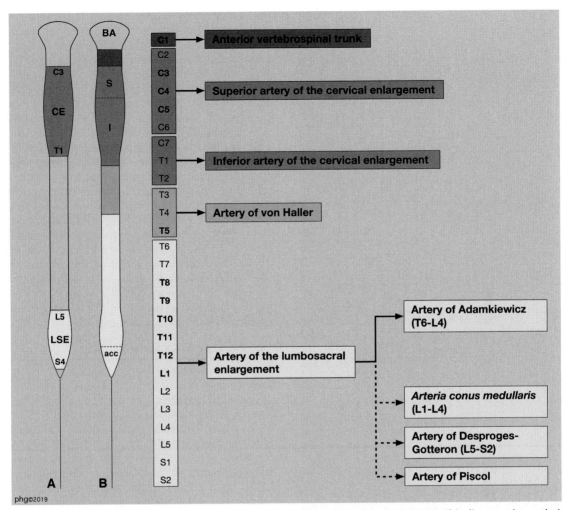

Fig. 10. Origin and labeling of anterior RMAs. The ASA is supplied by 5 constant RMAS. This diagram shows their vertebral levels of origin (numbered column) and approximate territories (spinal cord outline B). The most common levels of origin of each RMA are indicated in bold, with the exception of the inferior artery of the cervical enlargement, for which this information is not currently known. The cervical enlargement (CE) and lumbosacral (LSE) enlargement are illustrated in spinal cord outline A. The spinal cord outline is based on the data published by Ko and colleagues[85]. (1) the anterior vertebrospinal trunk comes from the VA (V4 segment) at C1, (2) the superior artery of the cervical enlargement arises from the VA between C2 and C6, (3) the inferior artery of the cervical enlargement originates from the supreme intercostal artery between C7 and T2, (4) the artery of von Haller arises from the left side of the aorta between T3 and T5, and (5) the artery of the lumbosacral enlargement most often originates between T6 and L4 on the left side (artery of Adamkiewicz). Accessory arteries are indicated by dotted arrows; under normal conditions, their territories rarely extends beyond the tip of the conus medullaris. acc, accessory; BA, basilar artery; I, inferior; S, superior. (*Data from* Ko HY, Park JH, Shin YB, Baek SY. Gross quantitative measurements of spinal cord segments in human. *Spinal Cord.* 2004;42(1):35-4; © 2019 Philippe Gailloud.)

and C5; it supplies a variable but relatively limited portion of the cervical cord. The inferior artery of the cervical enlargement is, in general, dominant. It comes from the supreme intercostal artery (C7-T2) but may also originate from the subclavian artery (C6), from a second thoracic ISA of aortic origin, or from a VA formed by a persistent seventh cervical ISA **(Fig. 11).**

The artery of von Haller

The artery of von Haller is a constant upper thoracic anterior RMA, most often found between T3 and T5 on the left side.[31,35] Its small caliber matches its limited territory, but the artery of von Haller may, as a variant, be the only source of supply for the lower thoracic and lumbosacral cord. It represents an endovascular pitfall, notably during bronchial procedures.[36,37]

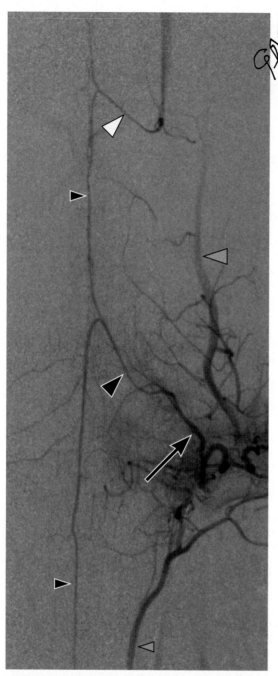

Fig. 11. Superior and inferior arteries of the cervical enlargement. The superior and inferior arteries of the cervical enlargement have been considered as variants of a single vessel but the author's experience suggests that they are independent and constant branches. This selective angiogram of the supreme intercostal artery (*arrow*) in a 27-year-old woman opacifies the inferior artery of the cervical enlargement at C7 (*large black arrowhead*) and, by reflux through the ASA (*small black arrowheads*), a superior artery of the cervical enlargement originating from the VA at C5 (*large white arrowhead*). In this case, the supreme

The artery of the lumbosacral enlargement

The artery of the lumbosacral enlargement, or artery of Adamkiewicz, is the main source of spinal cord supply. It most often originates between T6 and L4 on the left side but may, in theory, arise from lower lumbar or sacral ISA[32,38,39] (**Fig. 12A**). Accessory branches include the arteria conus medullaris[40] between L1 and L4, and the artery of Desproges-Gotteron between L5 and S2.[41] An artery of Piscol is a variation in which the descending ramus connects with the ASA, whereas the ascending ramus ends as a sulcal artery.[42] Contrary to an artery of Adamkiewicz of caudal origin (**Fig. 12B**), accessory branches have a territory limited to a portion of the conus medullaris (**Fig. 12C**); they are commonly associated with an artery of Adamkiewicz of cranial origin (T6-T9); conversely, a cranial accessory branch often accompanies an artery of Adamkiewicz of low origin. An accessory RMA can be injured by a lateral lumbar disc herniation,[41] a transforaminal injection,[43] or a spine manipulation.[44]

The Spinal Cord Vascularization

The extrinsic arterial vascularization

Several longitudinal arterial chains can be individualized within the arterial network covering the surface of the spinal cord (ie, the vasocorona)[45,46]: the ASAs, the anterolateral spinal arteries, the lateral spinal arteries, the PlatSAs, and the PmedSAs. The ASAs and PlatSAs are primary chains connected directly to the anterior and posterior RMAs. The anterolateral spinal arteries, lateral spinal arteries, and PmedSAs are secondary chains supplied by transverse branches of the primary chains (**Fig. 13**).

Developmental anatomy Medial branches stemming from the primitive ISAs contribute to the formation of a pair of paramedian anastomotic chains on the anterior surface of the neural tube. The more or less complete coalescence of these chains over the midline forms a single ventromedial channel corresponding to the basilar artery cranially and the ASA caudally.

Similar branches extending over the lateral and posterior surface of the neural tube form paired dorsolateral anastomotic chains. These chains remain separate despite being richly

intercostal artery is an isolated branch of the subclavian artery; the deep cervical artery (*large gray arrowhead*) and the T2 ISA (*small gray arrowhead*) are separate vessels opacified through anastomotic connections. Also note the duplication of the cervical ASA at C5. (© 2019 Philippe Gailloud.)

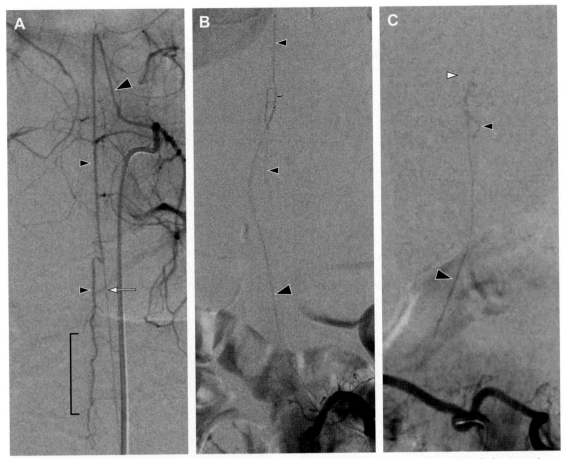

Fig. 12. The artery of the lumbosacral enlargement. (*A*) Left T9 injection in a 10-year-old girl documenting a robust RMA, the artery of Adamkiewicz (*large arrowhead*). A small L1 anterior RMA (*arrow*) is opacified by reflux via the ASA (*small arrowheads*); it may regress completely before adulthood or persist as an accessory vessel (arteria conus medullaris). The sulcal arteries are visible at the level of the conus medullaris (*bracket*). (*B*) Left L4 injection in a 79-year-old man showing an artery of Adamkiewicz of caudal origin (*large arrowhead*) supplying the lower thoracic and lumbosacral territory normally covered by an artery of the lumbosacral enlargement (*small arrowheads*). (*C*) Right L4 injection in a 59-year-old man opacifying an accessory anterior RMA (*large arrowhead*) that only participates in the supply of a portion of the ASA (*small black arrowhead*) limited to the tip of the conus medullaris; the ascending ramus (*white arrowhead*) appears to end as a sulcal branch (artery of Piscol). (© 2019 Philippe Gailloud.)

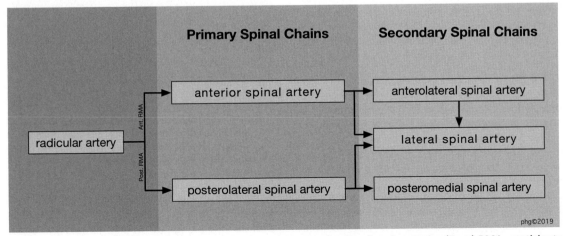

Fig. 13. Diagram of primary and secondary spinal arteries. Anterior (Ant.) and posterior (Post.) RMAs participate in the formation of the primary chains, the ASA, and the PlatSA. The secondary chains are not directly connected to RMAs; they are formed by transverse branches of the primary chains. The left and right PmedSAs are interconnected by a dense posterior plexus (not illustrated). (© 2019 Philippe Gailloud.)

interconnected across the midline; each has a lateral and a medial component lying in front and behind the line of emergence of the dorsal nerve roots, the PlatSAs, and PmedSAs.

The anterior spinal artery The ASA extends from the medulla oblongata to the tip of the conus medullaris, beyond which it continues as the artery of the filum terminale. The ASA forms through the selection of a preferential path within a primitive ventral arterial mesh.[47] Partial persistence of this mesh leads to the formation of focal or extensive duplications, in particular at the cervical level (see **Fig. 11**). Thoracic and lumbosacral duplications are, on the other hand, rare (**Fig. 14**). The ASA caliber varies between 0.2 mm at the thoracic level and 1.2 mm in the lumbosacral region.[48] Some segments may regress with age, notably at the upper cervical and midthoracic levels, where short interruptions are possible.[49,50]

The posteromedial and posterolateral spinal arteries The posterior RMAs supply the PlatSAs, which send small rami to the PmedSAs through the posterior nerve rootlets. The PmedSAs and PlatSAs alternate between plexiform channels and individual branches of variable, often inversely proportional, calibers. Multiple anastomoses connect the left and right PmedSAs across the midline (posterior plexus).[51] The upper cervical PlatSA is prominent, likely because of the large volume of white matter at that level.[52,53]

The periconal arterial anastomotic circle The ASA provides small arcuate arteries (rami cruciate) near the tip of the conus medullaris; these vessels course laterally and posteriorly to connect with the PSAs and form the periconal arterial anastomotic circle[8,54–56] (**Fig. 15**). Through this anastomosis, which is the only functionally significant connection between the anterior and posterior spinal circulations,[57] the distal ASA supplies the terminal segment of the PSAs.[58]

The intrinsic arterial vascularization
The sulcal arteries vascularize the central gray matter (centrifugal system), whereas the PSAs and the vasocorona supply most of the surrounding white matter via small perforating branches (centripetal system).[59] The 2 systems are interconnected by intramedullary anastomoses but remain functionally independent.[40]

Between 200 and 300 sulcal arteries arise from the ASA[8,59]; they travel down the anterior median fissure to penetrate the gray commissure, where they take the name of sulcocommissural arteries.[59] Their density is higher at the lumbosacral than at the cervical or thoracic

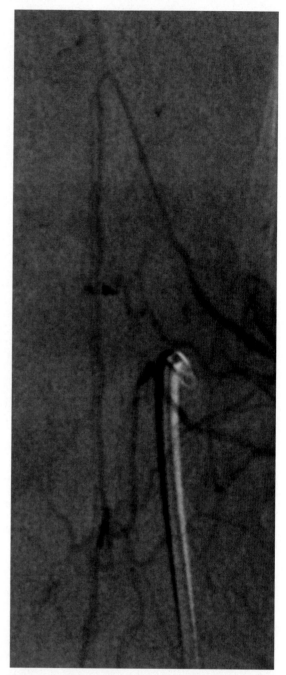

Fig. 14. Duplication of the thoracic ASA. This left T10 angiogram documents a duplication of the thoracic ASA in an 18-year-old woman, resulting from the focal persistence of paired primitive paramedian spinal chains. (© 2019 Philippe Gailloud.)

levels.[60–62] These variations are caused by the pronounced elongation of the thoracic and cervical cord segments during development.[63] The thoracic sulcal arteries are smaller, and their ascending and descending terminal rami cover

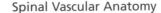

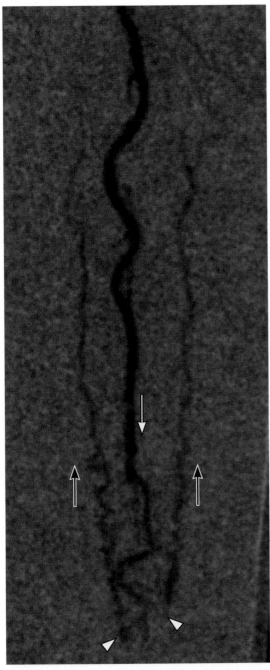

Fig. 15. The periconal arterial anastomotic circle. This magnified view of a left T9 angiogram in a 7-year-old boy documents anastomoses between the ASAs and PSAs via small arcuate branches (*arrowheads*). The flow is craniocaudal in the ASA (*white arrow*) and caudocranial in the PSAs (*black arrows*). (© 2019 Philippe Gailloud.)

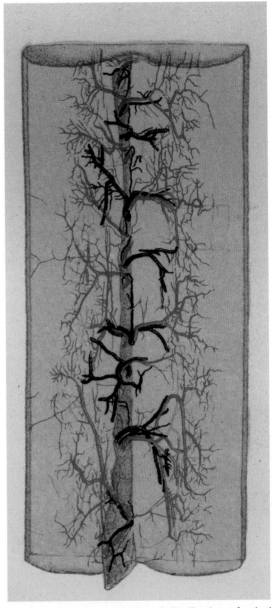

Fig. 16. Branching pattern and distribution of sulcal arteries and veins. Sulcal arteries generally have a unilateral distribution, irregularly alternating between the left and right sides. On the other hand, most sulcal veins have bilateral drainage territories. (*From* Kadyi H. *Über die Blutgefässe des Menschlichen Rückenmarkes.* Lemberg: Gubrynowicz & Schmidt; 1889.)

longer distances within the anterior median fissure, particularly in tall individuals. These features may represent an anatomic substrate for the increased sensitivity of the thoracic cord to ischemia.[62,64,65]

Most sulcal arteries have a unilateral territory but bilateral trunks also exist.[50,61,62] Trunks with multiple ipsilateral branches are less frequent.[61] The predominantly unilateral distribution of sulcal branches is consistent with the paired origin of the ASA. Left and right branches do not strictly alternate: 2 or 3 successive arteries may aim for the same hemicord, particularly at the thoracic level[66] (**Fig. 16**). Damage to a single sulcal artery can thus result in a limited unilateral infarct or be more extensive, longitudinally and/or transversally. Each limb of an ASA duplication provides sulcal branches for the ipsilateral hemicord.[66,67] The cervical predominance of the sulcal syndrome suggests that the occlusion of 1 limb of a duplicated ASA is a more likely mechanism than the loss of a single sulcal artery.[68]

Spinal collateral pathways

The development of collateral spinal cord supply relies on the enlargement of osseous and muscular anastomoses (**Fig. 17**), on the recruitment of alternate RMAs, and on the periconal arterial anastomotic circle. Collateral pathways influence the extent and severity of ischemic injuries, but their availability depends on the patient's age and the site, type, and timing of the arterial injury. The principles once established by Lazorthes remain valid[40]:

1. "The nearer the arterial obstruction is to the aortal origin and the farther it is removed from

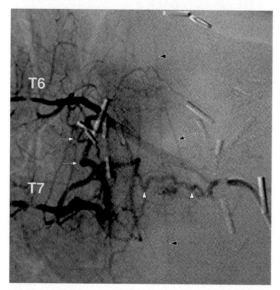

Fig. 17. Muscular and osseous collateral pathways. Right T6 ISA angiography in a young woman with prior spine tumor surgery. The only documented contribution to the thoracolumbar ASA (*black arrowheads*) was provided by a left T7 RMA (artery of Adamkiewicz, *black arrow*). Both T7 ISAs had been surgically ligated at their aortic origin; the artery of Adamkiewicz was supplied instead by the right T6 ISA via a combination of muscular (right T6 to right T7, *white arrows*) and retrocorporeal (right T7 to left T7, *small arrowheads*) anastomoses. These anastomotic pathways are most potent in children and young adults. (© 2019 Philippe Gailloud.)

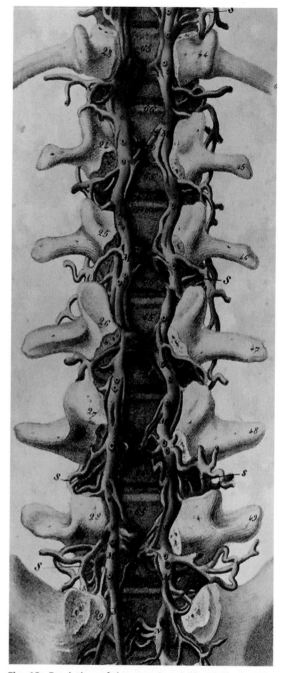

Fig. 18. Depiction of the anterior epidural plexus. The left and right anterior longitudinal veins are linked across the midline at the level of the basivertebral foramina; they connect laterally, through each neural foramen, with the EVVP. (*From* Breschet G. Recherches Anatomiques Physiologiques et Pathologiques sur le Système Veineux. Première Livraison. Paris: Rouen Frères, Libraires-Éditeurs; 1829.)

the spinal cord, the greater the possibilities of anastomotic substitution."

2. "The slower the obstruction is in establishing itself, the greater the chances of effective intervention by the substitution pathways, whereas a sudden obstruction takes the substitution pathways by surprise."

Spinal watershed zones

Axial watershed zone The axial watershed zone lies at the interface between the centripetal and centrifugal intrinsic circulations. The zone at risk is theoretically circular[40]; when combined with the increased gray matter vulnerability to

ischemia, it produces the snake-eye pattern typical of minimal or early ischemic injuries.[69] More severe lesions can damage the entire gray matter yet still spare the white matter.[70]

Longitudinal watershed zones Longitudinal watershed zones sit at the junction between adjacent radiculomedullary territories. They predominantly involve the anterior circulation as the plexiform nature of the posterior circulation offers a better protection against ischemia. Their topography depends on the number, size, and location of the contributing anterior RMAs, and the mechanism of injury (eg, single-branch occlusion vs hypotensive episode).

Posterior lumbosacral watershed zone The ASA supplies the most caudal portion of the PSAs via the periconal arterial anastomotic circle. This

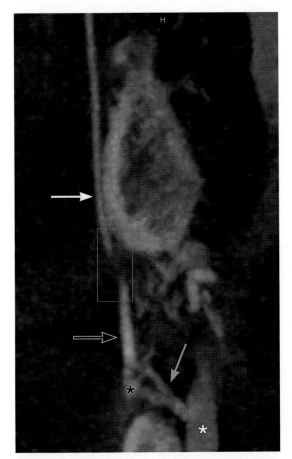

Fig. 19. The RMV and the antireflux mechanism. Coronal reconstruction of a 3-dimensional angiogram obtained in a 36-year-old woman, depicting the distal segment of a left L1 RMV. The intradural (*white arrow*) and extradural (*black arrow*) portions of the vein are delimited by its passage through the thecal sac. The short segment of RMV traveling within the 2 layers of the dura (*square*) corresponds to the antireflux mechanism; its narrowed lumen is below angiographic resolution. The RMV ends in the epidural plexus (*black asterisk*); the venous blood is drained toward the EVVP (*white asterisk*) by the transverse veins of the intervertebral venous plexus (*gray arrow*). (© 2019 Philippe Gailloud.)

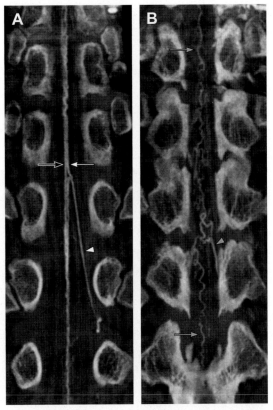

Fig. 20. The perimedullary venous system. Coronal reconstructions of a 3-dimensional angiogram (flat panel catheter angiotomography) obtained in a 25-year-old woman. The anterior perimedullary venous system (*A*) is more continuous and less sinuous that the posterior system (*B*). The AMSV (*white arrow*) courses along or deep to the ASA (*black arrow*); it drains into a left L1 RMV (*white arrowheads*). The PMSV (*gray arrows*) is partly well-delineated and partly plexiform. A posterior L1 RMV is seen (*gray arrowhead*). (© 2019 Philippe Gailloud.)

configuration establishes a longitudinal watershed zone along the dorsal aspect of the conus medullaris, the posterior lumbosacral watershed zone.[56]

THE SPINAL VENOUS SYSTEM

The spinal venous system is divided into 4 compartments:

1. The intrinsic spinal venous system
2. The extrinsic spinal venous system
3. The internal vertebral venous plexus (IVVP)
4. The external vertebral venous plexus (EVVP).

The antireflux mechanism is a valve-like structure formed by the passage of the radiculomedullary veins (RMVs) through the thecal sac; it demarcates the intradural and extradural compartments. The EVVP is not discussed further in this article.

The Internal Vertebral Venous Plexus

The IVVP comprises anterior and posterior longitudinal veins with numerous lateral and transverse anastomotic connections. The anterior longitudinal veins are attached to the vertebral bodies by the basivertebral veins and pressed against the vertebral wall by the posterior longitudinal ligament (**Fig. 18**). Their location is sensu stricto, not epidural.

The size and configuration of the posterior longitudinal veins are more variable. Breschet[71] distinguished between posterior longitudinal veins, present at the dorsal level only, and posterior epidural plexus, extending over the whole spine. Walther[72] simplified this notion by suggesting that the posterior longitudinal veins alternate plexiform and individualized configurations. The posterior longitudinal veins and plexus are not attached to the lamina but to the dorsal aspect of the thecal sac, with which they can move.

The neural foramen contains the intervertebral plexus, a venous ring made by the anterior and posterior longitudinal veins interconnected cranially and caudally by transverse anastomoses. The intervertebral plexus is a valve-free connection between the IVVP and EVVP.

The Radicular and Radiculomedullary Veins

RMVs are more numerous than RMAs: studies have found 11 to 40 anterior RMVs and 12 to 42 posterior RMVs.[73] These variations are likely explained by an age-related reduction in the number of RMVs, and by the use of different

A   **B**

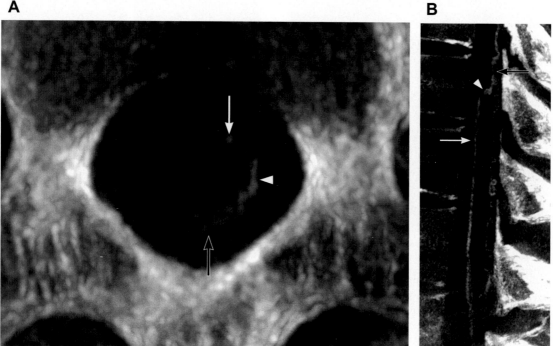

Fig. 21. Perimedullary venous anastomoses. Axial (*A*) and coronal (*B*) reconstructions of a 3-dimensional angiogram (flat panel catheter angiotomography) obtained in a 54-year-old woman. The anterior perimedullary venous system (*white arrow*) drains, in this case, toward the posterior perimedullary venous system (*black arrow*) via a left pial anastomosis (*arrowhead*). (© 2019 Philippe Gailloud.)

investigation techniques and anatomic definitions (RMVs vs radicular veins).

Dominant RMVs are most often found at the lumbosacral level[49]; they are more constant and prominent posteriorly.[74] Tadié and colleagues[74] identified 1 or 2 posterior RMVs and 1 anterior RMV at the thoracolumbar level, and 2 or 3 posterior RMVs in the midthoracic region, including a fairly constant 1 at about T6-T7.[74]

The antireflux mechanism

After observing that substances injected into the IVVP did not penetrate the intradural circulation, early anatomists postulated the existence of valves at or near the point of termination of RMVs in the epidural plexus.[64] Valves have now been ruled out, but modern investigators have discovered various mechanisms with a valve-like function.[75] The antireflux mechanism is principally a focal narrowing of the RMV as it crosses the thecal sac.[74,76–79] The caliber of this transdural segment roughly decreases from 950 to 130 μm, a relative stenosis of about 85% (Fig. 19). Additional factors may include an intraluminal dural fold and a focal increase in muscular fibers.[79]

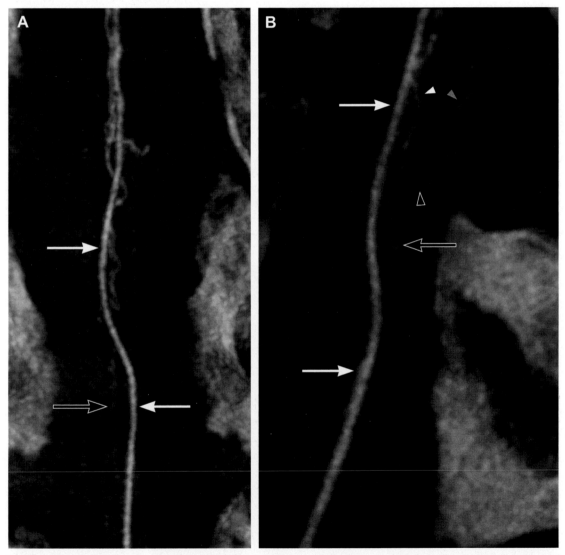

Fig. 22. The periconal venous anastomotic circle and the vein of the filum terminale. Coronal (*A*) and sagittal (*B*) reconstructions of a 3-dimensional angiogram obtained in a 74-year-old man. The vein of the filum terminale (*black arrow*) is a small midline vessel coursing along the filum terminale. The white arrows point to a lower lumbar or sacral RMV. The anterior (*white arrowhead*) and posterior (*gray arrowhead*) perimedullary venous systems are interconnected around the tip of the conus medullaris by the periconal venous anastomotic circle (*black arrowhead*). (© 2019 Philippe Gailloud.)

The antireflux mechanism controls the direction of the blood flow within the RMV. It protects the perimedullary network from pressure surges reaching the IVVP (eg, sneezing, pregnancy). The antireflux mechanism, combined with the near vertical course of lower thoracic and lumbosacral RMVs in the standing and sitting positions, appears to represent a risk factor for stagnation and thrombosis, which likely play a role in the development of spinal dural arteriovenous fistulas.[80]

The radicular veins

Numerous small veins course along the nerve roots from the venous plexuses of the spinal ganglia to the longitudinal spinal veins. Up to 3 true radicular veins accompany each nerve root. They flow toward the perimedullary venous system, are generally not connected with the IVVP, and do not contribute to the spinal cord drainage.[74,75]

The Perimedullary Venous System

The perimedullary venous network includes several longitudinal anastomotic chains, which lie alongside or deep to their arterial counterpart.[75] The anteromedian spinal vein (AMSV) and the posteromedian spinal vein (PMSV) are dominant; they are flanked by smaller anterolateral and posterolateral spinal veins. The AMSV is a relatively constant and straight channel extending from the skull base to the filum terminale (**Fig. 20**).[74] It receives tributaries from the anterior spinal nerve rootlets and connects cranially with the venous network of the brainstem. It can also drain into the posterior perimedullary system via a perimedullary thoracolumbar anastomosis.[74]

The lower thoracic and lumbar PMSV is a constant, sinuous, and usually dominant perimedullary venous channel.[74] It collects tributaries from dorsal and lumbar nerve rootlets, from the cauda equina, and from the anterior and posterior aspects of the spinal cord. Between T2 and T10, the posterior venous system has a plexiform appearance; its tortuosity increases with age.[74] Small or absent in the midthoracic region,[49] the PMSV is again clearly discernible at the cervical level, often as a duplicated channel.[74] The upper thoracic and cervical PMSV collects tributaries from dorsal nerve rootlets.

The perimedullary venous (coronary) network interconnects the longitudinal spinal trunks. However, large anastomoses are infrequent and their function unclear; they may represent an alternate drainage pathway protecting the spinal cord during transient, posture-related flow impairment. They occasionally drain one perimedullary venous system into the other (**Fig. 21**). The venous network surrounding the tip of the conus medullaris is similar to the periconal arterial anastomotic circle (**Fig. 22**).

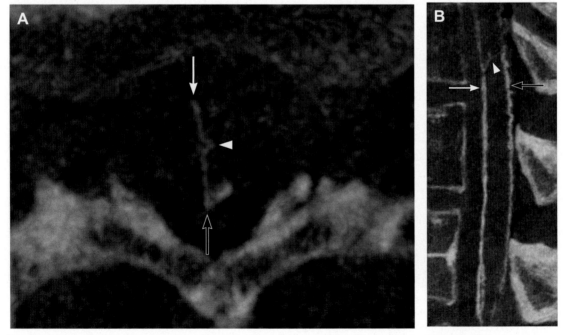

Fig. 23. Transmedullary venous anastomoses. Axial (*A*) and coronal (*B*) reconstructions of a 3-dimensional angiogram (same patient as **Fig. 22**). The anteromedian (*white arrow*) and posteromedian (*black arrow*) spinal veins are connected by a transmedullary anastomosis (median anteroposterior type) (*arrowhead*). (© 2019 Philippe Gailloud.)

The Intrinsic Venous System

The intramedullary venous network has a central and a peripheral compartment. The sulcal veins drain the median and anterior portion of the spinal cord into the AMSV[81]; they typically have bilateral territories. Sulcal veins establish longitudinal anastomoses, both at the level of the central gray matter and within the anteromedian fissure.[81]

The short peripheral veins follow a radial course ending in the coronary plexus; those within the anterior and posterior radicular fasciculi are, in general, more robust.[49] The larger, more constant septal veins drain into the PMSV.

Two main types of transmedullary venous anastomoses are recognized: a centrodorsolateral type[65] and a more common median anteroposterior type[50,76] **(Fig. 23)**. Both can become conspicuous when associated with a vascular malformation.

REFERENCES

1. Broman I. Über die Entwicklung und "Wanderung" der Zweige der Aorta Abdominalis beim Menschen. Anatomische Hefte 1908;36:407–550.
2. Evans HM. The development of the vascular system. In: Keibel F, Mall FP, editors. Manual of human embryology, vol. 2. Philadelphia: J.B. Lippincott; 1912. p. 570–708.
3. Gailloud P. Multiple thoracic bilateral intersegmental arterial trunks. Eur J Anat 2017;21:149–55.
4. Chiras J, Merland JJ. The dorsospinal artery. A little known anatomical variant. Its importance in spinal angiography. J Neuroradiol 1979;6(2):93–100.
5. Clavier E, Guimaraems L, Chiras J, et al. Isolated dorsospinal artery supplying anterior spinal artery. Neuroradiology 1987;29(2):213.
6. Lefournier V, Bessou P, Gailloud P, et al. Direct emergence of the dorsospinal artery from the aorta supplying the anterior spinal artery: report of two cases. AJNR Am J Neuroradiol 1998;19(10):1961–2.
7. Siclari F, Fasel JH, Gailloud P. Direct emergence of the dorsospinal artery from the aorta and spinal cord blood supply. Case reports and literature review. Neuroradiology 2006;48(6):412–4.
8. Kadyi H. Über die Blutgefässe des Menschlichen Rückenmarkes. Lemberg (Ukraine): Gubrynowicz & Schmidt; 1889.
9. Charpy A. Vaisseaux des Centres Nerveux. In: Poirier P, Charpy A, editors. Traité d'Anatomie Humaine. Paris: Masson et Cie, Éditeurs; 1899. p. 549–610.
10. Maillot C, Koritke JG. Origins of the posterior spinal artery trunk in man. C R Assoc Anat 1970;149: 837–47 [in French].
11. Padget DH. Designation of the embryonic intersegmental arteries in reference to the vertebral artery and subclavian stem. Anat Rec 1954;119:349–56.
12. Parkinson D, Reddy V, Ross RT. Congenital anastomosis between the vertebral artery and internal carotid artery in the neck. Case report. J Neurosurg 1979;51(5):697–9.
13. Chan PN, Yu SC, Boet R, et al. A rare congenital anastomosis between the vertebral artery and internal carotid artery. AJNR Am J Neuroradiol 2003; 24(9):1885–6.
14. Gailloud P, Gregg L, Pearl MS, et al. Ascending and descending thoracic vertebral arteries. AJNR Am J Neuroradiol 2017;38(2):327–35.
15. Krassnig M. Von der Arteria vertebralis thoracica der Säuger und Vögel. Anat Hefte 1913;49(3):523–609.
16. Dubreuil-Chambardel L. Traité des variations du système artériel. Variations des artères du membre supérieur. 1st edition. Paris: Masson et Cie; 1926.
17. Gailloud P. The supreme intercostal artery includes the last cervical intersegmental artery (C7) - angiographic validation of the intersegmental nomenclature proposed by Dorcas Padget in 1954. Anat Rec (Hoboken) 2014;297(5):810–8.
18. Pearl MS, Gest TR, Gailloud P. Superior rectal artery origin from the median sacral artery–angiographic appearance, developmental anatomy, and clinical implications. Clin Anat 2014;27(6):900–5.
19. Dubreuil-Chambardel L. Variations des Artères du Pelvis et du Membre Inférieur. Paris: Masson et Cie; 1925.
20. Willis TA. Nutrient arteries of the vertebral bodies. J Bone Joint Surg Am 1949;31A(3):538–40.
21. Willis T. Cerebri anatome, cui accessit nervorum descripto et usus. London: Typis Tho. Roycroft; Impensis Jo. Martyn & Ja. Allestry; 1664.
22. Chiras J, Morvan G, Merland JJ. The angiographic appearances of the normal intercostal and lumbar arteries. Analysis and the anatomic correlation of the lateral branches. J Neuroradiol 1979;6(3): 169–96.
23. Ratcliffe JF. The arterial anatomy of the adult human lumbar vertebral body: a microarteriographic study. J Anat 1980;131(Pt 1):57–79.
24. Crock HV, Yoshizawa H. The blood supply of the lumbar vertebral column. Clin Orthop Relat Res 1976;115:6–21.
25. Schiff DC, Parke WW. The arterial supply of the odontoid process. J Bone Joint Surg Am 1973; 55(7):1450–6.
26. Althoff B, Goldie IF. The arterial supply of the odontoid process of the axis. Acta Orthop Scand 1977; 48(6):622–9.
27. Lasjaunias P, Moret J, Theron J. The so-called anterior meningeal artery of the cervical vertebral artery. Normal radioanatomy and anastomoses. Neuroradiology 1978;17(1):51–5.

28. Greitz T, Lauren T. Anterior meningeal branch of the vertebral artery. Acta Radiol Diagn (Stockh) 1968; 7(3):219–24.

29. Minne J, Depreux R, Francke JP. Peri-odontoid arteries. C R Assoc Anat 1970;149:914–20 [in French].

30. Haffajee MR. A contribution by the ascending pharyngeal artery to the arterial supply of the odontoid process of the axis vertebra. Clin Anat 1997; 10(1):14–8.

31. Von Haller A. Iconum anatomicarum quibus aliquae partes corporis humani delineatae traduntur. Fasciculus VII - Arteriae cerebri Medullae spinalis Oculi. Göttingen (Germany): Widow of Abram Vandenhoeck; 1754.

32. Adamkiewicz A. Die Blutgefässe des menschlichen Rückenmarkes. II. Theil. Die Gefässe der Rückenmarks-Oberfläche. Sitzungsberichten der Kaiserlichen Akademie der Wissenschaften, Mathematisch-naturwissenschaftliche Classe 1882;85:101–30.

33. Tanon L. Les artères de la moelle dorso-lombaire. 1st edition. Paris: Vigot Frères, Editeurs; 1908.

34. Crock HV, Yamagishi M, Crock MC. The Conus medullaris and cauda equina in man. An Atlas of the arteries and veins. New York: Springer Verlag; 1986.

35. Gailloud P. The artery of von Haller: a constant anterior radiculomedullary artery at the upper thoracic level. Neurosurgery 2013;73(6):1034–43.

36. Cheng SJ, Hsueh IH, Po HL, et al. Watershed infarction of spinal cord after the embolization of bronchial artery: a case report. Zhonghua Yi Xue Za Zhi (Taipei) 1996;57(4):293–6.

37. Mesurolle B, Lacombe P, Qanadli S, et al. [Angiographic identification of spinal cord arteries before bronchial artery embolization]. J Radiol 1997;78(5): 377–80.

38. Doppman J, Chiro GD. The arteria radicularis magna: radiographic anatomy in the adult. Br J Radiol 1968;41(481):40.

39. Djindjian R, Hurth M, Houdart E. Angiography of the spinal cord. Baltimore (MD): University Park Press; 1970.

40. Lazorthes G, Gouaze A, Zadeh JO, et al. Arterial vascularization of the spinal cord. Recent studies of the anastomotic substitution pathways. J Neurosurg 1971;35(3):253–62.

41. Desproges-Gotteron R. Contribution à l'étude de la sciatique paralysante [Thesis] 1955. Paris.

42. Piscol K. Die Blutversorgung des Rückenmarkes und ihre klinische Relevanz. New York: Springer-Verlag; 1972.

43. Wybier M. Transforaminal epidural corticosteroid injections and spinal cord infarction. Joint Bone Spine 2008;75(5):523–5.

44. Balblanc JC, Pretot C, Ziegler F. Vascular complication involving the conus medullaris or cauda equina after vertebral manipulation for an L4-L5 disk herniation. Rev Rhum Engl Ed 1998;65(4):279–82.

45. Mettler FA. Neuroanatomy. 1st edition. St Louis (MO): The C.V. Mosby Company; 1942.

46. Noeske K. Über die arterielle Versorgung des menschlichen Rückenmarkes. Morphologisches Jahrbuch 1958;99(3):455–97.

47. Evans HM. On the development of the aortae, cardinal and umbilical veins, and the other blood vessels of vertebrate embryos from capillaries. Anat Rec 1909;3(9):498–518.

48. Romanes GJ. The arterial blood supply of the human spinal cord. Paraplegia 1965;2:199–207.

49. Lazorthes G, Gouaze A, Djindjian R. Vascularisation et circulation de la moelle épinière. Paris: Masson & Cie; 1973.

50. Thron A. Vascular anatomy of the spinal cord. Neuroradiological investigations and clinical syndromes. New York: Springer-Verlag; 1988.

51. Gillilan LA. The arterial blood supply of the human spinal cord. J Comp Neurol 1958;110(1):75–103.

52. Lasjaunias P, Vallee B, Person H, et al. The lateral spinal artery of the upper cervical spinal cord. Anatomy, normal variations, and angiographic aspects. J Neurosurg 1985;63(2):235–41.

53. Parke WW, Settles HE, Bunger PC, et al. Lumbosacral anterolateral spinal arteries and brief review of "accessory" longitudinal arteries of the spinal cord. Clin Anat 1999;12(3):171–8.

54. Mayer JCA. Anatomische Beschreibung der Blutgefässe des menschlichen Körpers. Berlin: G.J. Decker; 1788.

55. Henle J. Handbuch der Gefässlehre des Menschen. Braunschweig: Friedrich Vieweg und Sohn; 1868.

56. Gailloud P, Gregg L, Galan P, et al. Periconal arterial anastomotic circle and posterior lumbosacral watershed zone of the spinal cord. J Neurointerv Surg 2014;7(11):848–53.

57. Henle J. 1st edition. Handbuch der systematischen Anatomie des Menschen: Gefässlehre, vol. 3. Braunschweig: Druck und Verlag von Friedrich Vieweg und Sohn; 1868.

58. Bolton B. The blood supply of the human spinal cord. J Neurol Psychiatry 1939;2(2):137–48.

59. Adamkiewicz A. Die Blutgefässe des menschlichen Rückenmarkes. I. Theil. Die Gefässe der Rückenmarkssubstanz. Sitzungsberichten der Kaiserlichen Akademie der Wissenschaften, Mathematisch-naturwissenschaftliche Classe 1881;84:469–502.

60. Lazorthes G, Poulhes J, Bastide G, et al. La vascularisation artérielle de la moelle. Recherches anatomiques et applications à la pathologie médullaire et à la pathologie aortique. Neurochirurgie 1958;4: 3–19.

61. Zhang Z-A, Nonaka H, Hatori T. The microvasculature of the spinal cord in the human adult. Neuropathology 1997;17(1):32–42.

62. Hassler O. Blood supply to human spinal cord: a microangiographic study. Arch Neurol 1966;15(3):302.

63. Lazorthes G, Poulhes J, Bastide G, et al. Recherches sur la vascularisation artérielle de la moelle. Applications à la pathologie médullaire. Bull Acad Natl Med 1957;141(21–23):464–77.

64. Suh T, Alexander L. Vascular system of the human spinal cord. Arch Neurol Psychiatry 1939;41:659–77.

65. Herren RY, Alexander L. Sulcal and intrinsic blood vessels of the human spinal cord. Arch Neurol Psychiatry 1939;41(4):678–87.

66. Clemens HJ, von Quast H. Untersuchugen über die Gefässe des menschlichen Rückenmarkes. Acta Anat (Basel) 1960;42:277–306.

67. Turnbull IM. Microvasculature of the human spinal cord. J Neurosurg 1971;35(2):141–7.

68. Weidauer S, Nichtweiss M, Hattingen E, et al. Spinal cord ischemia: aetiology, clinical syndromes and imaging features. Neuroradiology 2015;57(3):241–57.

69. Hundsberger T, Thomke F, Hopf HC, et al. Symmetrical infarction of the cervical spinal cord due to spontaneous bilateral vertebral artery dissection. Stroke 1998;29(8):1742.

70. Kepes JJ. Selective necrosis of spinal cord gray matter. A complication of dissecting aneurysm of the aorta. Acta Neuropathol 1965;4(3):293–8.

71. Breschet G. Recherches Anatomiques Physiologiques et Pathologiques sur le Système Veineux. Première Livraison. Paris: Rouen Frères, Libraires-Éditeurs; 1829.

72. Walther C. Recherches Anatomiques sur les Veines du Rachis. Paris: Asselin et Houzeau; 1885.

73. Jellinger K. Zur Orthologie und Pathologie der Rückenmarksdurchblutung. New York: Springer; 1966.

74. Tadié M, Hemet J, Freger P, et al. Morphological and functional anatomy of spinal cord veins. J Neuroradiol 1985;12(1):3–20.

75. Dommisse G. The arteries and veins of the human spinal cord from birth. 1st edition. London: Churchill Livingstone; 1975.

76. Crock HV, Yoshizawa H. The blood supply of the vertebral column and spinal cord in man. New York: Springer-Verlag; 1977.

77. Tadié M, Hemet J, Aaron C, et al. Les veines radiculaires de drainage de la moelle ont-elles un dispositif de securite anti-reflux? Bull Acad Natl Med 1978; 162(6):550–4.

78. Tadié M, Hemet J, Aaron C, et al. Le dispositif protecteur anti-reflux des veines de la moelle. Neurochirurgie 1979;25:28–30.

79. van der Kuip M, Hoogland PV, Groen RJ. Human radicular veins: regulation of venous reflux in the absence of valves. Anat Rec 1999;254(2): 173–80.

80. Gailloud P. The arrow-tipped loop is a marker of radiculomedullary vein thrombosis linked to the anti-reflux mechanism-angiographic anatomy and clinical implications. Neuroradiology 2014;56(10): 859–64.

81. Gillilan LA. Veins of the spinal cord. Anatomic details; suggested clinical applications. Neurology 1970;20(9):860–8.

82. Hochstetter F. Uber die Entwicklung der A. Vertebralis beim Kaninchen, nebst Bemerkungen über die Entstehung des Ansa Vieussenii. Morphol Jahrb 1890;16:572–86.

83. His W. Anatomie Menschlicher embryonen. III. Zur Geschichte der Organe. Leipzig (Germany): Verlag von F.C.W. Vogel; 1885.

84. Schmeidel G. Die Entwicklung der Arteria vertebralis des Menschen. Morphol Jahrb 1933;71:315–435.

85. Ko HY, Park JH, Shin YB, et al. Gross quantitative measurements of spinal cord segments in human. Spinal Cord 2004;42(1):35–40.

Rapid On-site Evaluation of Spine Lesions

Israh Akhtar, MD*, Varsha Manucha, MD

KEYWORDS

- Spinal • Paraspinal • Vertebra • Rapid on-site evaluation (ROSE) • Cytology
- Fine-needle aspiration (FNA) • Core needle biopsy (CNB)

KEY POINTS

- Fine-needle aspiration (FNA) and core needle biopsy are currently the primary diagnostic modalities that clinicians and oncologists use to assess the nature of a mass lesion.
- Any superficial or deep-seated lesion occurring anywhere in the body, including bone and soft tissue, can undergo this procedure to pathologically characterize it.
- The outcomes of FNA, performed either alone or in combination with core biopsy, are best when performed and interpreted by skilled individuals. The roles of interventional radiologists and cytologists are pivotal in ensuring adequacy of the specimen and leading the clinical team in making the diagnosis and avoiding repeat diagnostic procedures or a more invasive open surgical biopsy.

INTRODUCTION

Fine-needle aspiration (FNA) and core needle biopsy (CNB) are currently the primary diagnostic modalities that clinicians and oncologists use to assess the nature of a mass lesion. This application applies most frequently to thoracic and abdominal organs, but any superficial or deep-seated lesion occurring anywhere in the body, including bone and soft tissue, can undergo this procedure to pathologically characterize it. Not only is the technique simple, safe, rapid, and cost-effective, it also gives cytologists an opportunity to triage the specimen upfront, thereby providing an accurate diagnosis integrated with results of ancillary tests, including microbiology, molecular studies, cytogenetics, and flow cytometry. The outcomes of FNA, performed either alone or in combination with core biopsy, are best when performed and interpreted by skilled individuals. The roles of interventional radiologists and cytologists are pivotal in ensuring adequacy of the specimen and in leading the clinical team in making the diagnosis and avoiding a repeat diagnostic procedures or a more invasive open surgical biopsy.

RAPID ON-SITE EVALUATION

FNA is a procedure by which a sample of cells is aspirated from a mass lesion by applying suction through a fine needle (22–25 gauge) attached to a syringe. CNB involves extracting a cylindrical piece of tissue from a mass lesion using a large (11–15 gauge), hollow needle.[1,2] FNA/CNB of deep-seated visceral mass lesions, soft tissue/ bone lesions, and deep-seated head and neck lesions are best performed under image guidance (ultrasonography or computed tomography) under local anesthesia or with conscious sedation. A cytology team comprising a cytopathologist or cytotechnologist may be called at the time of the procedure to evaluate the adequacy of the specimen. This process is called rapid on-site evaluation (ROSE).

The interventional radiologist, under image guidance, directs the needle into the mass lesion or an area of radiological abnormality, and the material

Disclosure: No disclosures.
Department of Pathology, University of Mississippi Medical Center, 2500 North State Street, Jackson, MS 39216, USA
* Corresponding author. 2500 North State Street, Jackson, MS 39216.
E-mail address: iakhtar@umc.edu

Neuroimag Clin N Am 29 (2019) 635–642
https://doi.org/10.1016/j.nic.2019.07.009
1052-5149/19/Published by Elsevier Inc.

so obtained, which is either an aspirate of the lesion or a CNB, is given to the cytologist. The cytologist prepares smears of FNA, and touch imprints (TIs) of CNB are prepared by gently removing the CNB from the biopsy needle and then rolling or dragging it onto a glass slide. The TI or FNA smear is air-dried and stained with modified Giemsa stain (Diff-Quik) and an immediate assessment of the adequacy and diagnostic yield is made by cytologist, using a microscope. Additional CNBs are obtained and TIs prepared if the initial material is not deemed adequate or representative of the lesion. This interpretation takes not more than a couple of minutes and is performed between each pass made by the interventional radiologist. The most commonly used stain for immediate assessment is Diff-Quik, but, based on the preference of the pathologist, hematoxylin-eosin and rapid Papanicolaou stain can also be used.[3,4] After a smear or TI is assessed, the remainder of the material is rinsed in Roswell Park Memorial Institute medium (RPMI) in order to make a cell block or core biopsy section, on which, subsequently, ancillary testing is performed. Molecular testing can be performed on the same paraffin-fixed block. An overall yield greater than 12% in adequacy rates has been reported when ROSE is performed, compared with when ROSE is not performed.[5,6]

Smears from FNA or TIs from CNB can give equally good results on on-site examination, depending on whether the lesion has been accurately targeted by the radiologist (**Fig. 1**). Valuable information on the morphology of the cell can be obtained through imprint cytology. The diagnostic concordance rate between the morphologic findings in TI and CNB is reportedly high, ranging from 88% to 90%.[2] FNA helps in targeting small lesions, whereas CNB is performed in osteoblastic and mixed-density osseous lesions. Depending

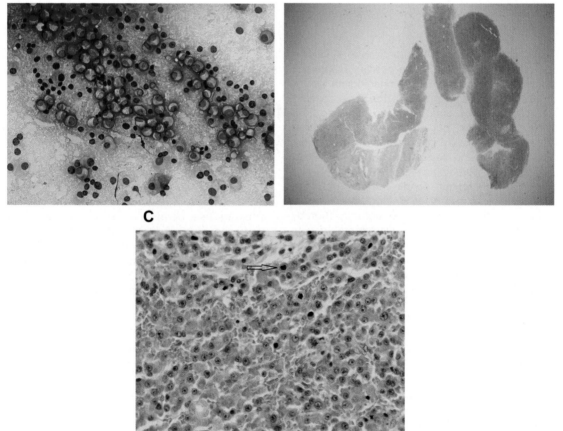

Fig. 1. (*A*) Plasma cell myeloma. Abnormal plasma cells in loosely cohesive clusters, in FNA smear (Diff-Quik, original magnification ×40). (*B*) CNB of plasma cell myeloma. Low power showing generous sample taken by the radiologist (hematoxylin-eosin, original magnification ×4). (*C*) Abnormal plasma cells in marrow spaces, completely replacing marrow. Arrow shows mitotic figures (hematoxylin-eosin, original magnification ×40).

on the nature of the lesion targeted, cytologists ask for more tissue if ancillary studies, such as immunohistochemistry or molecular testing, will be have to be performed. On an average, 2 to 3 dedicated passes should be sufficient; however, if cellularity on the slide is suboptimal, more samples are required. Judiciously triaging the specimen is a critical role that cytologists play in the management of patients.

COST-EFFECTIVENESS OF RAPID ON-SITE EVALUATION

Sample adequacy is an important aspect of overall FNA cytology performance. FNA effectiveness is augmented by an increasing number of needle passes, but increased needle passes are associated with higher costs and greater risk of adverse events. ROSE improves effectiveness of FNA when the per-pass adequacy rate is low. ROSE is unlikely to be cost-effective in sampling environments in which the per-pass adequacy is high.[7]

Recent developments in advanced imaging techniques, molecular testing, and targeted therapies have coincided with a rapid increase in the number of FNA procedures being performed. Concurrently, the demand for ROSE has also increased, outstripping the capacity of available cytopathologists at some institutions. ROSE assessors (eg, cytotechnologists) may be a cost-effective alternative to cytopathologists when the per-pass adequacy rate is moderate (60%–80%) or when the number of needle passes is limited.[7,8] Telecytology is increasingly being used to circumvent these problems because it increases the efficiency of ROSE through the transmission of static images, videomicroscopy, or whole scanned slides to pathologists for remote review.[9–11]

UTILITY OF CYTOLOGY IN VERTEBRAE AND SPINE

The lesions encountered in spinal and paraspinal areas can be both benign and malignant. Bones and vertebral column are the most favored sites for metastasis after lung and liver.[12–14] Approximately two-thirds of patients with cancer develop bone metastasis[15] (Fig. 2).

The incidence of skeletal metastasis from autopsy studies is 73% (range, 47%–85%) in breast cancer, 68% (range, 33%–85%) in prostate cancer, 42% (range, 28%–60%) in thyroid cancer, 36% (range, 30%–55%) in lung cancer, 35% (range, 33%–40%) in kidney cancer, 6% (range, 5%–7%) in esophageal cancer, 5% (range, 3%–11%) in gastrointestinal tract cancers, and 11% (range, 8%–13%) in rectal cancer.[15] Given the

high prevalence of breast, prostate, and lung cancer, they are responsible for more than 80% of cases of metastatic bone disease (Fig. 3). Primary hematopoietic malignancies common to this are non-Hodgkin lymphoma, multiple myeloma, and anaplastic large cell lymphoma.[16]

Nonneoplastic conditions that commonly affect the spine include osteoporotic fractures, discitis/osteomyelitis, degenerative disc disease, amyloidosis, extramedullary hematopoiesis, and Paget disease.[16] Obtaining cytologic material in infectious/inflammatory lesions allows rapid identification of organisms and initiation of treatment in many cases. Common infectious disorders include tuberculosis, blastomycosis, cryptococcosis, and bacterial abscess.[16,17]

Although in some cases an accurate assessment of the size, extent, and diagnosis of the lesion can be provided by imaging, a final decision regarding patient management depends on histologic diagnosis. FNA is a safe and a cost-effective alternative to an invasive surgical biopsy and has proved to be an effective means of establishing a definitive diagnosis of vertebral and paravertebral lesions, allowing appropriate patient management.

The most frequent indication for performing FNA of the spinal and paraspinal region is to evaluate patients with documented history of malignancy and presenting with new radiographically suspicious spinal and paraspinal lesions.[18–20] In patients with no known primary malignancy, FNA can be helpful in establishing an initial diagnosis of malignancy and to initiate a search for the occult primary malignancy.

It was as early as 1935 when Robertson and Ball[21] first reported the usefulness of diagnosing destructive spinal lesions by needle biopsy. Spinal and paraspinal lesions can be a diagnostic challenge because of their low frequency of occurrence and the limited cellularity that these specimens yield. Familiarity with the cytomorphologic features of different benign and malignant lesions occurring in this area is critical for the diagnosis. Evaluation of the adequacy of aspirated material is crucial in rendering a definitive diagnosis. However, ROSE on FNA of bony lesions is challenging because the aspirated specimens are generally bloody and tend to produce a low-cellular-yield sample.[22] The rate of unsatisfactory specimens is between 15.3% and 19%.[23,24] Irrespective, many studies have established the usefulness of FNA in all regions of the spine from cervical vertebrae to sacrum, with accuracy of more than 75%.[16,18] However, the accuracy rate depends on the skill of the radiologist in deciding the optimal route of approach at various anatomic

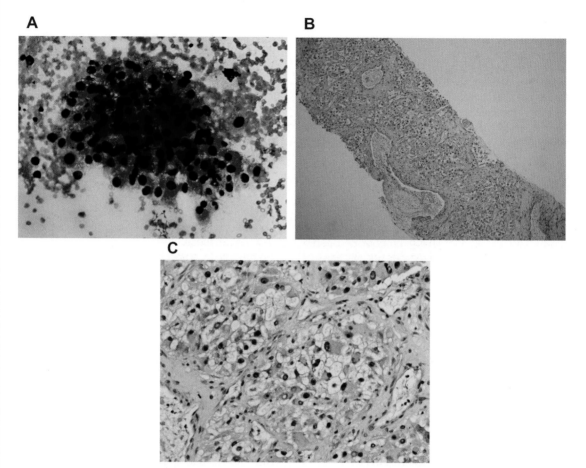

Fig. 2. (*A*) Metastatic renal cell carcinoma. Touch imprint showing cluster of malignant cells with finely vacuo-lated cytoplasm (Diff-Quik, original magnification ×40). (*B, C*) CNB showing clear cell renal cell carcinoma (hema-toxylin-eosin, original magnification ×20 [*B*], ×40 [*C*]).

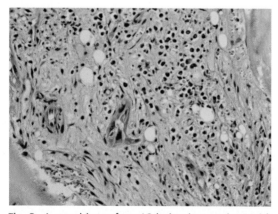

Fig. 3. A core biopsy from L2 lesion in a patient with history of lung adenocarcinoma. Rare malignant gland seen in marrow space, surrounded by trilineage marrow elements (hematoxylin-eosin, original magnification ×40).

levels.[19] The overall sensitivity of the procedure in spinal and vertebral lesions has been reported to be in the range of 93.3% to 96%, specificity 94.5% to 100%, positive predictive value 95.6% to 100%, and negative predictive value 90.7% to 92%,[16,24] which is comparable with the values in soft tissue and bone lesions[25] (**Table 1**).

Table 1
Sensitivity, specificity and predictive value of rapid on-site evaluation in bone, soft tissue, and overall

	Overall	Soft Tissue	Bone
Sensitivity (%)	96	97	93
Specificity (%)	98	98	100
PPV (%)	99	99	100
NPV (%)	92	94	86

Abbreviations: NPV, negative predictive value; PPV, positive predictive value.

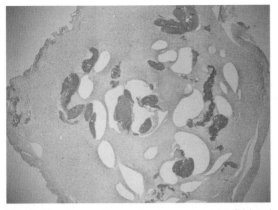

Fig. 4. Nondiagnostic specimen composed of blood only. Cell block shows only blood, no diagnostic cells are seen (hematoxylin-eosin, original magnification ×100).

Assessment of adequacy by on-site evaluation of the cytologic material is an important step in rendering a correct diagnosis and triaging the aspirate for special studies. Cell block material and core biopsies obtained at the time of FNA can be complementary in making a more reliable diagnosis.[16] Similarly, obtaining cytologic material in infectious/inflammatory lesions allows rapid identification of organisms and initiation of treatment in many cases.

For tumors causing spinal cord compression, such as lymphoma and small cell carcinoma, immediate on-site assessment is critical in order to initiate treatment.[16] Studies have also shown the reliability of FNA in diagnosing primary bone neoplasms and nonneoplastic lesions of the vertebral column, such as degenerative joint disease, osteoporotic fractures, Paget disease of the bone,

Table 2
Diagnostic categories when radiologist is confident about the placement of needles in a radiologically obvious lesion

Diagnostic Category	Definition	Criterion
Nondiagnostic	A specimen that provides no useful diagnostic information about the nodule, cyst, or mass identified by imaging studies	Blood, skeletal muscle, or fat (see **Fig. 4**)
Negative for malignancy	The specimen contains adequate cellular or extracellular material to evaluate or define a lesion identified on imaging studies	Bone marrow elements that confirm bone placement of needle or an inflammatory exudate that explains a suspected inflammatory lesion (**Fig. 5**)
Atypical cytology	1. Specimens displaying cytomorphologic aberrations greater than those clearly secondary to inflammation or repair but insufficient for assignment to the suspicious for malignancy category 2. Specimens nearly meeting criteria for assignment to the neoplasm category but lacking sufficient criteria for definitive diagnosis as a type of neoplasm	Hypocellular specimens with a few cells that are not entirely diagnostic of the radiologically detected lesion (neoplastic or not)
Suspicious for malignancy	The specimen shows some but insufficiently developed characteristics of a malignancy, including metastasis or lymphoma Although the attributes raise a strong suspicion, they are qualitatively and/or quantitatively insufficient for a frank diagnosis based purely on cytomorphology	Cytology raises a strong suspicion but qualitatively and/or quantitatively is insufficient for a definite diagnosis of malignancy (**Fig. 6**)
Positive for malignancy	Specimens that manifest unequivocally malignant cytologic attributes of either primary or metastatic neoplasms	Unequivocally cytologic features of either primary or metastatic neoplasm (**Fig. 7**)

amyloidosis, and fungal and mycobacterial infections.[16] The common benign neoplasms/lesions encountered in this area are giant cell tumor, osteoblastoma, schwannoma, and aneurysmal bone cyst.[16]

CYTOLOGIC DIAGNOSTIC CRITERIA

Aspirates from bone are usually bloody and hypocellular[22] (**Fig. 4**). As stated earlier, criteria to establish adequacy depend on the confidence of the radiologist about placement of the needle in targeted lesion. In general, cytopathologists use 5 diagnostic categories.

Definitions and criteria for each category for FNA of spine/bone lesions are detailed in **Table 2**. In the presence of a radiologically obvious lesion, even if the radiologist is certain of the location of the needle, if the aspirate contains only blood or rare fragments of bone and cartilage or fragments of skeletal muscle and fibroconnective tissue, with absent or rare marrow elements, it should be considered unsatisfactory/inadequate for diagnosis. It is common for cytologists to be under a lot of pressure from radiologists to render a definitive diagnosis at the time of ROSE. Cytologists should not give a definitive diagnosis if the aspirated material is hypocellular or inadequate for interpretation in order to avoid a false-negative diagnosis. Radiologists must also communicate clinical and radiologic findings at the time of ROSE with the cytologist in order to facilitate the diagnostic process.[7] Practical tips for interventional radiologists that can help aid sample procurement and triaging are listed in **Table 3**. It is pertinent that interventional radiologists, with assistance of cytology teams, procure adequate tissue at the time of FNA/biopsy so that the patients do not have to undergo additional testing for determination of eligibility for targeted

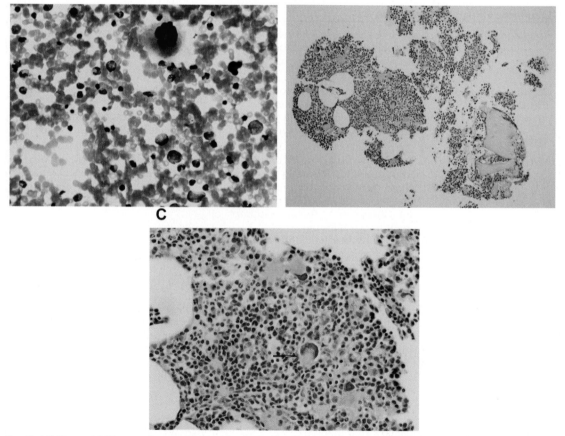

Fig. 5. (*A*) Normal trilineage bone marrow elements. Touch imprint shows megakaryocyte, (the large multinucleated cell), and white blood cell precursors in background (Diff Quik, original magnification ×20). (*B, C*) CNB showing trilineage marrow elements with megakaryocytes (*arrow*) (hematoxylin-eosin, original magnification [*B*] ×10, [*C*] ×40).

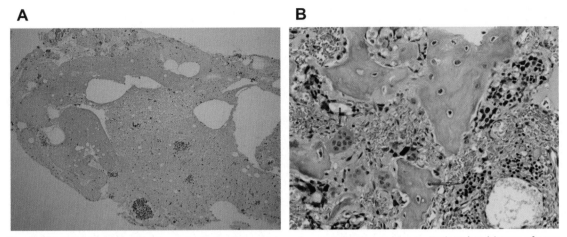

Fig. 6. (*A*) Cell block contains few atypical cells suspicious for metastatic carcinoma. Patient has history of prostate carcinoma. (*B*) Corresponding core biopsy showing tumor cells consistent with metastatic carcinoma (*arrow*). Also seen are osteoclast giant cells (*arrow*) (hematoxylin-eosin, original magnification ×60).

therapy or immunotherapy or even to participate in a clinical trial. Clearly, in the current era the clinical quest begins after the diagnosis, and adequate tissue procurement is paramount.

COMPLICATIONS

The average complication rate of spinal FNA has been reported to be from nil to 0.7% in various series, the commonest complications being pneumothorax, hematoma, and vascular or neural injuries.[19] Most complications, although infrequent, are acute. Transient radiculopathy and quadriparesis have also been reported following FNA of vertebral lesions.[17] Compared with open biopsy, FNA is associated with a lower risk of tumor seeding.[12] No infectious or neurologic sequelae are encountered.[17]

In conclusion, image-guided FNA of spinal and paraspinal lesion is a simple, cost-effective procedure[23] with diagnostic accuracy of up to 96.4%.[26] Interventional radiologists are pivotal in acquiring tissue, and, with the help of cytopathologists, play a vital role in acquiring adequate tissue, increasing diagnostic yield, and decreasing the number of nondiagnostic core biopsies. Effective triaging of the specimen, besides giving a timely and accurate diagnosis, directs the treating physician in the management of patients, avoiding unnecessary surgical exploration in most cases and starting treatment at the earliest opportunity.

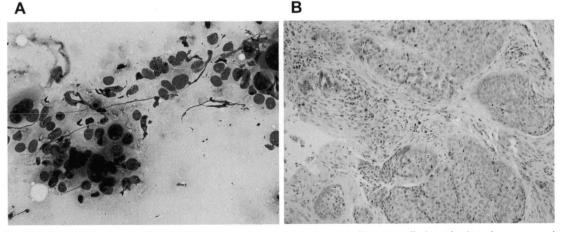

Fig. 7. (*A*) Paraspinal mass. Metastatic squamous cell carcinoma. Malignant cells in cohesive clusters, touch imprint (Diff-Quik, original magnification ×40). (*B*) CNB of paraspinal mass with metastatic squamous cell carcinoma (hematoxylin-eosin, original magnification ×40).

Table 3
Practical tips for effective triage of specimens

Infection	Send Sample for Culture
Suspected hematopoietic malignancy	Take additional passes for flow cytometry in RPMI, not formalin
Suspected metastasis from lung	Additional passes for molecular testing
Suspected metastasis from breast carcinoma	Additional tissue for prognostic markers
Suspected metastasis from colon	Additional tissue for microsatellite instability test and molecular markers

REFERENCES

1. Tehranzadeh J, Tao C, Browning CA. Percutaneous needle biopsy of the spine. Acta Radiol 2007; 48(8):860–8.
2. Leung CT, Dorota R, Natasha R, et al. Impact of touch preparations on core needle biopsies. Cancer Cytopathol 2014;122(11):851–4.
3. Silverman JF, Frable WJ. The use of Diff-Quik stain in the immediate interpretation of fine-needle aspiration biopsies. Diagn Cytopathol 1990;6:366–9.
4. Yang GC, Alvarez II. Ultrafast Papanicolaou stain. An alternative preparation for fine needle aspiration cytology. Acta Cytol 1995;39:55–60.
5. Schmidt RL, Walker BS, Howard K, et al. Rapid on-site evaluation reduces needle passes in endoscopic ultrasound-guided fine-needle aspiration for solid pancreatic lesions: a risk-benefit analysis. Dig Dis Sci 2013;58:3280–6.
6. Schmidt RL, Witt BL, Matynia AP, et al. Rapid on-site evaluation increases endoscopic ultrasound-guided fine-needle aspiration adequacy for pancreatic lesions. Dig Dis Sci 2013;58:872–82.
7. Schmidt RL1, Howard K, Hall BJ, et al. The comparative effectiveness of fine-needle aspiration cytology sampling policies: a simulation study. Am J Clin Pathol 2012;138(6):823–30.
8. Schmidt RL, Walker BS, Cohen MB. When is rapid on-site evaluation cost-effective for fine-needle aspiration biopsy? PLoS One 2015;10(8):e0135466.
9. Marotti JD, Johncox V, Ng D, et al. Implementation of telecytology for immediate assessment of endoscopic ultrasound-guided fine-needle aspirations compared to conventional on-site evaluation: analysis of 240 consecutive cases. Acta Cytol 2012;56:548–53.
10. Khurana KK, Kovalovsky A, Masrani D. Feasibility of telecytopathology for rapid preliminary diagnosis of ultrasound-guided fine needle aspiration of axillary lymph nodes in a remote breast care center. J Pathol Inform 2012;3:36.
11. Pantanowitz L, Wiley CA, Demetris A, et al. Experience with multimodality telepathology at the University of Pittsburgh Medical Center. J Pathol Inform 2012;3:45.
12. Menon S, Gupta N, Srinivasan R, et al. Diagnostic value of image guided fine needle aspiration cytology in assessment of vertebral and paravertebral lesions. J Cytol 2007;24-2:79–81.
13. Tampieri D, Weill A, Melanson D, et al. Percutaneous aspiration in cervical spine lytic lesions: Indications and technique. Neuroradiology 1991;33:43–7.
14. Kattapuram SV, Khurana JS, Rosenthal DI. Percutaneous needle biopsy of the spine. Spine 1992;17:561–4.
15. Coleman RE, Roodman S, Body S, et al. Clinical features of metastatic bone disease and risk of skeletal morbidity. Clin Cancer Res 2006;12(20):6243s–9s.
16. Akhtar I, Flowers R, Siddiqi A, et al. Fine Needle Aspiration Biopsy of Vertebral and Paravertebral Lesions. Retrospective Study of 124 Cases. Acta Cytol 2006;50:364–71.
17. Mchaughlin RE, Miller WR, Miller CW. Quadriparesis after needle aspiration of the cervical spine. J Bone Joint Surg Am 1976;584:1167–8.
18. Agarwal PK, Goel MM, Chandra T, et al. Predictive value of fine needle aspiration cytology of bone lesions: specimen adequacy, diagnostic utility and pitfalls. Arch Pathol Lab Med 2001;125:1463–8.
19. Kang M, Gupta S, Khandelwal N, et al. CT- guided fine needle aspiration biopsy of spinal lesions. Acta Radiol 1999;40:474–8.
20. Collins BT, Chen AC, Wang JF, et al. Improved laboratory resource utilization and patient care with the use of rapid on-site evaluation for endobronchial ultrasound fine-needle aspiration biopsy. Cancer Cytopathol 2013;121:544–51.
21. Robertson RC, Ball RP. Destructive spinal lesions: diagnosis by needle biopsy. J Bone Joint Surg Am 1935;17:749–56.
22. Alder O, Rosenberger A. Fine needle aspiration biopsy of osteolytic metastatic lesions. Am J Roentgenol 1979;133:15–8.
23. Gupta RK, Cheung YK, Ansari AGA, et al. Diagnostic value of image guided needle aspiration cytology in assessment of vertebral and intervertebral lesions. Diagn Cytopathol 2002;27:191–6.
24. Saad RS, Clary KM, Lin Y, et al. Fine needle aspiration biopsy of vertebral lesions. Acta Cytol 2004;48:39–46.
25. Khalbuss WE, Teot LA, Monaco SE. Diagnostic accuracy and limitations of fine-needle aspiration cytology of bone and soft tissue lesions: a review of 1114 cases with cytological-histological correlation. Cancer Cytopathol 2010;118(1):24–32.
26. Mondal A, Misra DK. CT-guided needle aspiration (FNAC) of 112 vertebral lesions. Indian J Pathol Microbiol 1994;37:255–61.